LIPPINCOTT'S
Cancer
Chemotherapy
Handbook

D1113697

LIPPINCOTT'S
Cancer Chemotherapy Handbook

SECOND EDITION

Delia C. Baquiran, MSN, MSB, RN
Chemotherapy Trainer
Oncology Nursing Society
Oncology Projects Consultant
New York, New York

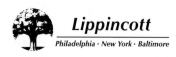

Lippincott
Philadelphia · New York · Baltimore

Acquisitions Editor: Margaret Zuccarini
Editorial Assistant: Helen Kogut
Senior Project Editor: Erika Kors
Senior Production Manager: Helen Ewan
Senior Production Coordinator: Nannette Winski
Art Director: Carolyn O'Brien
Cover Design: Becky Baxendell
Manufacturing Manager: William Alberti
Indexer: Greystone Indexing
Compositor: Peirce Graphic Services, Inc.
Printer: R. R. Donnelley and Sons, Crawfordville

Edition 2

9 8 7 6 5 4 3 2 1

Library of Congress Cataloging-in-Publication Data

Baquiran, Delia C.
    Lippincott's cancer chemotherapy handbook / Delia C. Baquiran.—2nd ed.
    p. ; cm.
    Includes bibliographical references and index.
    ISBN 0-7817-2646-8 (alk. paper)
    1. Cancer—Chemotherapy—Handbooks, manuals, etc. I. Title: Cancer
chemotherapy handbook. II. Title.
    [DNLM: 1. Neoplasms—drug therapy—Handbooks. QZ 39 B222L 2001]
RC271.C5 B37 2001
616.99'4061—dc21   00-048151

Care has been taken to confirm the accuracy of the information presented
and to describe generally accepted practices. However, the authors, editors,
and publisher are not responsible for errors or omissions or for any consequences from application of the information in this book and make no war-
ranty, express or implied, with respect to the content of the publication.

The authors, editors, and publisher have exerted every effort to ensure
that drug selection and dosage set forth in this text are in accordance with
the current recommendations and practice at the time of publication. However, in view of ongoing research, changes in government regulations, and
the constant flow of information relating to drug therapy and drug reactions,
the reader is urged to check the package insert for each drug for any change
in indications and dosage and for added warnings and precautions. This is
particularly important when the recommended agent is a new or infre-
quently employed drug.

Some drugs and medical devices presented in this publication have Food
and Drug Administration (FDA) clearance for limited use in restricted research
settings. It is the responsibility of the health care provider to ascertain the FDA
status of each drug or device planned for use in his or her clinical practice.

*To Alanya Cara, my wonderful daughter and
"bestest" friend who continues to inspire
and keep me in awe!*

*To all cancer patients and families, profiles of
love, hope, and courage for the valuable lessons
you have taught me.*

Reviewers

Lois S. Doane, MSN, RN, OCN, AOCN
Oncology Clinical Nurse Specialist
University of Tennessee Medical Center
Knoxville, Tennessee

Barbara G. Lubejko, MS, RN, OCN
Nurse Educator
The Johns Hopkins Oncology Center
Baltimore, Maryland

Jeanette Adams McNeill, DrPH, AOCN, ANP
Department Chair, Target Populations, Track Director-Oncology
University of Texas-Houston, School of Nursing
Houston, Texas

Christine Miaskowski, RN, PhD, FAAN
Professor and Chair
University of California, School of Nursing
San Francisco, California

Susan A. Rokita, MS, CRNP
Oncology Clinical Nurse Specialist
Penn State Geisinger Health System
Hershey, Pennsylvania

Constance Ziegfeld, MS, RN
Assistant Director of Nursing
Johns Hopkins Oncology Center
Baltimore, Maryland

Preface

"Cancer is one of the most curable chronic diseases in this country today." *(Vincent J. R. DeVita)*

Great strides have been made to achieve therapeutic benefits for the cancer population. For some cancers, these have resulted in a cure; for others, they have resulted in prolonged survival or improved quality of life. Over the years, the use of chemotherapy has been one of the mainstays in the treatment of cancer. Quantum leaps in the field of biotherapy have been made, making this modality a major player, too, in cancer therapy. It joins the ranks of chemotherapy, surgery, and radiation in the cancer armamentarium.

To achieve optimum treatment goals, the clinician has to be very knowledgeable about therapeutic options for the patient. Since chemotherapy and biotherapy can benefit the patient, keeping up to date will afford patients the best chance possible in managing their cancer.

The second edition of Lippincott's Cancer Chemotherapy Handbook builds on the wealth of updated information on all the chemotherapeutic and biological response modifiers that are available today.

TEXT ORGANIZATION

Presented in a concise, organized format, the book is divided into three parts:

Part One includes seven chapters that present information on the basics of chemotherapy (cell life cycle, treatment strategies, classification of chemotherapeutic agents), biologic response modifiers, clinical trials, patient education, and guidelines for safe handling of chemotherapeutic agents and assessing and managing side effects and toxicities.

Part Two presents chemotherapeutic drug monographs alphabetically organized for quick access in the clinical setting.

Part Three includes details on the indications and clinical considerations for frequently used combination regimens.

Appendices include an extensive resource guide to the National Cancer Institute's publications for cancer patients and the public, sample patient education material, the Yellow Pages for Cancer Patients and Caregivers, and the National Cancer Institute's Toxicity Scale.

FEATURES AND BENEFITS

This handbook is the **most current pocket resource available,** providing up-to-date information on *all* drugs used in chemotherapy, including **difficult-to-access information on biologic response modifiers and regimens in current use**.

- Handy pocket size permits easy portability for use in any setting: hospital, clinic, home, free-standing treatment centers.
- Drug monographs promote consistent presentation of drug-related information, including pediatric dosing considerations.
- Alphabetically organized drug monographs ensure quick and easy access to information on individual drugs.
- Separate section on managing toxic effects of chemotherapy provides guidelines for minimizing unpleasant side effects and possibly life-threatening toxicities.
- Appendices include extensive resources for information and services helpful to cancer patients, their families, and the nurses caring for them.

My experience in chemotherapy dates from the 1970s, when the mainstay of cancer therapy revolved around 5FU, adriamycin, leucovorin, and methotrexate. Thirty years later, many more drugs have been developed and approved by the Federal Drug Administration. I have been very fortunate to work with expert clinical nurses and oncologists, committed scientists, dedicated pharmacists, and other health care providers. Their contributions to the body of knowledge available for effecting better patient care management are reflected in this edition.

Delia C. Baquiran, MSN, MSB, RN
New York, New York

Acknowledgments

I wish to thank my reviewers and my "informal critique team," my colleagues, who were not lacking for encouragement and helpful comments. I hope I did justice to your suggestions. I am grateful to Margaret Zuccarini and Erika Kors, my editors, for their patient understanding when I couldn't meet my deadlines, and to Helen Kogut, editorial assistant, for her kind support of this project. Many thanks to Maia B. Ermita and Janice B. Torres for their research assistance and help with proofreading.

And lastly, to Jean Gallagher, my coauthor in the first edition, and to Janet Gordils Perez for their valuable contributions, without which this second edition would not have been possible.

Contents

I.

Cancer Chemotherapy

1

Overview of Chemotherapy

Chemotherapy is the use of cytotoxic agents to destroy cancer cells. Chemotherapy dates back to the 1500s, when heavy metals were used systemically to treat cancers, and severe toxicity and limited cure were reported. Since then, a vast spectrum of antineoplastic drugs has been discovered to achieve *cure, control,* and *palliation* of many cancers. The new and improved changes in the drug approval process of the Food and Drug Administration have speeded the entry of novel drugs that have made chemotherapy a vital part of the cancer armamentarium. Chemotherapy remains the primary treatment for some malignancies and an adjunct to other treatment modalities (surgery, radiation, and immunotherapy). Unlike surgery and radiation, chemotherapy is distinguished by its systemic effects. Most of the drugs are transported by the bloodstream; most do not cross the blood–brain barrier and therefore cannot reach the central nervous system.

To achieve the above goals, chemotherapeutic drugs (as single agents or in combination) may be used in the following strategies:

Adjuvant: A short course of high-dose, usually combination drugs is given after radiation or surgery to destroy residual tumor cells.

Consolidation: Chemotherapy is given after induction therapy has achieved a complete remission; the regimen is repeated to increase the cure rate or to prolong patient survival.

Induction: This term is commonly used in the treatment of hematologic malignancies. It refers to the use of usually a combination of high-dose drugs to induce a complete response when initiating a curative regimen.

Intensification: After complete remission is achieved, the same agents used for induction are given at higher doses, or different agents are given at high doses to effect a better cure rate or a longer remission.

Maintenance: Single or combination, low-dose cytotoxic drugs are used on a long-term basis in patients who are in complete remission to delay regrowth of residual cancer cells.

Neoadjuvant: Adjuvant chemotherapeutic drugs are used during the pre- or perioperative period.

Palliative: Chemotherapy is given to control symptoms, provide comfort, and improve quality of life if cure is impossible.

Salvage: A potentially curative high-dose regimen is given to a patient whose symptoms have recurred or whose treatment has failed with another regimen.

The human body is composed of an intricate network of nondividing and dividing cells organized into various tissues that perform specific functions. Nondividing cells, such as striated muscle cells and neurons, are highly differentiated and do not need to replicate to maintain their function. Dividing cells, such as germ, epithelial, and bone marrow stem cells, must replicate to maintain their function.

The body regulates all replication of dividing cells by maintaining a balance between the birth and death of cells. The body's maintenance of this homeostasis depends on the synthesis of trigger proteins, or signals, in response to cell death. This synthesis stimulates the entry and movement of dividing cells through the process of cell division.

▼ The Cell Cycle

The *cell cycle* is the cornerstone of cell division and proliferation. Both normal and malignant cells undergo this process, which may last for approximately 25 to 30 hours (Fig. 1-1). There are five phases to the process. In the first phase, *Gap 0* (G_0), a cell can stay in a dormant or latent state for months or even years until stimulated to move forward in the cycle. Because certain cells divide more rapidly than others, some rest in the G_0 phase for a brief period, whereas others bypass

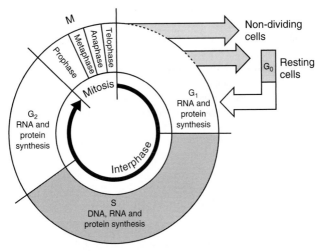

Fig. 1-1. The cell life cycle.

the G_0 phase and enter the second phase, the *Gap 1* (G_1) phase, directly if the body needs the immediate production of a certain cell. The G_1 phase occurs after mitosis, the birth of two daughter cells. During this phase, the cell synthesizes RNA and the proteins needed for DNA synthesis. The time a cell spends in this phase varies and can last from hours to days, depending on the cell type. After RNA and protein syntheses occur, the cell then enters the third phase, the *synthesis* (S) phase, when RNA, protein, and DNA syntheses occur and DNA replicates.

DNA is an essential nucleic acid composed of deoxyribose, a phosphate, and four nitrogenous bases: adenine, guanine, cytosine, and thymine. Adenine and guanine are the purines, and cytosine and thymine are the pyrimidines. Chemical reactions occur between the two purines and also between the two pyrimidines, leading to the formation of the double-stranded DNA helix, which serves as the genetic template of the cell.

Generally, the S phase lasts 8 to 12 hours. The cell then enters the fourth phase, *Gap 2* (G_2), when more RNA and protein syntheses take place in preparation for mitosis. This phase tends to last 2 to 4 hours; then the cell enters the fifth or *mitosis* (M) phase. The M phase consists of the following orchestrated subphases: prophase, metaphase, anaphase, and telophase (see Fig. 1-1). As the cell progresses through these subphases, the cytoplasm and nucleus divide so that replication of the cell results in the birth of two daughter cells.

It is not clearly understood how the body maintains normal cellular homeostasis. What has been postulated is that the body possesses a feedback system that signals a cell to enter the G_1 phase of the cell life cycle in response to cell death. In patients with cancer, this feedback system is dysfunctional, and the cancer cell enters the cell cycle independently of the body's feedback system.

▼ Cancer Cell Characteristics

Every cell in the body has a genetically programmed clock that directs the timing of its reproductive activity. Cancer is a disease in which the cells fail to respond to the homeostatic mechanism that controls the cellular birth and death processes. Although the growth of cancer cells is dysfunctional and uncontrolled, the cancer cells undergo the different phases of the cell cycle that normal cells do.

Four basic features differentiate the cancer cell from the normal cell:

- Uncontrolled cell proliferation
- Decreased cellular differentiation
- Inappropriate ability to invade surrounding tissue
- Ability to establish new growth at ectopic sites

Cancer cells have the same chemical structures as normal cells; the critical change appears to be in growth and differentiation. Cell production in cancer is not proportional to cell loss; production of new cells occurs at a faster rate than is needed to compensate for the loss of cells.

CELLULAR KINETICS

Most chemotherapeutic drugs exert cytotoxic activity primarily on macromolecular synthesis or function. This means that they interfere either with the synthesis of DNA, RNA, or proteins or with the appropriate functioning of the preformed molecule. When this interference happens, a proportion of the cells die. Chemotherapy works on the principle of first-order kinetics, which postulates that the number of tumor cells killed by an antineoplastic agent is proportional to the dose used. This is a constant percentage of the total number of malignant cells present. Figure 1-2 is a visual representation of the cell kill theory. For example, if a tumor containing 1 million cells is exposed to a drug that has a 90% cell kill rate, the first chemotherapy dose will destroy 90%, or 900,000, of the cancer cells. The second dose will kill another 90% of the remaining cells (90,000), and 10,000 cells will survive. Because only a portion of the cells die, expected

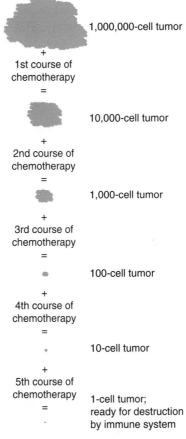

1,000,000-cell tumor

\+
1st course of
chemotherapy
=

10,000-cell tumor

\+
2nd course of
chemotherapy
=

1,000-cell tumor

\+
3rd course of
chemotherapy
=

100-cell tumor

\+
4th course of
chemotherapy
=

10-cell tumor

\+
5th course of
chemotherapy
=

1-cell tumor;
ready for destruction
by immune system

Fig. 1-2. Cell kill theory. A set percentage of cells is killed after each dose of chemotherapy. The percentage killed is dependent upon the drug therapy. In the above example, each course of chemotherapy kills 90% of cells in a cancerous tumor.

doses of chemotherapy must be repeated to reduce the population of cancer cells until just one cell remains. It is hoped that the body's immune response will kill the final cell.

▼ Classification of Chemotherapeutic Agents

Antineoplastic drugs are classified according to their mode of action and the phase of the cell cycle in which the drug is active. This classification is not absolute; it is likely that more than one mechanism is involved. Multiple intracellular sites might be implicated and not confined to specific cycle events. However, it is always the rapidly dividing cells that are most sensitive to these drugs. Chemotherapeutic drugs that are most effective during a particular phase of the cycle are known as *cell cycle–specific drugs.*

CELL CYCLE–SPECIFIC AGENTS: ANTIMETABOLITES, VINCA ALKALOIDS, EPIPODOPHYLLOTOXINS, TAXANES, CAMPTOTHECINS

Most cancers have proliferating and resting cells. Proliferating cells must be in cycle for phase-specific agents to cause their death. Because not all cells are in cycle at the same time, cycle-specific chemotherapy is administered in divided doses or as a continuous infusion. These methods of administration facilitate the lysis of cells as they enter certain phases of the cycle. The number of cells in cycle is referred to as the *growth fraction.* Cell cycle–specific drugs therefore reduce the growth fraction of the tumor.

Antimetabolites

Antimetabolites are synthetically formulated to mimic the naturally produced metabolites, purines, pyrimidines, or folates essential for the synthesis of nucleic acids and DNA. This results in cell death. They exert their effects during the S phase of the cell life cycle and are most effective against tumors that have a high growth fraction. Relatively quiescent tissues have low growth fractions of about 0.01, whereas rapidly proliferating cells such as those of the gastrointestinal tract, mucosal epithelium, and the hair follicles have growth fractions of about 0.1.

Capecitabine	5-Fluorouracil
Cytosine arabinoside	Gemcitabine
Deoxycoformycin	6-Mercaptopurine
Floxuridine	Methotrexate
Fludarabine	Thioguanine

Mitotic Inhibitors

Mitotic inhibitors interfere with the formation of the mitotic spindle, causing metaphase arrest. They are primarily known as M-phase active, but they may also have activity in G_2 and S. These drugs are the vinca alkaloids, the epipodophyllotoxins, and the taxanes.

Vinca alkaloids, also called plant alkaloids, are extracts of the periwinkle plant. They bind to microtubular proteins, which are key to forming the mitotic spindle of the dividing cells. This binding arrests mitosis, which eventually causes cell death. The vincas act mainly in the M phase; however, high doses can also disrupt RNA and protein synthesis. *Epipodophyllotoxins* were isolated from the mandrake plant (May crab apple). They act in the premitotic phase, G_2 and S, and interfere with topoisomerase II enzyme reaction. *Taxanes* cause mitotic arrest by forming abnormal spindle fibers and mitotic asters.

VINCA ALKALOIDS	EPIPODOPHYLLOTOXINS	TAXANES
Vinblastine	Etoposide	Docetaxel
Vincristine	Teniposide	Paclitaxel
Vindesine		
Vinorelbine		

Camptothecins

Camptothecins (the name is derived from the Chinese tree *Camptotheca acuminata*) are a new subcategory of cell cycle– specific drugs. They act in the S phase and inhibit topoisomerase I, a nuclear enzyme necessary for maintaining DNA structure. Inhibition of this enzyme results in single-stranded DNA breaks and subsequently cell death. The camptothecins are:z

Irinotecan
Topotecan

CELL CYCLE–NONSPECIFIC AGENTS: ALKYLATING AGENTS, NITROSOUREAS, ANTITUMOR ANTIBIOTICS, HORMONES, HORMONE ANTAGONISTS

Antineoplastic agents that are effective through all phases of the cell cycle and are not limited to a specific phase are called *cell cycle–nonspecific drugs*. These drugs directly affect the DNA molecule and display no specificity for cells that are dividing. They are considered more toxic than their cell cycle–specific counterparts because their destructive action does not differentiate between normal and malignant cycling cells. Their toxicities are felt throughout the cell cycle. Nonspecific agents are given in bolus doses because they cause death independently of the proliferative state of the cell. These agents also reduce the number of cells that make up a tumor, which is known as the *tumor burden.*

Alkylating Agents

Alkylating agents alter DNA structure through the poorly understood process of alkylation (H^+ ion alkyl substitution), which results in cross-linking and strand breaking of DNA and destruction of its template. Destruction of the DNA genetic template terminates replication of the information needed for cellular division and leads to cell lysis. The alkylating agents are described as *radiomimetic* because they mimic the actions of radiation therapy on the cells. The alkylating agents are as follows:

Busulfan	Ifosfamide
Carboplatin	Melphalan
Chlorambucil	Mechlorethamine hydrochloride
Cisplatin	Thiotepa
Cyclophosphamide	Uracil mustard
Dacarbazine	

Nitrosoureas

Nitrosoureas are alkylating agents that also destroy DNA so that synthesis can no longer occur, but they are unique in that they are lipid-soluble and cross the blood–brain barrier into the central nervous system. The nitrosoureas are:

Carmustine	Streptozocin
Lomustine	

Antitumor Antibiotics

Most *antitumor antibiotics* are isolated from fermented broths of various *Streptomyces* bacteria. The focal point of their cytotoxicity is the DNA. These drugs interfere with DNA-directed RNA synthesis by intercalating between the base pairs of DNA and generating toxic oxygen-free radicals, causing single- or double-stranded DNA breaks. The antitumor antibiotics are as follows:

Dactinomycin

Daunorubicin

Doxorubicin

Idarubicin

Mitomycin-C

Mitoxantrone

Plicamycin

Hormones and Hormone Antagonists

Hormones and *hormone antagonists* (*antihormones*) are a diverse group of drugs that are beneficial in cancer therapy. Some hormones alter the cellular environment and affect the permeability of the cell membrane in ways that will affect cell growth. These drugs, which are hormonal or hormone-like agents, inhibit tumor proliferation by blocking or antagonizing the naturally occurring substance that stimulates tumor growth.

Androgens: testosterone propionate, methyltestosterone, fluoxymesterone

Antiandrogens: flutamide

Antiestrogens: tamoxifen

Aromatase inhibitors: aminoglutethimide

Estrogens: diethylstilbestrol, estradiol

Glucocorticoids: prednisone, hydrocortisone, dexamethasone

Gonadotropin inhibitors: leuprolide, goserelin

Progestins: megestrol acetate

MISCELLANEOUS AGENTS

Bleomycin

Hydroxyurea

L-asparaginase

Procarbazine

Bleomycin and L-asparaginase fit into this category because they do not exert their effects during the S or M phases of the cycle, as do the antimetabolites or the vinca alkaloids. Bleomycin exerts its effect during G_2 and L-asparaginase during G_1. Procarbazine and hydroxyurea are miscellaneous cell cycle–nonspecific agents.

▼ Combination Chemotherapy

According to the Gompertzian model of tumor growth, tumors in their early stages grow rapidly because they have a high growth fraction. Eventually, as the tumor burden increases, its growth plateaus and the growth fraction decreases. Growth fraction and tumor burden are therefore inversely related. Cell cycle–specific and cell cycle–nonspecific drugs are given in combination, because cell cycle–specific drugs reduce a tumor's growth fraction and cell cycle–nonspecific drugs reduce the tumor burden.

Many antineoplastic agents are dose-limiting because of their overall cytotoxicity. The limits imposed by the toxicities on the different organ systems led to the use of combination drugs to achieve better therapeutic outcomes. Combination therapy involves the use of two or more drugs proven effective against a tumor type. The development of this strategy is one of the major advances in cancer treatment in the past 20 years. Combination therapy is superior to single-drug therapy because of higher tumor response rates and increased duration of remissions. Many regimens in current use (see Unit III) have been shown to increase the response rate by two to four times. Two or more drugs can be given simultaneously or in sequence. The response rates and survival rates are more dramatic because they accomplish the following:

- Maximum cell kill within the range of toxicity tolerated by the host
- A broader range of coverage of resistant cell lines in the heterogeneous population
- Minimal or slow development of new resistant cell groups

When designing successful drug combinations, the following principles should be used:

- Selected drugs should be proven partially effective against the tumor when used alone.
- The drugs that are combined should not have overlapping toxicities.
- The dosage and schedule should be maximized.
- The combination drugs should be administered at consistent intervals.
- Drugs that can produce synergy should be selected.

To ensure lysis of proliferating and resting cells, combination chemotherapy is administered in courses (also referred to as cycles). The number of courses used in treatment varies depending on the type of cancer, the chemotherapy agents used, and the patient's response to therapy.

2

Biologic Response Modifiers

Janet Gordils–Perez

Biologic therapy is the fourth modality in the treatment of cancer, after surgery, chemotherapy, and radiation. Biologic therapy produces anticancer effects either through the actions of the natural immune defense system or by the administration of natural substances. Biologic therapies for the treatment of cancer are referred to as *biologic response modifiers* (BRMs). These substances, which are naturally produced in small quantities in the body, can now be produced in large quantities through recombinant DNA technology. Some may function to boost the host immune system to protect the body from foreign substances such as tumor cells (Dudjak & Fleck, 1991; Wujcik, 1993).

With recent developments in hybridoma technology (Fig. 2-1), researchers can now produce virtually unlimited amounts of identical monoclonal antibodies (mAbs) by cloning these hybrid cells and maintaining them indefinitely in tissue culture (Jorde, 1994; McCance et al., 1994). Recombinant DNA techniques (Fig. 2-2) combine parts of the DNA of two or more different organisms, which can be induced in culture to produce limitless amounts of human proteins. In this way, synthetic proteins identical to those naturally occurring in limited quantities in the body can now be reproduced in large quantities (Old, 1996; Tomaszewski et al., 1995a). The development of hybridoma technology and recombinant DNA techniques has increased the application of BRMs in clinical use for the diagnosis and treatment of cancer.

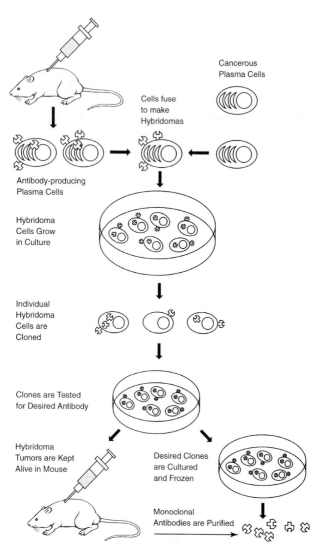

Fig. 2-1. Using hybridoma technology to make monoclonal antibodies. (Reprinted with permission from Schindler, L. W. [1988]. *Understanding the immune system* [NIH Publication No. 88–529]. Washington, DC: U.S. Department of Health and Human Services.)

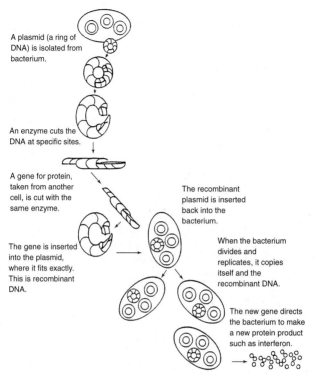

A plasmid (a ring of DNA) is isolated from bacterium.

An enzyme cuts the DNA at specific sites.

A gene for protein, taken from another cell, is cut with the same enzyme.

The gene is inserted into the plasmid, where it fits exactly. This is recombinant DNA.

The recombinant plasmid is inserted back into the bacterium.

When the bacterium divides and replicates, it copies itself and the recombinant DNA.

The new gene directs the bacterium to make a new protein product such as interferon.

Fig. 2-2. Recombinant DNA technique. (Reprinted with permission from Schindler, L. W. [1988]. *Understanding the immune system* [NIH Publication No. 88–529]. Washington, DC: U.S. Department of Health and Human Services.)

▼ Biologic Response Modifiers

The National Cancer Institute's Division of Cancer Treatment Subcommittee on Biological Response Modifiers has defined BRMs as agents or approaches that alter the relationship between host and tumor by changing the host's immune response to tumor cells, which results in a therapeutic effect (Farrell, 1996). BRMs include mAbs, cytokines, and other biologic agents such as tumor necrosis factor (TNF). Many BRMs are under investigation in clinical trials. The Food and Drug Administration (FDA) has approved more than 25

BRMs for use in medical treatment; Table 2-1 reviews those approved by the FDA for the treatment of cancer.

There are three ways in which BRMs function: by direct cytotoxic activity on tumor cells (e.g., TNF), by restoring, strengthening, or modulating the host's tumor-immune response (e.g., bacillus Calmette-Guerin, cytokines), and by modifying other biologic effects, such as by interfering with the tumor cell's survival and metastatic abilities (e.g., mAbs) (Engelking & Wujcik, 1994; Tomaszewski et al., 1995b).

Biologic therapy for cancer treatment can be divided into active and passive approaches and further subdivided into nonspecific and specific biotherapy. Active biotherapy attempts to use substances that elicit an immune response capable of eliminating or retarding tumor growth through immunization of cancer patients. Vaccines such as anti-idiotype mAbs are used to induce active specific immunity. Passive biotherapy uses substances that supplement components of the host's immune system. Passive specific biotherapy includes the use of mAbs; passive nonspecific biotherapy uses cytokines (Rosenberg, 1993a).

▼ Monoclonal Antibodies

Many tumor cells express substances on their surface that are unique to tumor cells. These substances may be absent or found in small quantities in normal cells, making tumor cells antigenically different from normal cells. These substances are known as tumor-associated antigens (Kwok, 1990). Monoclonal antibodies are glycoproteins made to target these tumor-associated antigens. They are produced to recognize and bind to antigens expressed by a particular tumor and elicit an immune response.

Antibodies are immunoglobulins produced by plasma B cells in response to antigens. They are divided into five subclasses (IgA, IgD, IgE, IgG, IgM), depending on the heavy polypeptide chain they contain. Each class performs a role in the immune response. Monoclonal antibodies are usually of the IgG or IgM subclass.

Monoclonal antibodies can be used alone (unconjugated) or in combination (conjugated) with cytotoxic agents, toxins, radioisotopes, or biologic agents. Unconjugated mAbs have shown antitumor activity in clinical trials. The FDA has ap-

Table 2-1. FDA-Approved Biologic Response Modifiers

Biologic Agent	Year Approved	Clinical Application
Interferon-alfa	1986	Hairy cell leukemia
	1988	Kaposi's sarcoma
		Condyloma acuminata
	1991	Chronic hepatitis C
	1992	Chronic hepatitis B
	1995	Chronic myelogenous leukemia
		Adjuvant therapy for melanoma
	1997	Conjunction with chemotherapy in patients with follicular lymphoma
Interferon-beta	1992	Multiple sclerosis
Interferon-gamma	1991	Chronic granulomatous-related infection
	2000	Severe malignant osteopetrosis
Interleukin-2	1992	Renal cell carcinoma
	1998	Metastatic melanoma
Epoetin alfa	1989	Anemia related to chronic renal failure in patients on dialysis
	1991	Anemia with zidovudine-treated patients with HIV
	1993	Anemia associated with cancer chemotherapy
	1999	Anemia in patients undergoing surgery
Muromonab-CD3	1986	Acute allograft rejection in renal transplant patients
		Steroid-resistant acute allograft rejection in cardiac and hepatic transplant patients
Satumomab-pendetide	1993	Detection of colorectal and ovarian cancer
G-CSF	1991	Nonmyeloid cancers after mylosuppressive treatment
		After autologous bone marrow transplantation in patients with nonmyeloid cancers
		Severe chronic neutropenia

(continued)

Table 2-1. FDA-Approved Biologic Response Modifiers *(Continued)*

Biologic Agent	Year Approved	Clinical Application
	1998	Acute myeloid leukemia patients receiving induction or consolidation chemotherapy Transplantation of autologous peripheral blood progenitor cells
GM-CSF	1991	Nonmyeloid cancers in patients undergoing autologous bone marrow transplantation Acute myelogenous leukemia after chemotherapy Engraftment delay or failure after bone marrow transplant
	1996	Myeloid reconstitution after allogeneic bone marrow transplantation Transplantation of autologous peripheral blood progenitor cells
Oprelvelkin	1997	Nonmyeloid cancers after myelosuppressive treatment at risk of severe thrombocytopenia
Rituximab	1997	Relapsed or refractory low-grade or follicular, B-cell non-Hodgkin's lymphoma
Trastuzumab	1998	Metastatic breast cancer whose tumors over-express HER2 protein
Denileukin diftitox	1999	Persistent or recurrent cutaneous T-cell lymphoma

Abbreviations: G-CSF, granulocyte colony-stimulating factor; GM-CSF, granulocyte macrophage colony-stimulating factor.

Data from Rieger, P. T., & Haeuber, D. (1995). A new approach to managing chemo-related anemia: Nursing implications of epoetin alfa. *Oncology Nursing Forum, 22,* 71–81; Abernathy, E. A. (1996). Biotherapy. In R. McCorkle, M. Grant, M. Frank-Stromberg, & S. B. Baird (Eds.), *Cancer nursing: A comprehensive textbook* (2nd ed.). Philadelphia: Saunders; U.S. Food and Drug Administration (2000). Product Approval Information [on-line]. Available by e-mail: www.fda.gov.

proved two unconjugated mAbs for the treatment of cancer. Rituximab (Rituxan) was approved in 1997 for the treatment of non-Hodgkin's lymphoma. It is administered as a weekly intravenous infusion at a dose of 375 mg/m^2 for 4 consecutive weeks. The most common side effects occurred during the first infusion. These included fever, chills, rigors, myalgia/arthralgia, urticaria, nausea, diarrhea, and mucosal congestion (Kosits & Callaghan, 2000). Trastuzumab (Herceptin) was approved in 1998 as a single agent for the treatment of patients with metastatic breast cancer whose tumors overexpress the HER2 proteins and who have received one or more chemotherapy treatments, or in combination with paclitaxel for those who have not received chemotherapy. The initial loading dose is administered at a dose of 4 mg/kg over a 90-minute intravenous infusion. The maintenance dose is 2 mg/kg over 30 minutes. The most common side effects include chills, fever, nausea, vomiting, pain, rigors, headache, dizziness, dyspnea, hypotension, rash, and asthenia (Herceptin package insert, 1998).

Researchers are developing potentially more effective therapy by conjugating mAbs to cytotoxic agents, toxins, or radioisotopes (Jurcic et al., 1997). Monoclonal antibodies conjugated to cytotoxic agents include doxorubicin, daunorubicin, and methotrexate (Kwok, 1990). In theory, chemoimmunoconjugates target cancer cells and bypass normal cells; therefore, maximum doses of cytotoxic agents can be administered and chemotherapy-related side effects can be minimized (Gdicke & Riethmller, 1995; Groenwald et al., 1995).

Immunotoxin therapy has been developed to deliver toxins to the tumor cell to cause cell death. The toxins used are extremely potent bacterial or plant products. The most common bacterial toxins include diphtheria toxin and *Pseudomonas* exotoxin A. Ricin, gelonin, and saponin are plant products. A single molecule is sufficient to kill a cell (Scheinberg & Chapman, 1995). In 1999, Denileukin diftitox (Ontak) was the first genetically engineered recombinant DNA-derived cytotoxic fusion protein approved by the FDA for the treatment of patients with persistent or recurrent cutaneous T-cell lymphoma. Ontak is composed of fragments A- and B- of the diphtheria toxin that are genetically linked to recombinant interleukin-2 (IL-2). It targets cells expressing the IL-2 receptor and directs the cytocidal action of the diphtheria toxin to malignant cutaneous T-cell lymphoma. This inhibits protein synthesis and causes cell death. The recommended dose is 9 or 18 μg/kg/day administered intravenously over 15 minutes for 5 consecutive days every 21 days. Ontak is usually well tolerated; however, side effects include chills, fever, infection, pain, headache, flulike syndrome, dizziness, chest pain, hypotension, tachycardia, nausea, vomiting, diarrhea, and hypoalbuminemia (Ontak package insert, 1999).

Conjugation of mAbs to radioisotopes has both diagnostic and therapeutic applications. Satumomab pendetide has been approved for diagnostic use in the detection of colorectal and ovarian cancer (Cytogen, 1993). Monoclonal antibodies coupled with radioisotopes (^{131}I, ^{123}I, ^{111}In, ^{99m}Tc) (Scheinberg & Chapman, 1995) are used to image and localize tumors and monitor progression of disease. Serial images assist in identifying tumor sites shown by specific areas of radioactive uptake. Therapeutically, radioactive isotopes (predominately ^{131}I) are conjugated to an antibody that is produced to target and attach to a specific tumor antigen; the radioactive isotope can then internally irradiate the target and adjacent cancer cells (Groenwald et al., 1995). Radioimmunoconjugates for therapy involve higher doses of radiation than those used for radioimmunodetection.

Monoclonal antibodies have also been used in combination with cytokines to enhance cytotoxic effects. These cytokines include IL-2, interferon, granulocyte macrophage colony-stimulating factor (GM-CSF), macrophage colony-stimulating factor (M-CSF), and TNF (Jurcic et al., 1997). Cytokines have been shown to enhance effector cell–mediated antibody-dependent cellular cytotoxicity, which can augment the efficacy of mAbs (Gdicke & Riethmller, 1995). Most trials have involved patients with melanoma. Few antitumor responses have been observed, except in a trial using mAb R24 against GD3 ganglioside in combination with IL-2, in which 10 of 32 patients had partial responses (Baquiran et al., 1996; Scheinberg & Chapman, 1995).

Monoclonal antibodies have been used *ex vivo* to remove residual tumor cells from the bone marrow of patients undergoing autologous transplant and to decrease the incidence of graft-versus-host disease by removing T lymphocytes from donor marrow before allogeneic transplant (Scheinberg & Chapman, 1995). Monoclonal antibodies have been shown to be effective in the detection and treatment of both solid tumors and hematologic malignancies.

TOXICITIES

Toxicities associated with mAbs are minimal. However, anaphylaxis may occur. Serious toxicities are usually associated with rapid infusions and high doses and may occur only in the first few administrations. Immediate access to emergency medications, oxygen equipment, and an emergency cart is essential in the management of an allergic reaction or anaphylaxis. A skin test or a test dose may be administered before the initial dose to assess for hypersensitivity reactions. Prophylactic medications (acetaminophen and diphenhydramine hydrochloride) may be necessary to prevent allergic reactions. Other potential side effects include fever, chills, rigors, hypotension, dyspnea, pruritus, rash, nausea and vomiting, diarrhea, arthralgia, and myalgia (Bodey et al., 1996).

Monoclonal antibodies combined with cytokines can produce toxicities associated with the particular cytokine. For example, mAbs used with IL-2 can cause hypotension, fever, and renal and pulmonary toxicities (Gdicke & Riethmller, 1995), and chemoimmunoconjugates may cause nausea and vomiting or myelosuppression.

▼ Cytokines

Cytokines are naturally occurring substances released from stimulated cells of the immune system. They have a major role in mediating the activity of the immune system and can alter the growth and metastasis of cancer cells. Cytokines include interferons, colony-stimulating factors, interleukins, and TNF (Groenwald et al., 1995). The production or administration of one cytokine induces the production and response of other cytokines. Table 2-2 lists cytokines with their cell source and potential clinical applications.

INTERFERONS

Interferons are a family of glycoproteins produced by the body in response to viral infections and biologic inducers. Research has demonstrated that interferons can interfere with viral replication and also have antiproliferative and immunomodulatory biologic properties. There are three primary types of interferons: alpha, beta, and gamma (Gantz et al., 1995; Post-

Table 2-2. Cytokines With Their Cell Source and Potential Clinical Applications

Cytokine	Cellular Source	Effects and Potential Applications
Interleukins		
IL-1	Macrophages/monocytes; endothelial cells, keratinocytes, astrocytes, B cells, T cells, kidney mesangial cells	May have use as an anticancer agent, a proinflammatory agent, or a hematopoiesis stimulant.
IL-2	T cells, NK cells, B cells	Used in tumor immunotherapy: expands LAK and TIL populations in vivo, promotes TIL growth in in vitro. Causes regression in transplantable murine tumors and human melanoma and renal cell cancer.
IL-3	NK cells, mast cells, T cells, eosinophils	Aids myeloid cell expansion in vivo; may have use in treating bone marrow failure. IL-3 antagonists may be useful in treating leukemia and allergic diseases.
IL-4	Stromal cells, T cells, mast cells	Stimulates B-cell growth and antibody production. May have use as an antitumor or anti-inflammatory agent.
IL-5	T cells, activated mast cells	A major eosinophil-stimulating factor in vivo. May have use as an antitumor agent. Stimulates B-cell antibody production.
IL-6	T cells, monocyte/macrophages, fibroblasts	Anti-IL-6 may be useful in treating arthritis or osteoporosis.
IL-7	Stromal cells, spleen, thymus	Promotes B-cell and T-cell development. May have use as an immunostimulant. Required for lymphopoiesis.
IL-8	Monocytes, fibroblasts, endothelial cells, kera-	Induces neutrophil infiltration in vivo. Present in patients

	Source	Function
	tinocytes, tumor cells, neutrophils, T cells, NK cells, granulocytes, phagocytes	with psoriasis, rheumatoid arthritis, and gout.
IL-9	T cells	May be an in vivo–enhancing factor during hematopoiesis.
IL-10	T cells, B cells, mast cells, macrophages, keratinocytes	A cytokine suppressor and an immunosuppressor in vivo. May have use as an anti-inflammatory agent.
IL-11	Stromal cells	Important in hematopoiesis; enhances immune responses.
IL-12	B lymphoblastoid cells, macrophages/monocytes	Activates T cell and NK cells. May have use as an antitumor or anti-infective agent.
IL-13	Activated T cells	Inhibits HIV replication and is anti-inflammatory in vitro. No in vivo information is available to date.
Hematopoietic Growth Factors		
EPO	Renal cells, hepatocytes, tumor cells	Controls production of erythrocytes. Increases hematocrit in animals. Used in treating anemia.
M-CSF	Stromal cells, macrophages, fibroblasts, T cells, B cells	May downregulate immunologic and inflammatory reactions. May have use in hemopoietic recovery and treatment of leukemia. Stimulates hemopoietic progenitors to form macrophages.
G-CSF	Fibroblasts, macrophages, endothelial cells, stromal cells	Leads to elevated neutrophil counts in vivo. Stimulates hemopoietic progenitors to form granulocytes. Used for non-myeloid cancers after myelosuppressive treatment, after autologus bone marrow transplantation in patients with nonmyeloid cancers, severe neutropenia, and acute myeloid leukemia receiving induction or consolidation chemotherapy.

(continued)

Table 2-2. Cytokines With Their Cell Source and Potential Clinical Applications *(Continued)*

Cytokine	Cellular Source	Effects and Potential Applications
GM-CSF	T cells, macrophages, fibroblasts, endothelial cells, mast cells	An immunopotentiating factor; aids growth and survival of mature red blood cells. Involved in lung surfactant removal. Used for nonmyeloid cancers in patients undergoing autologous bone marrow transplantation, acute myelogenous lukemia after chemotherapy, engraftment delay or failure after bone marrow transplantation of autologous and peripheral blood progenitor cells.
Stem cell factor	Fibroblast cells	Promotes stem cell proliferation and development. May have use in treatment of HIV infection.
Tumor Necrosis Factors		
TNF-alpha	Macrophages, NK cells, mast cells, monocytes, T cells, neutrophils	An antitumor agent; exhibits antiviral, antibacterial, and antimalarial activities. Antagonists may be useful in treating arthritis and septicemia. Major mediator of inflammation. Induces tumor necrosis.
TNF-beta	NK cells, T cells, B cells, myelomas	An inflammatory cytokine that is cytotoxic for tumors in vivo. Activates neutrophils, macrophages, and fibroblasts.

		Plays a role in wound healing and may have antimalarial activity. Has immunosuppressive effects and thus may prevent rejection of transplanted organs.
Interferons		
IFN-alpha	Leukocytes, B cells, macrophages, T cells	Inhibits viral replication. Has antitumor, antibacterial, and antiparasitic activity in vivo. Used in treating hepatitis, herpes, Kaposi's sarcoma, hairy cell leukemia, chronic myelogenous leukemia, melanoma, follicular lymphoma.
IFN-beta	Fibroblasts, epithelial cells	Has considerable antiviral and immunomodulatory effects in vivo. Used in treating multiple sclerosis.
IFN-gamma	NK cells, T cells	Activates macrophages and monocytes. Microcidal and tumorcidal in vivo. May have use as an antitumor agent, in fighting infection, and in treating arthritis. Appears effective against chronic granulomatous disease.

Abbreviations: IL, interleukin; NK cells, natural killer cells; LAK cells, lymphokine-activated killer cells; TIL, tumor-infiltrating lymphocytes; EPO, erythropoietin; M-CSF, macrophage colony-stimulating factor; G-CSF, granulocyte colony-stimulating factor; GM-CSF, granulocyte macrophage colony-stimulating factor; TNF, tumor necrosis factor; IFN, interferon.

Adopted with permission from Casciari, J. J., Sato, H., Durum, S. K., Fiege, J., & Weinstein, J. N. (1996). Reference databases of cytokine structure and function. In H. M. Pinedo, D. L. Longo, & B. A. Chabner (Eds.), *Cancer chemotherapy and biological response modifiers* (Annual 16, pp. 315–346). Amsterdam: Elsevier Science B.V.

25

White, 1996b). Alpha interferon is produced mainly by leukocytes in response to viral, bacterial, or tumor cell stimulation. Beta interferon is derived by fibroblasts and epithelial cells in response to viruses and foreign nucleic acids. Gamma interferon is produced by T lymphocytes and natural killer cells as an integral component of the immune response (Gantz et al., 1995; Hood & Abernathy, 1996).

Interferons influence the immune system by binding to a cell surface receptor and inducing a cascade of biologic events (antiviral, antiproliferative, immunomodulatory). Interferons have antiviral characteristics: they can protect an infected cell from invasion by another virus and can indirectly inhibit viral DNA replication, which hinders the spread of the virus to other cells (Skalla, 1996). Interferons demonstrate antiproliferative effects by inhibiting the growth and division of cancer cells. They also stimulate the expression of human lymphocyte antigens and tumor-associated antigens of tumor cell surfaces, making the tumor cell more apparent (Groenwald et al., 1995). Interferons influence immunomodulatory biologic effects by directly interacting with T lymphocytes to stimulate or inhibit the production of other cytokines. These cytokines can then signal natural killer cells and other lymphocytes to recognize and destroy cancer cells.

The interferons have overlapping but clearly distinct biologic activities and therefore cannot be interchanged.

Toxicities

The toxicities associated with alpha interferon are dose- and route-dependent. The most common side effects are flulike syndrome and fatigue. Flulike syndrome includes fever, chills, malaise, myalgia, and headache. Fatigue is usually the dose-limiting side effect. Tolerance to toxicities may develop with subsequent doses, and toxicities generally subside with a dose adjustment or discontinuation. The interferon can be better tolerated if started at a low dose and escalated in small increments. It may be necessary to reduce the dose of the interferon because of its toxicities (Gantz et al., 1995).

HEMATOPOIETIC GROWTH FACTORS

Hematopoietic growth factors are naturally occurring hormone-like glycoproteins that regulate the proliferation, differentiation, and maturation of blood cells by binding to surface receptors of specific cells. Hematopoiesis (Fig. 2-3) is the process

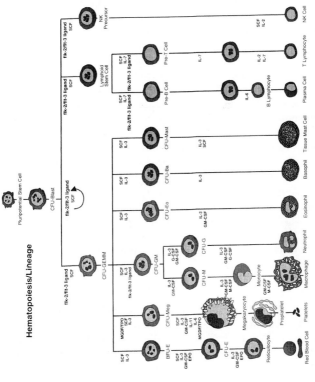

Fig. 2-3. Function of hematopoietic growth factors in hematopoiesis. (Reprinted with permission from Amgen Inc., Thousand Oaks, CA.)

of blood cell formation that occurs in the bone marrow. Each cell is derived from the pluripotent stem cell, the most primitive cell. The pluripotent stem cell can differentiate and mature into either a lymphoid or myeloid cell line. Mature functioning cells include lymphocytes, erythrocytes, platelets, neutrophils, eosinophils, basophils, and monocytes. Hematopoietic growth factors can target cells of a specific cell line, making them single-lineage growth factors, or can simultaneously regulate several cell lines, classifying them as multilineage growth factors. For example, granulocyte colony-stimulating factor (G-CSF) is a single-lineage growth factor that affects only granulocytes. However, GM-CSF is a multilineage growth factor that affects granulocytes, monocytes, and macrophages. Hematopoietic growth factors have been produced through genetic engineering technology by cloning them in mammalian, bacterial, or yeast host cells (De La Pena et al., 1996b; Pitler, 1996).

Hematopoietic growth factors have played a major role in preventing infection in cancer patients by shortening the duration of neutropenia in those receiving chemotherapy. Patients can better tolerate the standard treatment regimen and may be able to tolerate higher doses of chemotherapeutic agents, which may improve therapeutic outcomes. Four hematopoietic growth factors (G-CSF, GM-CSF, erythropoietin, IL-11) have been approved by the FDA, and many other growth factors are being studied in clinical trials. These include M-CSF, stem cell factor, megakaryocyte growth and development factor, IL-3, and GM-CSF/IL-3 fusion protein (PIXY 321) (Parkinson, 1996).

G-CSF

G-CSF is produced by macrophages, endothelial cells, fibroblasts, neutrophils, and bone marrow stomal cells (Gabrilove & Golde, 1997). They increase the number of granulocytes, particularly neutrophils. Filgrastim is a recombinant human G-CSF produced in *Escherichia coli.* It is commercially available as Neupogen. Filgrastim was first approved to decrease the incidence of infections in patients with nonmyeloid malignancies receiving myelosuppressive chemotherapy. Recently, it received regulatory approval for use in patients with nonmyeloid cancers undergoing autologous bone marrow transplantation, patients with severe chronic neutropenia, patients undergoing peripheral blood progenitor cell collection, and patients with acute myeloid leukemia receiving induction or consolidation chemotherapy. Filgrastim is administered intravenously or subcutaneously at dosages ranging from 5 to 10 μg/kg/day starting 24 hours after the last dose of chemotherapy and continuing until the absolute neutrophil count exceeds 10,000/μL (Amgen, 1998). The most common side effect is generalized bone pain, particularly in the lower back, pelvis, and sternum. The pain usually occurs within a 24-hour period as the neutrophil count begins to recover (Gabrilove & Golde, 1993).

GM-CSF

GM-CSF is naturally secreted by endothelial cells, mast cells, fibroblasts, B lymphocytes, and T lymphocytes. It stimulates the growth and differentiation of hematopoietic cells and enhances the function of mature neutrophils, granulocytes, eosinophils, monocytes, and macrophages (Gabrilove & Golde, 1997). Sargramostim is a genetically engineered form of GM-CSF produced through recombinant DNA technology. It is commercially available under the trade name Leukine. Sargramostim has been approved for myeloid recovery in patients undergoing autologous bone marrow transplantation with nonmyeloid cancers, in patients who have undergone allogeneic or autologous bone marrow transplantation in whom engraftment is delayed or has failed, in older adult patients with acute myelogenous leukemia to accelerate neutrophil recovery and reduce the incidence of severe and life-threatening infections after induction chemotherapy, and to accelerate myeloid recovery in patients undergoing allogeneic bone marrow transplantation from HLA-matched related donors. It is usually administered at a dose of 250 μg/m²/day. It may be administered as a subcutaneous injection or as an intravenous infusion at least 24 hours after cytotoxic chemotherapy or radiation therapy (Immunex, 1998). Flulike syndrome, including fever, bone pain, fatigue, myalgia, and headache, is a common side effect. Erythema and pain at the injection site has also been reported. A first-dose reaction characterized by hypotension, tachycardia, flushing, pain, shortness of breath, nausea, and vomiting has been seen with intravenous administration. This phenomenon may be observed with subsequent administrations (De La Pena et al., 1996*b*).

Erythropoietin

Erythropoietin (EPO) is naturally produced by the kidneys and liver in response to decreased red blood cell production or hypoxia. EPO stimulates the production of erythrocyte progenitors to proliferate, differentiate, and mature into erythrocytes. Epoetin alfa is a biosynthetic form of EPO derived from cultures of genetically modified mammalian cells using recombinant DNA technology. It is commercially available under the trade names Epogen and Procrit. It was first approved for use in the treatment of anemia related to chronic renal failure. It was later approved for use in patients with human immunodeficiency virus infection who experience zidovudine-induced anemia, patients with anemia associated with cancer chemotherapy, and patients with anemia who are scheduled to undergo elective surgery. Epoetin alfa is usually administered at a dosage of 50 to 150 units/kg three times a week until the target hematocrit (30% to 36%) is achieved and maintained. Anemic surgical patients receiving epoetin alfa should receive 300 units/kg/day for 10 days before surgery, on the day of surgery, and for 4 days after surgery. If possible, all patients should take oral iron supplements to maintain adequate blood levels for erythropoiesis. Epoetin alfa is usually well tolerated; however, side effects include fever, myalgia, rashes, and headaches. Patients must be closely monitored for an increase in blood pressure. Epoetin alfa is contraindicated in patients with uncontrolled hypertension (Amgen, 1998; De La Pena et al., 1996*b;* Ortho Biotech, 1998).

INTERLEUKINS

Interleukins are regulatory substances produced by lymphocytes and monocytes (Groenwald et al., 1995). They bind to target cells to transmit messages between leukocytes. Interleukins demonstrate a wide range of biologic effects that enhance the immune response. The three main biologic characteristics of interleukins are that they modulate the immune system by altering the communication between tumor cells and immune cells; regulate the immune system by augmenting, restoring, or restraining immune activity; and stimulate hematopoiesis. Interleukins work interdependently with various immune cells (De La Pena et al., 1996*a*).

IL-2 is the most studied interleukin. It is being investigated as a single agent and in combination with other BRMs or chemotherapeutic agents (De La Pena et al., 1996*a;* Lotze & Rosenberg, 1991; Rosenberg, 1993a). IL-2 is a cytokine produced by stimulated T lymphocytes. It exerts antitumor activity by inducing immune effector cells such as lymphokine-activated killer, natural killer, or T cells; secreting other cytokines such as IL-1, interferon gamma, or TNF; or affecting tumor vasculature, leading to tumor necrosis. IL-2 plays a role in both humoral and cell-mediated immunity (De La Pena et al., 1996a; Lotze, 1991; Parkinson, 1996).

In 1992, a recombinant form of IL-2 (aldesleukin [Proleukin]) was approved by the FDA for the treatment of renal cell carcinoma. In 1998, it was approved for the treatment of adults with metastatic melanoma. Standard therapy is 600,000 IU/kg every 8 hours by a 15-minute intravenous infusion for a total of 14 doses. After 9 days of rest, the schedule is repeated for another 14 doses, for a maximum of 28 doses per cycle. Patients may be retreated if response or stable disease is noted after 4 weeks. The patient will have a rest period of at least 7 weeks from the date of discharge before retreatment. Low doses of aldesleukin are well tolerated; however, multisystem toxicities are observed with higher doses (Chiron, 1998). Three major side effects are capillary leak syndrome, flulike syndrome, and skin changes. Capillary leak syndrome occurs because of the shift of fluid from the intravascular to the extravascular space. This syndrome is characterized by hypotension, hypoperfusion, edema, oliguria, dyspnea, and tachycardia. Flulike syndrome includes fatigue, malaise, myalgia, arthralgia, headache, and fever with chills. Patients experiencing skin changes report flushing, erythematous rash, pruritus, stomatitis, dry scaly skin, or inflammation at the administration site. Toxicities are dose- and schedule-dependent and are reversible once therapy is discontinued (De La Pena et al., 1996a).

In 1997, the FDA approved IL-11 (oprelvelkin [Neumega]) for the treatment of patients with nonmyeloid malignancies who are at high risk for severe thrombocytopenia. IL-11 directly stimulates the proliferation of hematopoietic stem cells and megakaryocyte progenitor cells and induces megakaryocyte maturation, resulting in increased platelet production. The suggested dose for adults is 50 μg/kg administered subcutaneously until the postnadir platelet count is 50,000/μL or more (Neumega package insert, 1997). Side effects include atrial arrhythmias, tachycardia, palpitations, dyspnea, fatigue, transient anemia, mild blurred vision, conjunctival redness, and papilledema (Rust et al., 1999).

TUMOR NECROSIS FACTOR

Tumor necrosis factor (TNF) is a natural substance produced by activated macrophages, T lymphocytes, and natural killer cells in response to the presence of tumor cells and infectious agents (Groenwald et al., 1995; Tomaszewski et al., 1995b). TNF has both cytotoxic and cytostatic effects. It stimulates the production of IL-1, IL-6, GM-CSF, and G-CSF and can cause tumor necrosis and hinder the development of new capillary networks in the tumor (Tomaszewski et al., 1995b). TNF binds to the surface of antigens on tumor cells to destroy the endothelial cells of the capillaries while sparing normal cells. TNF has been studied in various solid tumor malignancies, including melanoma and sarcoma; however, its use in clinical trials has been limited because of its toxicities, which include hypotension and adult respiratory distress syndrome. Other symptoms that can make therapy unpleasant are fevers, chills and rigors, muscle pain, fatigue, and headaches. The doses necessary to achieve therapeutic antitumor effects in humans have been intolerable. Strategies to inhibit TNF toxicity are being developed to allow the administration of doses that produce therapeutic responses (Groenwald et al., 1995; Parkinson, 1996).

▼ Additional Biologic Agents and Approaches

VACCINE THERAPY

Vaccine therapy has been studied in various malignancies such as breast, melanoma, colon, and lung cancers. The development of tumor vaccines is based on the idea that there are tumor-associated antigens on the cell surface of tumors not found on normal cells. The immune system can be taught, by active specific immunization with vaccines, to recognize these tumor-associated antigens, stimulate an immune response, and prevent the recurrence of cancer (Hoover & Hanna, 1991). Vaccines have been produced by immunization with autologous or allogeneic tumor cells using living cells, irradiated cells, or cell fragments. Immunologic adjuvants may be added to a vaccine to boost the immunogenicity of the vaccine. Two of the adjuvants used are bacille Calmette-Guerin and keyhole limpet hemocyanin (Livingston, 1991). Various types of cancer vaccines are used in clinical studies: whole-cell vaccines, cell lysate vaccines, viral oncolysate vaccines, shed antigen vaccines, ganglioside vaccines, anti-idiotype vaccines, and genetically engineered vaccines (Livingston, 1991; Schirrmacher, 1995). Vaccines may be administered intradermally, intralesionally, or subcutaneously.

Vaccine therapy is a promising approach in the treatment of cancer. It is well tolerated because of its low toxicity. The common side effect is a local reaction at the injection site consisting of erythema, pruritus, inflammation, or tenderness.

GENE THERAPY

Gene therapy is a technique in which new genetic material is inserted into a patient's cell to correct an inborn genetic error or to introduce a new biologic function to the cell (Rosenberg, 1992). Oncogenes and tumor suppressor genes play an important role in the development of cancer: oncogenes encode for elements that stimulate cell growth, and tumor suppressor genes counteract cell growth signals. Therefore, variations or activation of growth-promoting oncogenes and inactivation of tumor suppressor genes can lead to transformation of normal cells into cancer cells (McCance et al., 1994).

The clinical application of gene therapy in the treatment of cancer has been in enhancing the host's immune response. Clinical studies assessing gene therapy are highly experimental. Approaches in cancer therapy include direct targeting of cancer cells with genes that lessen their growth and manipulation of cells to augment existing immunotherapy or chemotherapy approaches. One approach of gene therapy in cancer treatment is to insert genes coding for cytokines directly into lymphocytes that can specifically recognize a patient's malignant tumor cells. Tumor-infiltrating lymphocytes have been used for this strategy. Another strategy is directly inserting genes into cancer cells to make them more easily recognizable by the body's immune system. Cancer cells express cytokine genes that make the tumors more antigenic, resulting in an antitumor immune response. Retroviral vectors are most commonly used to introduce new genes into human cells. Retroviral vectors carry the new genetic material into dividing cells such as tumor cells while sparing normal cells (Hwu, 1995).

Little toxicity has been reported with gene therapy; however, it is too early in clinical testing to determine the long-term effects.

▼ Handling and Preparation

It is not known whether BRMs have an effect on the person handling and preparing them. Most institutions have policies and procedures outlining the proper handling, preparation, and disposal of BRMs. Only nurses, physicians, and pharmacists with specialized training should prepare BRMs. Personnel should follow the manufacturer's recommendations for preparation and storage of commercially available agents. Research protocols and pharmaceutical companies provide guidelines for handling and preparing investigational agents.

Monoclonal antibodies conjugated with radioisotopes, toxins, or chemotherapeutic agents must be handled and prepared according to chemotherapy and radiation therapy guidelines. Time, distance, and shielding are the three main radiation safety precautions taken by personnel and family members.

Most BRMs must be stored in the refrigerator at 2° to 8°C (36° to 46°F) because they are unstable at room temperature. Vials should never be frozen. A cooler may be used to transport BRMs from the hospital to the home. However, BRMs should be thawed at room temperature before administration. Vials should not be shaken, because this may lead to excess foaming, resulting in dosing error or inactivation of the protein. BRMs are supplied in liquid or powder forms that may require reconstitution with a diluent. They are usually prepared immediately before administration by the pharmacist, nurse, or patient. Vials should be gently swirled or rotated to dissolve the powder in solution. Manufacturers provide the appropriate diluent for reconstitution. Caution should be taken when diluting the BRM to ensure the correct amount of diluent is used. BRMs from different manufacturers are not interchangeable.

▼ Patient and Family Education

Patient and family teaching relevant to biotherapy is an important function of the oncology nurse. Nurses may play a role in obtaining informed consent before initiation of treatment. Patients should be informed of the therapeutic benefits and risks of treatment in a manner suited to their ability to understand. Oncology nurses administering BRMs must clarify and reinforce information provided by physicians when necessary. Additional information about BRMs may be helpful for patients and family members so that they can better understand the treatment plan (Conrad & Horrell, 1995).

An individualized teaching plan should be developed for all patients receiving BRMs. Patients self-administering BRMs

Table 2-3. Management of Side Effects Associated With BRMs

System	Toxicity	Assessment	Intervention
Constitutional	Flulike syndrome Fatigue Fever Myalgia Headache Chills Arthralgia	Obtain a baseline assessment of performance status, level of fatigue, mental status, impact on quality of life and activities of daily living, and nutritional and hydration status	Monitor vital signs, including temperature. Administer antipyretics as ordered. Administer meperidine for chills and rigors. May need to premedicate with subsequent doses. May administer acetaminophen, indomethacin, and diphenhydramine. Encourage adequate nutritional and fluid intake. Encourage usual sleep pattern and rest periods during day. Assist patient in prioritizing activities according to energy level. May need to reduce dose or increase in small increments. Provide comfort measures and emotional support.

(continued)

Table 2-3. Management of Side Effects Associated With BRMs (*Continued*)

System	Toxicity	Assessment	Intervention
Cardiovascular	Capillary leak syndrome Hypotension Tachycardia Arrhythmias Myocardial ischemia	Perform a cardiovascular assessment. Assess for weight gain, orthostatic changes, ECG changes, and history of cardiac disease. Perform ongoing cardiovascular assessment as clinically indicated.	Monitor for decrease in urinary output and edema. Measure abdominal girth daily if ascites is present. Administer 5% albumin for capillary leak syndrome. Closely monitor IV hydration and electrolytes. Elevate extremities if peripheral edema is present. Closely monitor vital signs. Instruct patient to get out of bed slowly to prevent dizziness. Obtain baseline ECG. Instruct patient to report signs of dizziness, palpitation, and chest pain.
Central nervous system	Confusion Impaired memory Anxiety Impaired concentration Somnolence Mood changes	Assess for psychiatric history. Perform a neurologic and mental status assessment at baseline and when clinically indicated. Assess for subtle changes in mood, affect, and cognition.	May need to reduce or discontinue treatment as ordered. Instruct patient and family to report labile or inappropriate responses. Provide emotional support. Encourage expression of feelings.

System	Symptoms	Assessment	Interventions
	Depression Agitation Insomnia Disorientation		Obtain psychiatric consult if indicated. Instruct patient and family to report a change in mental status. Reorient patient when indicated. Instruct patients to avoid alcohol and drugs that may alter mental status.
Digestive	Anorexia	Obtain baseline and ongoing assessment of dietary intake, height, and weight.	Instruct patient to eat small, frequent meals. Encourage patient to eat meals high in calories and protein. Encourage supplements, such as Ensure.
	Diarrhea Nausea Vomiting	Assess bowel habits and nutritional status. Obtain current list of medications patient is taking. Inspect perineal skin.	Instruct patient to avoid spicy food. Instruct patient to observe consistency and number of stools per day. Encourage increase in fluid intake. Observe for signs of dehydration. Monitor fluid and hydration status. Monitor intake and output. Administer IV fluids as clinically indicated.
	Taste alterations	Obtain baseline and ongoing assessment of changes in taste.	Administer antidiarrhea medications or antiemetics as ordered. Encourage oral hygiene before and after meals.

(continued)

Table 2-3. Management of Side Effects Associated With BRMs *(Continued)*

System	Toxicity	Assessment	Intervention
	Mucositis	Assess oral cavity at regular intervals.	Obtain dietary consult for ideas in food preparation. Instruct patient to report oral discomfort. Instruct patient to avoid oral irritants such as alcohol, spices, and commercial mouthwash. Instruct patient to rinse with bicarbonate and nystatin swish.
Hematologic	Anemia Neutropenia Thrombocytopenia	Obtain complete blood count with differential and prothrombin time and partial thromboplastin time at baseline and at regular intervals. Assess for signs and symptoms of anemia, infection, and bleeding.	Monitor vital signs, including temperature. Administer blood products as ordered. Obtain blood cultures with febrile neutropenia. Teach patients the signs and symptoms of anemia, neutropenia, and thrombocytopenia. Teach patients neutropenic and thrombocytopenic precautions. Instruct patients to report any signs and symptoms associated with anemia, neutropenia, and thrombocytopenia.

Hepatic	Elevated liver enzymes and bilirubin	Obtain liver function tests at baseline and at regular intervals. Assess for symptoms associated with hepatic dysfunction. Obtain current list of medications patient is taking. May need to reduce or discontinue treatment as ordered. Teach patients signs and symptoms associated with hepatic dysfunction. Instruct patient to report generalized itching, yellowing of sclera or skin, darkening of urine, and changes in mental status.
Integumentary	Erythema Rash Flushing Pruritus Desquamation Dryness	Perform a daily skin assessment. Monitor injection sites for induration and erythema. Obtain skin disorder history if indicated. Administer antipruritic medications as ordered. Rotate injection sites. Instruct patient to avoid irritation to skin. Apply water-based, perfume- and alcohol-free lotion or cream. Instruct patient on proper skin care. Instruct patient to report any skin change and breakdown.
Pulmonary	Tachypnea Dyspnea Shortness of breath Cough Congestion	Obtain baseline assessment of pulmonary function, smoking history, and breath sounds. Perform ongoing pulmonary assessment as indicated. Obtain baseline chest x-ray. Monitor oxygen saturation by pulse oximeter. Administer oxygen as ordered. Keep head of bed elevated. Instruct patient to report congestion, sputum production, shortness of breath, and dyspnea.

(continued)

Table 2-3. Management of Side Effects Associated With BRMs *(Continued)*

System	Toxicity	Assessment	Intervention
Renal	Oliguria Increase in blood urea nitrogen and creatinine Fluid retention Weight gain	Obtain renal function tests at baseline and at regular intervals. Assess for fluid imbalance. Obtain weight at baseline and at regular intervals.	May need to reduce or discontinue treatment as ordered. Monitor intake and output and peripheral edema. Administer diuretics as ordered. Instruct patient to report changes in urinary output, peripheral edema, and weight gain.

Data from: Conrad, K. J., & Horrell, C. J. (1995). *Biotherapy: Recommendations for nursing course content and clinical practicum.* Pittsburgh: Oncology Nursing Press; Sandstum S. K. (1996). Nursing management of patients receiving biological therapy. *Seminars in Oncology Nursing, 12*(2), 152–162.

require verbal and written instructions on preparation and administration techniques as well as self-care measures. Audiovisual aids may be a useful tool to reinforce teaching. Patients must be instructed about the proper storage and disposal of BRMs. Patients should be provided all the necessary materials for self-administration (e.g., needles, syringes, alcohol swabs, and needle disposal container).

Nurses must review all possible side effects and symptom management with patients. Patients should be reassured that most toxicities are dose-, route-, or schedule-dependent and are reversible once the therapy is discontinued. Nurses, in collaboration with physicians and patients, can establish interventions to minimize toxicities.

▼ Management of Side Effects and Toxicities

Nurses administering BRMs should be certified in cardiopulmonary resuscitation. They must be able to assess for and manage the known and unexpected toxicities associated with BRMs. Emergency equipment must be readily available because of the risk of an anaphylactic response. Nurses should conduct ongoing assessments of the patient's response to treatment. Patients administering BRMs at home may keep a diary to track all toxicities and medications taken for symptom management.

Many potential side effects and toxicities are associated with BRMs. They produce a broad range of systemic toxicities (Table 2-3). The side effects are commonly dose-dependent and are reversible once the therapy is discontinued. The two most common side effects are flulike syndrome and fatigue. Flulike syndrome is characterized by fatigue, malaise, myalgia, arthralgia, headaches, and fever with chills. Toxicities may be minimized by administering acetaminophen before and at regular intervals after treatment. Patients experiencing fatigue report tiredness, exhaustion, weakness, lack of energy, and inability to concentrate (Engelking & Wujcik, 1994; Tomaszewski et al., 1995b). Patients should be instructed on conserving energy and planning rest periods throughout the day. Emphasis should be placed on proper nutrition and hydration. The management of fatigue related to BRMs and chemotherapy is discussed in Chapter 5.

3

Clinical Trials

The goals of clinical cancer research are to improve the therapeutic outcomes for cancer patients and to improve the quality of care. Important progress in cancer therapy has been possible because of clinical trials, but public confidence and support have waned because of past abuses and mistakes. However, without the benefit of experimentation, new and improved treatments will never be tested, and the important questions that need to be asked will never be answered. Good clinical trials need the support of both clinicians and patients. For this to happen, clinical trials must be carefully planned to ensure that the physical, moral, and ethical welfare of patients is safeguarded. This chapter deals with cancer drug development and the clinical trials system, from concept to implementation. It also deals with the mechanisms that protect the rights of human subjects and discusses the responsibilities of the nurse who takes care of them.

▼ Clinical Trials

According to federal regulations governing the protection of human subjects, research is "the systematic investigation, including research development, testing, and evaluation, designed to develop or contribute to generalized knowledge" (National Commission, 1991). Two historical events greatly affected the establishment of federal regulations to protect the rights of human subjects involved in research: the Nuremberg Trial in 1946 and the Tuskegee Disclosure in 1972. As a result, the Institutional Review Board (IRB) was created to monitor and review research, and the National Research Act (1994) established the National Commission for the Protection of Human Subjects of Biomedical and Behavioral Research. This group wrote the *Belmont Report,* which governs the ethical conduct of biomedical research.

The three principles on which the protection of human subjects is based are autonomy, beneficence, and justice. *Autonomy* requires respecting a person's self-determination and refraining from obstructing a person's actions unless those actions are clearly detrimental to others. It also includes protecting a person who has diminished autonomy. *Beneficence* refers to the principle of "doing no harm," as stated in the Hippocratic oath, and of maximizing possible benefits and minimizing possible risks. The principle of *justice* addresses fairness in the distribution of the benefits and burdens of scientific research.

▼ Drug Development

The process of translating the new knowledge gained from the bench (basic research) is long and expensive. Drug development starts with the acquisition and screening of chemical compounds. Screening is done on these compounds using animal or human cancer cells grown *in vitro,* transplanted animal tumors, and human xenografts. Then, animal toxicology studies and pharmacokinetic measurements are undertaken to provide vital information about the drug's metabolism, half-life, absorption, excretion, and clearance. These studies enable the scientist to formulate an initial dose and schedule that would be acceptable for testing in humans.

When the preclinical trial is completed, an investigational new drug application is filed with the Food and Drug Administration (FDA). Before it approves a research protocol, the FDA requires documentation stating that the research will be done according to ethical standards and giving the name of the IRB, if applicable, that will be responsible for monitoring and evaluating the study.

▼ Three Phases of Clinical Trials

Agents being tested progress through the phases of the clinical trial (Table 3-1). In a *phase I* setting, new drugs (alone or

Table 3-1. Phases of a Clinical Trial

Phase	Objective
I	Determine the maximum tolerated dose at a given dose and schedule. Define toxicities. Investigate pharmacokinetic activities of the agent.
II	Determine antitumor activity at a given dose and schedule. Validate toxicities.
III	Compare with standard therapies using randomized trials. Make recommendations for general use.
IV	Conduct postmarketing studies to identify other clinical applications for the drug. Generate more information about added benefits and risks.

in combination) are tested to assess toxicity and to determine the *maximum tolerated dose.* Another objective of a phase I study is to determine biochemical events associated with the new drug (Simon & Friedman, 1992). This is achieved by performing pharmacokinetic studies. The data that are gathered are helpful in assessing the activity or toxicity of a new agent. *Phase II* trials determine the antitumor activity of a drug or a combination of drugs against a particular cancer type. Patients in this phase usually receive 75% to 90% of the maximum tolerated dose to prevent any severe toxicity. The primary end point is tumor response, as evidenced by shrinkage in the tumor in patients with measurable disease. Once the antitumor activity of the new agent is established in a phase II study, the efficacy of the new treatment is compared with a current standard regimen. *Phase III* follows, and patients who are entered on this level are usually randomized. The sample sizes required are large, necessitating multi-institutional cooperative group trials. Randomization is important and is undertaken to prevent biases.

After these three phases are completed, a new drug application is submitted to the FDA. In 1992, it took the FDA an average of 19 months to approve a new drug. With the dramatic changes in health care, reforms to accelerate the approval process have been implemented. When the application is approved, the drug then becomes available in the market. It is estimated that it costs $50 to $70 million and takes approximately 6 to 12 years to develop a new drug.

Phase IV focuses on postmarketing studies and the collection of more data on the new treatment.

▼ The Research Protocol: From Concept to Implementation

A *research protocol* is a guideline ensuring the consistent administration of an experimental procedure or treatment. It includes these important components:

1. The *protocol summary* gives an overview of the research study, the goals, and a schema of the protocol.
2. The *objective* describes the scientific hypotheses to be addressed by the study. The outcomes of the study should always relate to the stated objectives.
3. The *background* section explains the rationale for pursuing the proposed study. It contains scientific facts regarding the disease and the results of recent laboratory experiments and clinical trials.
4. The *patient eligibility* describes the patient or subject population, inclusion and exclusion criteria, and other characteristics needed to be enrolled in the trial.
5. The *pretreatment evaluation* section outlines all baseline evaluations and laboratory and diagnostic screening to be completed to determine a patient's eligibility for the study.
6. The *treatment plan* reviews the protocol therapy. It includes information on drug administration, time frames, where the treatment is going to be given, and modifications in therapy.
7. *Evaluation during study* correlates with the treatment schema. It contains a calendar of tests, diagnostic procedures, and pharmacokinetic studies, if indicated, that must be performed while the patient is on the study.
8. *Criteria for therapeutic response,* or *end points,* are precisely stated criteria used to measure the success or failure of the treatment. The primary end point is usually the tumor response (Table 3-2). Other end points include disease-free survival, duration of response, quality of life, and treatment toxicity.
9. *Criteria for toxicity* include the methodology for grading toxicities related to treatment. Appendix D contains the National Cancer Institute toxicity scale, the most com-

Table 3-2. Tumor Response

Response	Description
Complete response (CR)	Disappearance of all clinical evidence of tumor by physical examination or radiologic studies with no appearance of new lesions. The response must last for a minimum of 4 weeks. The patient must be free of all cancer-related symptoms, and all abnormal biochemical parameters must return to normal.
Partial response (PR)	Fifty percent or greater decrease in the sum of the product of the diameters of measured lesions. No new lesions may appear. This improvement must continue for at least 4 weeks, during which there is no cancer-associated deterioration in weight, performance status, or symptoms. If there is no change in tumor size but the biochemical parameters decline by 80% or more, the patient will be considered stable.
Stable disease (STAB)	Patients who do not meet the criteria for partial response without signs and symptoms of progressive disease for a minimum of 3 months.
Progressive disease (PROG)	A greater than 25% increase in the total area of the bidimensionally measurable lesion(s). The appearance of new lesions or greater or significant deterioration that cannot be attributed to treatment or medical conditions will be considered disease progression.

mon toxicity scale used in clinical trials. This section also defines adverse drug reactions and reporting mechanisms that are in accordance with the safety reporting guidelines of the FDA (21 CFR 312.32).

10. *Criteria for removal from study* specify the circumstances under which a patient may be taken off the study, such as disease progression, noncompliance, or loss to follow-up.

11. *Pharmacologic information* describes the drug or drugs to

be given and data about formulation, stability, mechanism of action, availability, route of administration, and side effects.

12. *Protection of human subjects* describes the major expected toxicities from the treatment, potential benefits to the patient or society, alternative treatments, incremental costs as a result of participation, and procedures for protecting the privacy and confidentiality of patients.

13. *Biostatistical considerations* include information about sample size, expected time for accrual, randomization procedures if appropriate, stopping rules, and study duration.

14. *Informed consent procedures* outline the requirements of the IRB for obtaining patient consent, the consent process, including who may register the patient, documentation of the informed consent, and how the privacy and confidentiality of the patient will be ensured.

▼ Informed Consent

The Department of Health and Human Services defines informed consent as "the knowing consent of an individual or his legally authorized representative so situated as to be able to exercise free power of choice without inducement or any element of force, fraud, deceit, distress, or any other form of constraint or coercion" (Varrichio & Vassak, 1989). It is a legal and ethical prerequisite for patients participating in research studies. Current regulations protecting human rights are described in the *Common Rule*, which specifies that an informed consent must include:

1. A statement that the study involves research, an explanation of the purposes of the study, the expected duration of the participation of the subject, and a description of the procedures to be followed

2. A description of any reasonably foreseeable risks or discomforts

3. A description of any potential benefits to the subject or to others from the research

4. A disclosure of appropriate alternative treatments that the subject might want to consider

5. A statement describing the extent to which confidentiality of the subject will be maintained
6. Explanations regarding whether compensation or treatments are available if injury occurs
7. A statement that the participation of the subject is voluntary, that refusal to participate involves no penalty or loss of benefits to which the subject is otherwise entitled, and that the subject may withdraw at any time without prejudicing his or her care in the future
8. An explanation of whom to contact for answers and questions about the study and the subject's rights.

▼ The Economics of Clinical Trials

Participation in clinical research is one of the best opportunities for finding a cancer cure. Recent reports, however, show that only 3% of adult cancer patients and 1.5% of senior citizens with cancer are enrolled in clinical trials. Economic concerns, specifically the denial of coverage by third-party payors, are considered a disincentive for patients. Most health plans still deny coverage of investigational treatments. The patient must also consider the additional costs of tests and treatments required by the protocol, as well as travel costs. The physician and the nurse responsible for obtaining informed consent from the patient must make the patient aware of these added costs, because preauthorization from the patient's health plan may be needed before enrollment into the protocol. For the institution conducting the clinical investigation, there are research costs for personnel who will be responsible for the various aspects of the research, such as patient accrual, enrollment, follow-up, monitoring, data collection, and analysis.

In December 1999, New Jersey became the first state where insurers voluntarily agreed to ensure coverage of all costs for routine care for patients enrolled in clinical trials sponsored by the National Institute of Health, the Department of Defense, and the Veterans Administration. Several states have followed this mandate. There is federal support and pending legislation that will provide insurance reimbursement for participation in clinical trials. It is hoped that these initiatives will encourage enrollment in clinical research of patients who would otherwise shy away because of the added costs.

▼ Institutional Review Board

Any research institution receiving federal research funds must have an IRB. The IRB is composed of several members with a primary concern in a scientific area and in a nonscientific area, and one lay person unaffiliated with the institution. The IRB plays a key role in ensuring the protection of human research subjects. It ensures that the rights and welfare of human subjects are protected, that informed consents are obtained, and that the confidentiality and integrity of research subjects and data are maintained. The IRB is required to monitor ongoing research activities and to keep documentation of IRB minutes, all research proposals, scientific findings and evaluations, and correspondence with investigators, federal and regulatory agencies, and industrial sponsors of research.

▼ Role of the Nurse in Clinical Trials

There are various practice implications for a nurse working with patients enrolled in clinical trials. The degree of involvement and responsibility may vary depending on the nurse's primary function—either as the direct caregiver or as the research nurse who is intimately involved with the research project itself. These responsibilities fall into three categories—patient care, data management, and education and protocol development:

PATIENT CARE

- Assists in the recruitment and accrual of patients into a protocol
- Screens patients and facilitates entry into a protocol
- Ensures that informed consent is properly obtained
- Assesses, manages, and documents symptoms, toxicities, and responses of the patient to the regimen
- Administers drugs or treatments as required by the protocol
- Conducts pharmacokinetic studies and handles specimens according to the protocol
- Helps coordinate all necessary tests, diagnostic procedures, and treatments to be given in a safe, timely, and appropriate manner.

DATA MANAGEMENT

- Collaborates with members of the research team in collecting and maintaining the integrity of patient data
- Assists with biostatistical analysis of the data
- Develops and reviews documentation sources such as flow sheets, patient diaries, and calendars for obtaining quality data
- Secures case report forms, regulatory documents, and other written communication with the IRB, FDA, National Cancer Institute, and pharmaceutical companies in an organized manner
- Assists and facilitates clinical trial audits when appropriate
- Participates in maintaining quality control measures to ensure objective and clean data

EDUCATION AND PROTOCOL DEVELOPMENT

- Educates the patient and family about the research study and makes appropriate referrals if necessary
- Participates in the development and revision of clinical protocols, making sure that the proposed treatment plan, schedule, and study requirements are attainable with respect to resources of the institution and the patient
- Educates self and other health care personnel about new clinical trials and changes, and updates them on the progress of current trials
- Collaborates with the research team in the planning, design, implementation, and monitoring of investigational studies
- Acts as a resource person to other caregivers in matters pertaining to protocols, such as amendments, protocol requirements, and compliance

4

Preparation, Administration, and Handling of Chemotherapy

▼ Ensuring Patient Safety: Preventing Chemotherapy Errors

The chemotherapy administration process provides many opportunities for various health care professionals to make mistakes. The error may occur anywhere in the chemotherapy administration system, from the moment the oncologist writes the chemotherapy order to the actual drug administration by the nurse. A breakdown in this multistep process can cause lethal consequences. When the error is not detected before it reaches the patient, the patient suffers the serious and toxic effects. In December 1999, the Institute of Medicine reported that 44,000 to 98,000 Americans die each year from preventable errors (LNN, Dec. 6, p. 190). A study by Edgar et al. (1994) found that of the 43 medication errors that resulted in death, 11 involved chemotherapy overdoses. The celebrated case of the *Boston Globe* reporter who died of a chemotherapy error in 1994 was a wake-up call for health care institutions to invest more time and effort in examining their medication administration system. Diligent analysis found that in most institutions, system failures were the primary cause of medication errors. Since then, system-based changes and guidelines have been implemented. Voluntary, rather than mandatory, error reports have risen dramatically because "no one feared punishment for honestly reporting mistakes" (Cohen, 2000). Studies of medication errors have found that poor staffing, breakdowns in communication, inadequate staff education, and poor drug information contribute to the problem.

In response to President Clinton's call for aggressive action to prevent medication errors, provisions have been made in the fiscal year 2001 budget. New spending in the amount of $16 million has been earmarked to address the problem. The Agency for Healthcare Research and Quality has been authorized to use $20 million in existing funds for research. These initiatives will focus on medical error prevention programs, patient safety research, reporting, and dissemination of information.

According to the Institute for Safe Medication Practices, a nonprofit organization that monitors and recommends safe medication practices, the following error-reduction strategies relating to chemotherapy administration have brought about positive changes in various institutions:

1. Only physicians who are experienced in the use of antineoplastic agents prescribe chemotherapy and manage the patient. In certain institutions where different levels of practitioners are allowed to write orders (oncology fellows, nurse practitioners), their orders are cosigned by the physician attending.

2. Chemotherapy is administered by professional staff members who are specially trained in chemotherapy administration. They should have completed an educational program according to their institutional policies and should comply with mandates for yearly competency requirements. In 1998, the Oncology Nursing Society developed a cancer chemotherapy course based on the society's cancer chemotherapy guidelines and recommendations for practice. The course describes a didactic content and a clinical practicum needed to prepare the nurse to care for patients undergoing chemotherapy in various settings.

3. Orders are verified by at least two health care professionals, preferably one RN and one pharmacist. This involves a double check of the patient's name, drug, dose calculation, route, frequency, total daily dose, and date of administration. Verbal orders for chemotherapy are not accepted.

4. The patient is identified positively by two health care professionals before drug administration. The patient's iden-

tity is verified by checking the identification band and the medical record number, and asking the patient to spell his or her name and give his or her address. In outpatient treatment centers, a photo attached to the patient's profile card or an identification band can help identify the patient.

5. Patient education is a key component of the chemotherapy treatment. Patients are taught about side effects and self-care management and about the proper handling and disposal of chemotherapy agents.

6. Treatment parameters are identified and assessed before drug administration.

7. The use of a bar-code system has been shown to decrease medication errors. Computerized order entry systems are helpful; preprinted order sets are a good alternative.

8. Professional staff are oriented to the chemotherapy process and are instructed to follow standardized guidelines for writing chemotherapy orders, such as:

   a. Use the drug's generic name, not the brand name, acronym, or abbreviation.

   b. Avoid decimals; round off to a whole number. If a decimal is required, use a zero before the decimal point (0.5 mg, not .5 mg).

   c. Never use trailing zeros. If the dose is 20 mg, write it as "20 mg," not "20.0 mg," because the extra zero might be mistakenly added to the dose.

   d. Refer to established maximum dose limits. If these are exceeded, specify the rationale and obtain necessary approvals as set by the institution.

   e. Maintain good communication with the nurses and pharmacists who are involved in the chemotherapy administration system. If the order is "challenged," the prescribing physician should not take it as an affront but as a helpful intervention to ensure the safety of the patient and the team.

9. Whenever new drugs or research protocols are started, diligent efforts are made to educate everyone involved about the protocol details and treatment regimen.

10. Hospital administrators should provide support for a multidisciplinary team of physicians, nurses, and pharmacists who are intimately involved in chemotherapy processes to work with a quality improvement professional. This team will analyze medication errors and recommend and promote institution-wide and system-based improvements to prevent errors.

▼ Calculating Chemotherapy Dosages

Most chemotherapy dosages are calculated based on body surface area (BSA) or weight (kg). The BSA, the external surface of the body, is expressed in square meters (m^2). The BSA is more commonly used for dosing calculations because it is a more accurate measure of fluid and tissue proportion. To determine the BSA, a nomogram, a slide rule, or a BSA conversion calculator can be used. Throughout the institution, only one method should be used consistently to avoid variances in calculation, which might lead to dosing errors.

A *nomogram* (Fig. 4-1) is a table of three columns that correlates a person's height and weight. The patient's height is located in the left column, the weight is found in the right column, and a ruler is used to draw a line between the two. The point at which the line intersects the middle column represents the patient's BSA. Because children differ in fluid and tissue proportions, a separate nomogram is used for children.

Chemotherapy doses are often ordered in milligrams per square meter (mg/m^2). To calculate the dose a patient will receive, the drug ordered in mg/m^2 is multiplied by the determined BSA:

$$\text{Dose} = (mg/m^2) \times m^2$$

If a patient with a BSA of $1.60\ m^2$ is ordered to receive paclitaxel $50\ mg/m^2$, the patient would be given $(50\ mg/m^2) \times (1.60\ m^2) = 80\ mg$ paclitaxel.

For obese patients, the ideal body weight (IBW) calculation may be used instead of the patient's actual weight. The formula most often used is the following:

IBW (female) = 45.5 kg + (2.3 kg × [height − 60 in])
IBW (male) = 50 kg + (2.3 kg × [height − 60 in])

Dosing based on the area under the curve, used in ordering carboplatin doses, is explained in Unit II.

▼ Pretreatment Assessment

Before a chemotherapy treatment is initiated, the health professional responsible for the administration of the agent must

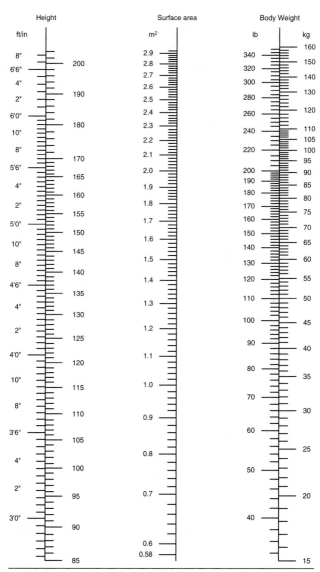

An estimate of a patient's surface area can be obtained by marking the patient's height and weight and drawing a line between these two points; the point at which this line intersects the middle scale represents the patient's surface area.
Note: Adapted from *Normal Laboratory Values, Scientific American Medicine* (Vol. 3) (p. 19), by D.C. Dale and D.D. Federman (Eds.), 1996, New York: Scientific American.

Fig. 4-1. Adult nomogram.

independently assess the patient. This pretreatment assessment and preparations must include the following:

1. The patient's physical, cognitive, and emotional state
2. The patient's knowledge of his or her disease and the treatment plan
3. The patient's previous experience with chemotherapy or other treatment modalities
4. History of drug allergies
5. Presence of written informed consent if the patient is enrolled in a research protocol, or if required according to institutional policy. Informed consent verifies that the patient has been educated about the drug to be received and its benefits and risks.
6. Patient education needs, how these are going to be met, outcomes to be achieved, and plans for follow-up
7. Laboratory parameters and accepted ranges for drug administration (e.g., blood urea nitrogen and creatinine for patients who are to receive nephrotoxic agents) and the patient's laboratory values before drug administration
8. A written physician's order that includes the following:
   - Patient's name and medical record number
   - Date the order was written and date of drug administration
   - Normalized chemotherapy dose calculated in mg/m^2 or a unit of measurement, and the total *daily* dose to be given, not the total dose for the cycle
   - Route of administration
   - Frequency of administration
   - Length of time of administration
   - Medication orders for hydration, diuresis, anaphylaxis, emesis, and hypersensitivity reactions appropriate for the drug regimen
9. Readily available emergency equipment and medications should any adverse reactions, such as anaphylaxis, occur. A chemotherapy spill kit should also be within easy reach.
10. The patient's name, date, drug, and dose on the label on the prepared agent and order verification by a pharmacist
11. Good venous access and verification of the intended use, patency, and integrity of the vascular access device, according to institutional policy.

▼ Routes of Administration

After the pretreatment assessment is completed, the RN may administer the chemotherapy. As advances in chemotherapy occur, the routes of administration continue to evolve. The choice of drug route depends on the therapeutic intent. Peripheral and central lines are the most commonly used methods to administer chemotherapy. In the past 2 years, more oral cytotoxic agents have been discovered; oral administration makes it more convenient for patients to receive treatment at home and is less expensive but presents different challenges for the clinician. Alternative routes of drug delivery to specific sites in the body using devices or catheters are becoming more popular in clinical practice. This section discusses the methods of drug delivery, traditional and alternative routes, and practice implications for nurses.

ORAL

A wide variety of oral agents are now available. Capecitabine, a recent discovery, is an oral prodrug of 5-fluorouracil. A *prodrug* is a chemical precursor of an active agent that needs to be converted into an active agent to become effective. The conversion is accomplished by one or more enzymes found in the liver, tumor sites, or other tissues. Prodrugs are believed to provide more selective and intensive therapy for the target tumor.

Most oral cytotoxic agents are self-administered by the patient at home, so the practice implications for the nurse involve patient education, monitoring for compliance, drug accounting, and documentation. Most of these functions involve intervention and are often accomplished by timely and skillful telephone triage.

INTRAMUSCULAR/SUBCUTANEOUS

Few chemotherapeutic agents are given using these routes. Some examples are leuprolide (subcutaneous), leucovorin (intramuscular), granulocyte colony-stimulating factor (subcutaneous), and several vaccines in immunotherapy. The nurse should monitor the platelet count because of the potential for bleeding, rotate injection sites to avoid further trauma, assess for infection, and ensure there is enough muscle mass and tissue for absorption. Education is important so that the patient will follow these precautions.

IV SIDE ARM

The IV side arm method involves the instillation of an agent into the side port (also referred to as the Y site) of a free-flowing IV line using a syringe. This is a common technique for vesicant administration. In the absence of blood return, administration must be stopped immediately to avoid injury through extravasation. If more than one agent is to be administered using this method, at least 10 mL of IV solution should be allowed to infuse between agents.

IV PUSH

IV push involves the direct administration of an agent into a central venous access device (CVAD) or peripherally into a vein using a butterfly needle or angiocatheter.

IV PIGGYBACK

The IV piggyback method involves the administration of an agent using a secondary set that is "piggybacked" into a primary line.

CONTINUOUS INTRAVENOUS INFUSION

Chemotherapy may be given by continuous infusion by means of peripheral access or a CVAD. Continuous infusions vary in length from hours to days, depending on the drug and protocol. The drug is usually in 250 to 1,000 mL of IV solution. To ensure a consistent flow and timely delivery of the drug, the infusion is usually hooked up to a gravity pump.

INTRAPERITONEAL CHEMOTHERAPY

Intraperitoneal (IP) chemotherapy is administered directly into the peritoneal cavity through a temporary catheter, an external intraperitoneal catheter, or an implanted port (Fig. 4-2). This route is useful for the treatment of intra-abdominal malignancies. There is a significant pharmacokinetic advantage in IP chemotherapy because it allows a lower peritoneal

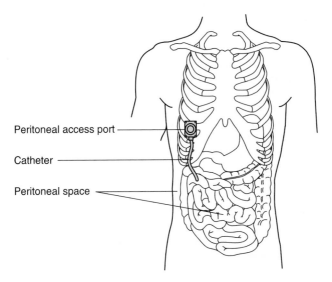

Fig. 4-2. Intraperitoneal port.

clearance than plasma clearance of certain neoplastics, thus exposing the tumor to higher drug concentrations. There is also decreased potential for systemic toxicity because the cytotoxic drugs are metabolized in the liver before entering the systemic circulation.

Nursing Implications

1. Assess the patient for signs or symptoms of intra-abdominal infection: fever, abdominal pain, or discomfort. If these signs exist, do not administer the drug.
2. Assess the patency of the implanted port before administration. Noncoring needles (19G), usually 1″ long for average-size patients, are adequate to access the rubber diaphragm of the port. Longer needles are needed for obese patients.
3. Teach the patient about the side effects that may occur during and after drug administration (abdominal distention, pain, cramps, nausea, vomiting, diarrhea, constipation, shortness of breath, esophageal reflux). These symptoms will subside about 48 hours after completion

of treatment. The patient should also be instructed to
turn from side to side every 30 minutes for 4 hours to
promote drug distribution.

4. Maintain the patient in a semi-Fowler's position.
5. Infuse the chemotherapy, which is added to 1 to 2 L
   normal saline at body temperature. Some patients report feeling cold during the infusion; blankets should
   be provided.
6. If severe abdominal pain occurs during the infusion of
   an agent that is either a vesicant or an investigational
   agent, stop the infusion and notify the physician.
7. Analgesics or antianxiety agents (e.g., meperidine or
   lorazepam) may be prescribed to relieve discomfort or
   anxiety during treatment.
8. Documentation should include date, time, drug, dosage,
   needle gauge and length, assessment of catheter patency, patient teaching and educational materials given,
   and patient's tolerance of treatment.

INTRAHEPATIC CHEMOTHERAPY

This route of administration is indicated in patients with colorectal metastasis to the liver. Intrahepatic chemotherapy is
administered in one of two ways: through a port catheter
placed in the common hepatic artery, with the port body subcutaneously placed below the rib cage, or with a pump
surgically implanted into a subcutaneous pocket in the abdominal wall (Almadrones et al., 1995). To administer
chemotherapy through an arterial port catheter, a noncoring
needle is used to access the device. To administer chemotherapy through a pump (by bolus or continuous infusion), a
special noncoring pump needle is used percutaneously to access the pump's flat, circular septum, which is connected to
a drug reservoir. Hepatic pump models include the
Medtronic, the Arrow, and the Infusaid pumps. By means of
percutaneous injection, the pump reservoir is filled with an
agent that is infused from the pump into a vein, an artery, or
a body cavity (Fig. 4-3). The charging fluid in a small inner
chamber is recharged intrinsically each time the pump is refilled. When not being used to administer chemotherapy,
this pump must be refilled every 2 weeks with an infusate solution to ensure that it remains charged and ready for use.
The remaining infusate must be withdrawn from the pump

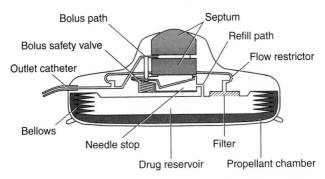

Fig. 4-3. Schematic drawing of the Arrow® implantable pump for intrahepatic chemotherapy administration.

before more infusate can be administered and before the agent can be administered into the reservoir. The pump should be manipulated only by qualified personnel, who should follow the manufacturer's instructions regarding proper use.

Flow rates range from 1 to 2 mL/day and are predetermined by the manufacturer. Flow rates increase at high altitudes, with fever, and with hypertension. Ambulatory hepatic infusion pumps can cause chemical hepatitis, chemical cholecystitis, and cholangitis.

Nursing Implications

1. Teach the patient how the pump works and precautions to take:
   a. Avoid rough physical activity that might cause a blow to the pump site.
   b. Do not place heating pads or hot-water bottles directly over the pump site. Avoid saunas or long baths. Increased temperature increases the pump's flow rate.
   c. Avoid deep-sea and scuba diving, because the increased pressure will affect the flow rate of the pump. Snorkeling and swimming are permitted.
   d. Notify the physician or nurse when traveling by air, because the medication might need to be adjusted.
2. Emphasize the importance of keeping appointments for medication refills.

3. Before initiating treatment, a flow study must be undertaken and documented on the chart. The flow study verifies catheter placement and regional perfusion.
4. Access the pump septum with the special needle for the particular model being used. This is crucial to preserve the integrity of the self-sealing refill port.
5. Do not aspirate the pump. Aspiration causes blood to be drawn into the catheter and can result in catheter occlusion.
6. Record the drug residual at every visit. The residual volume is used to calculate the delivery rate. It also serves as a check for proper pump function.
7. Document the date, time, infusate, amount, patient's response during and after the procedure, and patient teaching and educational materials given.

INTRATHECAL/INTRAVENTRICULAR

Drugs such as methotrexate, cytarabine, and thiotepa are commonly given by these methods. These routes are indicated in the management of patients who have leukemia and lymphomas of the central nervous system. An intrathecal catheter can be attached to an implanted port or pump. The Ommaya reservoir (Fig. 4-4) is an implanted ventricular device that allows the percutaneous injection of cytotoxic drugs directly into the lateral ventricles of the brain.

Nursing Implications

1. Teach the patient about the procedure, whether the patient is going to have a lumbar puncture or surgical placement of an Ommaya reservoir.
2. Assess the patient for signs and symptoms of increased intracranial pressure.
3. Observe the site for signs of infection.
4. Use preservative-free drug and diluents to prevent neurotoxicity.
5. Assess for proper function of the reservoir.

INTRAVESICAL

This method, used for the treatment of superficial bladder cancer and cancer *in situ*, involves the instillation of chemother-

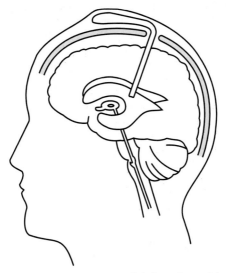

Fig. 4-4. Side inlet Ommaya reservoir in lateral ventricle.

apy (thiotepa, doxorubicin, or mitomycin) through a urinary catheter into the patient's bladder. The dwell time is 1 to 2 hours, after which the catheter is unclamped or removed to drain the medication. The patient is asked to void. All wastes should be treated or disposed of as chemotherapeutic wastes.

INTRAPLEURAL

Antineoplastic agents such as nitrogen mustard and bleomycin are injected through the patient's chest tube in this method. This is done to sclerose the pleural lining to prevent recurring pleural effusion from the malignancy. The pleural cavity is completely drained using a thoracotomy tube, followed by the instillation of the chemotherapeutic agent. The tube is clamped, and the patient is repositioned every 15 minutes for approximately 2 hours. The chest tube is then attached to suction for 18 hours. Most patients are anxious about this procedure and may complain of pain. Supportive measures are taken.

▼ Central Venous Access Devices (CVADs)

Before the development of CVADs, patients receiving chemotherapy needed to have multiple peripheral venous punctures for laboratory tests, therapy, and blood transfusions. Peripheral venous integrity gradually diminishes with frequent venipunctures, and CVADs provide a more reliable and less painful means to achieve the same purposes using the central circulation. CVADs are inserted into a major vein of the arm, chest, or neck or the femoral or portal circulation. They are constructed from a radiopaque material so proper placement can be assessed. Single-lumen or multilumen catheters are available in various sizes.

There are four categories of CVADs:
- Percutaneous catheters
- Tunneled catheters
- Implanted ports
- Peripherally inserted central catheters (PICCs)

Table 4-1 lists the indications, placement, disadvantages, advantages, potential complications, maintenance care, materials used, available sizes, and commonly used catheter manufacturers.

SELECTION

Ideally, selection should be based on input from the patient, the patient's family or significant other, the physician, the surgeon, and the nurse. Factors taken into account before selecting a device include the following:
- The treatment to be received
- The patient's cognitive and physical ability to perform catheter maintenance care
- The presence of a caregiver to provide maintenance care if the patient cannot do so
- Advantages and disadvantages of the devices available

ROUTINE CARE

CVADs require meticulous care to prevent complications. Routine care involves irrigation, cap changes, exit-site skin care, and dressing changes. Nurses must follow institutional procedures for each aspect of maintenance care.

Irrigation

- After each use, the catheter must be flushed with 5 to 10 mL normal saline, followed by irrigation with a heparin solution. (Groshong catheters are the only exception for irrigation with heparin; they contain a catheter tip valve that prevents the backflow of blood into the catheter.)
- When the catheter is not in use, each lumen must be flushed with heparin.
- The volumes of heparin used vary from 2 to 5 mL; the concentrations range from 10 to 100 units/mL.
- The frequency with which an unused catheter is to be heparinized varies from every day to once monthly, depending on the device and the institution.

Cap Changes

- Catheters that are not being used require a sterile injection cap or adapter.
- Injection caps or adapters are changed daily, every 3 days, or weekly, depending on the institution.
- To avoid unnecessary opening of the catheter, changing should be coordinated with irrigation.

Site Care

The site is assessed for signs of infection (redness, swelling, discharge, tenderness) and cleaned with an antiseptic solution, using a circular motion moving outward from the exit site.

Dressing Changes

- Generally, sterile technique is used in an inpatient setting and clean technique is used in the home environment.
- Institutional guidelines are followed for the frequency of changes (every day to once weekly) and the dressing used (occlusive or transparent, with or without gauze).
- If the dressing becomes wet, soiled, or loose, it needs to be changed more frequently.

SERUM SAMPLING

The volume of normal saline and concentrations of heparin used vary for serum sampling. Nurses must follow institu-

Table 4-1. Comparison of Central Venous Access Devices

Indication	Placement	Disadvantages	Advantages
Percutaneous Central Venous Catheter (23 to 16 g [1.9F to 4.8F])			
Short-term access for acute care	Under local anesthesia, the catheter is advanced though venous puncture into the subclavian or jugular vein and the tip is advanced into the superior vena cava. It is sutured in place.	Effect on body image. Requires maintenance care.	Cost-effective. Can be placed at patient's bedside. Single-, double-, and triple-lumen catheters available.
Tunneled Catheters (2.7F to 12.5F)			
Long-term use for frequent access	Under general anesthesia, two small incisions are made: one in the area lateral to the junction of the clavicle and first rib and the other on the chest wall. The catheter and its attached Dacron cuff are inserted	Effect on body image. Requires maintenance care. Limits contact sport participation. Limits swimming. Requires a physician to place and remove. Surgical procedure.	No needle puncture to access. Tunnel and Dacron cuff anchor the catheter in place and are barriers to infection. Double- and triple-lumen catheters are available. External portion can be easily repaired. Easy

Potential Complications	Common Maintenance Care	Materials Used	Available Catheters/ Manufacturers
Infection Occlusion Air embolism Breakage Dislodgement	Irrigate with 2 to 5 mL of a 10-unit/mL heparin solution daily to weekly. Before and after medications, flush with 5 to 10 mL normal saline. Remove old dressings using aseptic technique. Inspect the site for signs of infection. Clean the site with povidone–iodine solution from the catheter outward. Cover the site with an occlusive dressing. Change injection caps or adapters every 3 to 7 days.	Elastomeric hydrogel Silicone elastomer Polyurethane	Centrasil (Baxter) C-PICS (Cook) Per-Q Cath (Gesco)
Infection Occlusion Breakage Air embolism Dislodgement	Same as above	Silicone elastomer Silicone	Arrow (Arrow) Chemocath (HDC) Edwards (Edwards) Groshong (Bard) Hemed (Gish) Hickman Broviac (Davol/Bard) Leonard (Davol/Bard) Raaf (Quinton)

(continued)

Table 4-1. Comparison of Central Venous Access
Devices *(Continued)*

Indication	Placement	Disadvantages	Advantages
	through the chest wall incision and advanced up through a created subcutaneous tunnel and through the first incision, and threaded into the subclavian or jugular vein into the superior vena cava or right atrium.		to remove. Can conceal with clothing.
Implanted Ports (4F to 12F)			
Long-term use for frequent venous access	Dome-shaped, round, square, or hexagonal reservoir with attached catheter is inserted under anesthesia. Two incisions are made: one over the vein in which the catheter is to be placed and the other subcutaneously on the chest wall to create a pocket between the skin and muscle fascia for the reservoir to lie.	Needle puncture with noncoring (Huber) needle to access the rubber diaphragm of the reservoir beneath the subcutaneous tissue. Requires a physician to place and remove. Surgical procedure. Costly.	Not visible. Available in single and dual ports. Subcutaneous tunnel provides a barrier to infection. Minimal maintenance care. Minimal interference with activities.

Potential Complications	Common Maintenance Care	Materials Used	Available Catheters/ Manufacturers
Infection Occlusion Extravasation with needle dislodgement	Same as for percutaneous central venous catheter, except flush with 2 to 5 mL of 100 units/mL heparin solution after use and monthly when not used.	Silicone elastomer Polyure-thane	Cath Link 20 (Bard) Chemo Port (HDC) Groshong (Catheter-Technology Corp.) Hickman (Davol) Implantofix (Burron Medical) Infuse-A-Port (Strato) Life-Port (Strato) Omega Port (Norfolk Medica) P.A.S. Port (Pharmacia Deltec)

(continued)

Table 4-1. Comparison of Central Venous Access
Devices *(Continued)*

Indication	Placement	Disadvantages	Advantages
	The catheter attached to the port is advanced from the subcutaneous pocket through a created subcutaneous tunnel into a large vein, and its tip is placed in the inferior or superior vena cava, peritoneal cavity, or hepatic artery. The reservoir is sutured to the muscle fascia and the subcutaneous pocket is sutured closed.		

Peripherally Inserted Central Catheters (PICCs) (23 to 16 g [1.9F to 4.8F])

Indication	Placement	Disadvantages	Advantages
Short- to long-term use for venous access	Under local anesthesia, the catheter is advanced through a cephalic, basilic, or median cubital vein in the antecubital region and advanced through the right subclavian vein into the superior vena cava. It may or may not be sutured in place.	Effect on body image. May limit arm mobility. Limits contact sport participation and swimming. Requires maintenance care.	No needle puncture to access. Single- and dual-lumen catheters. Can conceal with clothing.

Potential Complications	Common Maintenance Care	Materials Used	Available Catheters/ Manufacturers
			Port-A-Cath (Pharmacia Deltec) Sea-Port (Harbor Medical)
Infection Occlusion Phlebitis Breakage Extravasation Dislodgement	Same as above. When changing dressing, pull upward toward patient's shoulder to prevent catheter dis-lodgement.	Elastomeric hydrogel Silicon elastromer Polyure-thane	Centrasil (Baxter) C-PKS (Cook) Groshong (Bard) Per-Q Cath (Gesco)

tional policy for the volume and concentration to use. The first sample of specimen from access devices that are flushed with heparin must be discarded to avoid sending a contaminated (heparinized) sample.

COMPLICATIONS AND MANAGEMENT

Infection, the most common catheter complication, is caused by migration of the bacteria from the exit site or the catheter hub up the outer catheter into the venous circulation. The organisms responsible for infections are streptococci, staphylococci, and *Candida* (Moosa et al., 1991). The diagnosis and management of catheter infections and other potential CVAD complications are listed in Table 4-2.

▼ Ambulatory Infusion Pumps

During the past several years, ambulatory external infusion pumps have become a practical and cost-effective means of administering chemotherapy. Eligibility criteria are as follows:

1. The patient or caregiver must be willing and able to learn about pump operations.
2. The patient must have sufficient visual acuity and manual dexterity.
3. The patient must have a CVAD for continuous chemotherapy infusion.
4. The patient must have readily available transportation to the ambulatory clinic for drug preparation and drug changeovers, or the patient's insurance plan must approve reimbursement for a visiting nurse service to manage pump care.

Patients who are to receive chemotherapy through an ambulatory infusion pump must be educated about:

1. Purpose and function of the pump
2. Operating procedures and troubleshooting techniques
3. Alarm systems (if applicable)
4. How to wear the pump
5. Type and number of batteries required (if applicable), and when and how to change them
6. The importance of periodically checking that clamps are open and tubing is free of kinks

Table 4-2. Potential Complications of Central Venous Access Devices

Definition	Prevention	Sequence in Which to Intervene
Air Embolism		
Air inadvertently introduced into a central venous device that causes an embolism. Clinical manifestations: cyanosis, difficulty breathing, chest pain, tachycardia, hypotension, respiratory failure.	Maintain secure connection of injection cap or adapter to the catheter hub. Maintain secure connection of IV tubing to the catheter hub and to the extension tubing. Have patient perform the Valsalva maneuver when changing IV tubing. Quickly change IV tubing at the catheter hub. Remove air from the IV tubing or syringes used.	1. Position patient on left side. 2. Position bed in Trendelenburg position. 3. Assess the catheter hub tubing connection and IV tubing connections. 4. Correct the source of air entry, if identified. 5. Administer oxygen. 6. Monitor vital signs. 7. Notify physician.
Breakage		
Damage or puncture to the external catheter that impairs the integrity of the catheter wall.	Avoid the use of hemostats or clamps having teeth. Use an extracorporeal clamp or plastic clamp affixed to the catheter. Avoid clamping the distal end of the catheter near the hub. Avoid using scissors when changing the catheter dressing.	1. If IV fluids are infusing, stop the infusion. 2. Immediately clamp the catheter above and below the break. 3. Obtain a repair kit specifically designed for the type and diameter of the catheter. 4. Consult institutional policy for repair of catheter breakage. If unavailable, use the pamphlet provided with the repair kit. 5. Set up a sterile field. 6. Don nonsterile gloves. 7. Clean the catheter break and areas of the catheter around the break with povidone–iodine swabs.

(continued)

Table 4-2. Potential Complications of Central Venous Access Devices *(Continued)*

Definition	Prevention	Sequence in Which to Intervene

Breakage *(continued)*

8. Remove gloves.
9. Place patient in a supine flat position.
10. Don sterile gloves.
11. Prepare a 5-mL syringe with heparin solution (concentration varies per institution).
12. Attach the injection cap or adapter to the catheter repair section.
13. Prime the catheter repair section with heparin solution.
14. Cut the catheter, using sterile scissors, above the catheter break and below the clamp above the break.
15. Insert the stylet of the catheter replacement section into the patient's remaining catheter. If glue is part of the manufacturer's repair kit: (a) fill the provided syringe with glue and attach the provided blunt needle to the syringe; (b) using the syringe, administer glue around the old and new catheter ends.
16. Slide the plastic sleeve attached to the new catheter repair section over the site at which the new catheter repair section is inserted into the patient's remaining catheter. If glue was used, insert the blunt needle of a syringe under each end

Table 4-2. Potential Complications of Central Venous Access Devices *(Continued)*

Definition	Prevention	Sequence in Which to Intervene
Breakage *(continued)*		of the sleeve and rotate the sleeve around to distribute the glue.
		17. Attach the syringe with heparin used to prime the catheter repair section and irrigate the catheter with the remaining amount of heparin.
		18. Secure the repaired catheter section to a tongue blade for 24 hours.
		19. Discard waste in a proper receptacle.
		20. Document the procedure.
Partial Dislodgement		
An increased amount of catheter length external to the exit site.	Secure by: a. applying an occlusive dressing. b. coiling the catheter on top of or beside occlusive dressing. c. providing children with extra length of IV tubing (to avoid tension on catheter while playing). d. wearing a tight-fitting shirt and pinning tape secured around a section of IV tubing to the shirt.	1. Measure the external length of the catheter. 2. Secure the external catheter in place using an occlusive dressing and/or tape. 3. Assess the catheter for flashback of blood in the IV tubing visually or by aspiration with a syringe. 4. Obtain a chest x-ray to verify catheter tip placement.

(continued)

Table 4-2. Potential Complications of Central Venous
Access Devices *(Continued)*

Definition	Prevention	Sequence in Which to Intervene
Total Dislodgement		
Catheter is completely external to the exit site.		1. Cover the exit sige with a sterile gauze pad. 2. Apply pressure over the site. 3. Apply a pressure dressing. 4. Notify physician.
Occlusion		
Inability to infuse or aspirate from a device.	Heparinize device after each use. (Groshong catheters are an exception; they do not require heparin.) Monitor IV infusions. Check that all catheter clamps are open. Check that there are no kinks in the catheter or IV tubing.	1. Use a 10-mL syringe to verify blood return. If without blood return from a port, verify noncoring needle placement by pressing on the noncoring needle until the needle makes contact with the back wall of the port. 2. Attempt to irrigate slowly with a 10-mL syringe filled with normal saline. If able to irrigate, proceed with treatment; if not, proceed to step 3. 3. Have the patient change positions and perform the Valsalva maneuver. 4. Attempt to irrigate again with 10 mL normal saline. 5. If unable to resistance is met, attempt to restore patency of the catheter lumen(s). 6. Consult institutional policy for declotting access devices using urokinase. (Urokinase triggers fibrinolysis.) If there is no policy to

Table 4-2. Potential Complications of Central Venous
Access Devices *(Continued)*

Definition	Prevention	Sequence in Which to Intervene
Occlusion *(continued)*		
		consult, follow the drug insert instructions for administration.
		7. Gently roll the vial of urokinase between both hands.
		8. Draw up 5000 units/ mL of urokinase into a 3-mL syringe.
		9. Clamp the catheter lumen with a clamp free of teeth or a clamp provided on the catheters.
		10. Attach a syringe with thrombolytic agent to the catheter hub.
		11. Unclamp the catheter lumen and slowly instill drug.
		12. Five minutes after instillation, attempt to aspirate blood.
		13. If unable to aspirate blood, allow thrombolytic agent to sit in the catheter and attempt to aspirate every 5 minutes for a total 30 minutes. If after 30 minutes aspiration attempts are unsuccessful, leave urokinase in the catheter for 60 minutes. If after 60 minutes aspiration attempt is successful, aspirate 5 mL of blood, then flush with 10 mL of normal saline, and resume treatment. If aspiration attempt is

(continued)

Table 4-2. Potential Complications of Central Venous Access Devices *(Continued)*

Definition	Prevention	Sequence in Which to Intervene
Occlusion *(continued)*		unsuccessful, urokinase may be instilled. If the patient complains of pain during the irrigation attempt or declotting procedure, stop the attempt, obtain a chest x-ray, and notify physician.

Clinical Manifestations of Infection	Prevention	Diagnosis	Interventions
Exit Site			
Redness Swelling Discharge Tenderness	Practice meticulous site care. Avoid getting exit sit wet. Practice site care should site or dressing get wet or soiled.	Positive exit-site culture. Positive catheter serum culture.	Practice meticulous site care. Give IV antibiotics for 10 to 14 days. Assess patient's and family members' catheter maintenance technique.
Tunnel			
Redness Tenderness Tracking	Maintain sterility when accessing a port with a noncoring needle. Maintain aseptic technique when attaching or removing a syringe or tubing to non-coring needle tubing.	Positive catheter serum culture.	Remove catheter. Give IV antibiotics for 10 to 14 days. Apply topical antibiotic ointment and occlusive dressing over removal exit site.

Table 4-2. Potential Complications of Central Venous Access Devices *(Continued)*

Clinical Manifestations of Infection	Prevention	Diagnosis	Interventions
Port Pocket			
Redness Swelling Warmth Tenderness/ pain Cellulitis	Same as above	Positive port serum culture. Positive port pocket fluid culture.	Give IV antibiotics for 10 to 14 days. Remove port if no response to antibiotics. Pack port pocket after removal with antibiotic ointment and sterile gauze; cover with occlusive dressing.
Systemic			
Fever Chills Hypotension Tachycardia Diaphoresis Pallor	Practice meticulous site care. Monitor counts for neutropenia. Maintain aseptic technique when connecting and disconnecting tubing or syringes.	Positive catheter serum culture. Positive peripheral serum culture. Positive catheter tip culture.	Give IV antibiotics. (If catheter has more than one lumen, administer through alternating lumens.) Monitor vital signs. Monitor complete blood count. Monitor urine output. Remove catheter if patient experiences chills or rigors or has no response to antibiotic and/or is neutropenic.

7. How to protect the pump from moisture during bathing
8. Proper care and monitoring of the access device to which the pump is connected.

The patient should contact a health professional immediately for any concerns or problems.

▼ Safe Handling and Disposal of Chemotherapy

PREPARATION OF CHEMOTHERAPEUTIC AGENTS

1. Prepare these agents using a Class II or III biological safety cabinet (also referred to as a vertical laminar airflow hood). These cabinets contain high-efficiency particulate air filters that pull air away from the face of the person preparing the drug. These cabinets should remain functioning 24 hours a day, 7 days a week and should be vented to the outside. They should be cleaned daily with a 70% alcohol solution, and they should be serviced every 6 months to ensure performance (Carmignani & Raymond, 1997; Gibbs, 1991; Gullo, 1988).
2. Wear long-sleeved, nonabsorbent gowns with elastic at the wrists and a back closure during drug preparation.
3. Wear a plastic mask and goggles in settings without a biological safety cabinet, such as a physician's office (Alexander, 1991).
4. Use a plastic absorbent pad to cover the work surface in the preparation area so that any droplet contamination is absorbed.
5. Prime IV lines for chemotherapy administration with D_5W or normal saline before drug administration. Do not prime with the chemotherapy drug.
6. Use hydrophobic filter needles to draw antineoplastic drugs from vials and ampules.
7. Use a sterile gauze pad to purge air from a chemotherapy-filled syringe, connect and disconnect IV tubing containing antineoplastic drugs, open chemotherapy vials and ampules, remove syringes from IV lines used for IV push administration, and remove empty chemotherapy bags or bottles from IV spikes (Gullo, 1988).
8. Use a needleless delivery system or Luer-Lok connections to prevent accidental disconnection.

9. Use powder-free latex gloves at least 0.007″ thick when handling chemotherapy agents. Personnel who have a latex allergy should use alternative products made with nitrile.

10. Wash hands before and after handling antineoplastic agents.

11. Never store food or beverages in a refrigerator used for storage of chemotherapy agents.

12. Avoid eating, drinking, applying cosmetics, or chewing gum in the drug preparation area (American Society of Hospital Pharmacists, 1993; Gullo, 1988).

13. Transport chemotherapy drugs in sealed bags to prevent spillage. Spill kits should be readily available, and personnel should be properly instructed in chemotherapy handling and exposure procedures.

14. Dispose of chemotherapy wastes in impervious, leak-proof containers.

15. Instruct patients who receive chemotherapy at home to store the drugs in areas where the proper temperature will be maintained and away from the reach of children.

16. Cover the toilet with a waterproof shield or pad before flushing (Gullo, 1988).

17. Wear gloves when handling body excreta of patients who have received these drugs within a 48-hour period (Carmignani & Raymond, 1997; Gullo, 1988; Laidlaw et al., 1984).

18. Dispose of equipment contaminated with antineoplastic drugs in labeled hazardous waste receptacles (Carmignani & Raymond, 1997). Chemotherapy wastes should be disposed of in approved landfills or incinerators (American Society of Hospital Pharmacists, 1993).

MINIMIZING EXPOSURE TO CHEMOTHERAPEUTIC AGENTS

Given the large number of health care personnel who handle antineoplastic agents, questions have arisen about possible long-term risks of exposure to these drugs. The teratogenic risk for health care professionals of child-bearing age is another concern. Advisory bodies have stated that if professionals follow the recommendations given while handling and disposing of these drugs, teratogenic risk is unlikely. The risk to those who handle chemotherapy and the body excreta of patients who have received these agents is unknown. Therefore, professionals must follow the precautions listed previously to minimize their exposure.

Health care workers can be exposed to chemotherapy by skin and mucous membrane *absorption, inhalation,* and *ingestion.* Skin and mucous membrane absorption and inhalation can occur while:

- Opening a vial or ampule of a chemotherapy agent
- Eliminating air from a syringe filled with a chemotherapy agent
- Disposing of IV bags, bottles, syringes, and tubing used in the administration of these agents
- Disposing of the body excreta of patients who have received these drugs

Ingestion can occur through hand-to-mouth contact with food, cosmetics, cigarettes, or equipment contaminated with chemotherapy (Gullo, 1988; Oncology Nursing Society, 1988).

Conflicting research findings regarding the long-term effects of exposure to chemotherapy agents led to the establishment of advisory bodies that address exposure issues and recommend safe practice techniques for the handling and disposal of these drugs (Alexander, 1991; Dunne, 1989; Gibbs, 1991). These advisory bodies are the Occupational Safety and Health Administration, the American Society of Hospital Pharmacy, the Oncology Nursing Society, and the National Study Commission on Cytotoxic Exposure.

The recommendations made by these advisory bodies serve as guidelines; institutional policies for chemotherapy handling, administration, and disposal may vary. Nurses must be familiar with their institution's policies and procedures and use them to minimize their exposure.

MEASURES FOR ACCIDENTAL EXPOSURE TO CHEMOTHERAPY

- Eye contact: Immediately rinse the affected eye or eyes with copious amounts of water for at least 15 minutes.
- Skin contact: Immediately wash the area with soap and water.
- Clothing contact: Immediately remove the article of clothing and wash areas where skin contact occurred

with soap and water. Place soiled clothing in a plastic bag until laundered, then wash the clothing twice separately from all other clothing. After laundering twice, put the machine through a wash cycle free of any clothing. In institutions, place clothing or linen soiled with antineoplastic agents in a contaminated linen receptacle.

• Bed linen contact: Immediately remove the linen and place it in a contaminated linen receptacle, then clean the mattress using a 70% alcohol solution. Once the alcohol dries, the bed may be remade with clean linens.

▼ Box 4-1. Contents of an Antineoplastic Spill Kit

NUMBER	ITEM
1	Gown with cuffs and back closure (made of nonpermeable fabric)
1 pair	Shoe covers
2 pair	Gloves
1 pair	Utility gloves
1 pair	Chemical splash goggles
1	Rebreather mask (National Institute of Occupational Safety and Health-approved)
1	Disposable dustpan (to collect broken glass)
1	Plastic scraper (to scoop materials into dustpan)
2	Plastic-backed absorbable towels
1 each	250-mL and 1-L spill-control pillows
2	Disposable sponges (one to clean up spill, one to clean up floor after removal of spill)
1	Sharps container
2	Large, heavy-duty waste disposal bags
1	Container of 70% alcohol for cleaning soiled area
1	Hazardous waste label

From *Controlling occupational exposure to hazardous drugs* (OSHA Instruction CPL 2-2, 20B) (pp. 21-1–21-34), by Occupational Safety and Health Administration (OSHA), 1994, Washington, D.C.: Author. Copyright 1995 by OSHA.

MANAGEMENT OF CHEMOTHERAPY SPILLS

The recommended sequence for handling a chemotherapy spill is as follows:

1. Don a pair of powder-free latex gloves.
2. Place an absorbent pad over the spill to contain it.
3. Rinse the absorbed spill area with water.
4. Clean the area with a detergent.
5. Dispose of all equipment used as chemotherapy waste (American Society of Hospital Pharmacists, 1990; Carmignani & Raymond, 1997).

To expedite the handling of a spill and to minimize patient and employee exposure, chemotherapy spill kits (Box 4-1) should be readily available.

5

Management of Toxic Effects of Chemotherapy

Chemotherapy, like any medication, has the potential to cause side effects. Unique to these agents, however, are the nature and extent of the injury they are capable of inflicting. Chemotherapeutic agents are highly toxic and have narrow therapeutic indices. Although these agents exhibit a certain degree of specificity for malignant cells, they cannot discriminate effectively between normal and malignant cells. Consequently, other rapidly proliferating cells, such as the bone marrow cells, the spermatogonia, and the gastrointestinal crypt epithelium cells, are very vulnerable. Cytotoxic agents can induce virtually every type of pathology on the organ systems. The clinical manifestations can vary in onset from acute to chronic and in severity from mild to severe. Most of these symptoms are reversible; some are cumulative and life-threatening.

The need to curb the growth of cancer cells most often outweighs the disadvantages produced by these side effects; patients and prescribers often choose to accept these expected but undesirable and often life-threatening side effects to curtail malignant cell growth, reduce the tumor burden, and increase the potential for cure.

New and improved drugs have entered the market at a rapid rate in the past 3 years. The "fast-track" approach by the Food and Drug Administration has allowed speedier approval of promising experimental drugs for cancer patients. More successful outcomes with this wide spectrum of cytotoxic agents have been achieved because barriers to high-dose chemotherapy and combination modalities can be minimized with the use of growth factors. The use of chemoprotectants has been favorable, and more sophisticated technology abounds. All of these factors contribute to better treatment options for oncology patients. However, with these benefits come attendant risks.

Chemotherapy-induced toxicities have important consequences for the clinician and the patient. Serious concern about the myriad adverse effects can limit the use of potentially effective drugs as primary agents or adjuvants for certain malignancies and as retreatment agents after primary use. Risks and quality-of-life issues can deter patients from complying with the treatment plan or seeking more aggressive regimens. The physical and psychological assault from the chemotherapy experience on an already burdened host can be extremely difficult. Therefore, astute management of these toxicities is of paramount importance so that the goals of cancer treatment will not be delayed. By understanding the pathophysiology of these toxicities, the nurse can develop strategies to minimize the distressing and sometimes life-threatening consequences of chemotherapy.

This chapter focuses on the more common chemotherapy-induced toxicities on the various body systems, their management, and patient education considerations. Oncology nurses play a pivotal role in managing these toxicities and in teaching the patient to implement self-care interventions at home.

▼ Cardiotoxicity

Bone marrow transplantation and the use of colony-stimulating factors are hematologic strategies used in the treatment of cancer, enabling dose intensification. These techniques increase the sensitivity of myocardial cells to chemotherapy, causing an increased potential for acute, chronic, and possibly irreversible cardiac damage. Adverse effects to the cardiac system are mostly associated with anthracycline therapy, particularly doxorubicin and daunorubicin. Cardiac alterations may be acute or chronic, and manifestations may vary from subtle ECG changes to life-threatening cardiomyopathies such as arrhythmias, congestive heart failure, and ischemia. Cardiotoxicity may be potentiated by concomitant mediastinal radiation and the use of other potentially cardiotoxic drugs, such as high-dose cyclophosphamide. Other risk factors are age (children and adults older than 50 years are more affected), preexisting cardiac disease, smoking, malnutrition, renal and hepatic impairment, and a history of hypertension.

The clinical presentation of cardiotoxicity resembles that of congestive heart failure. The patient has dyspnea and a nonproductive cough. Other manifestations are distended neck veins, ankle edema, tachycardia, and cardiomegaly. The use of the new cardiac protectant, dexrazoxane, in doxorubicin therapy for metastatic breast cancer may help diminish the incidence of cardiac toxicity. In severe cases, the chemotherapeutic agents should be discontinued and supportive measures provided (Table 5-1).

MANAGEMENT AND PATIENT EDUCATION

1. Monitor the patient's cardiac function by obtaining cardiac enzymes, multigated radionuclide angiography, and electrocardiograms before and throughout treatment.
2. Obtain baseline assessments of the peripheral and apical pulse, blood pressure, the presence of edema, and difficulty with breathing or chest pain.
3. Teach the patient to report signs and symptoms indicative of early cardiac problems, such as tachycardia, dyspnea, and dizziness.
4. Stress the importance of a low-salt diet, fluid restriction to 1 L/day, and rest periods if the patient develops congestive heart failure.
5. Administer cardioprotectants such as dexrazoxane if ordered.
6. Limit the cumulative chemotherapy dose according to guidelines, with dose reductions if the patient is receiving concomitant irradiation.
7. Instruct the patient about the importance of taking digoxin and diuretics and the associated side effects if these medications are ordered.
8. Teach the patient to avoid alcohol and tobacco because of their stimulant effect on the heart muscle.

Table 5-1. Cardiotoxic Agents

Agent	Characteristics	Toxicity	Interventions
Cyclophosphamide	ST-T wave changes Dyspnea Friction rub Fever Dull or sharp precordial pain	Hemorrhagic myocardial necrosis Pericarditis Congestive heart failure Myocarditis	Cardiac assessment Monitor IV infusion volume Avoid fluid overload
Dactinomycin Daunorubicin Doxorubicin	Transient ECG changes	Cardiac failure Cardiomyopathy Congestive heart failure (doxorubicin only)	Cardiac assessment Never exceed maximum lifetime doses of doxorubicin: 550 mg/m^2; daunorubicin: 600 mg/m^2 (450 mg/m^2 if prior mediastinal radiation therapy) Ongoing evaluation of cardiac status Possible use of cardioprotective agent Inotropic drugs to increase cardiac output Diuretics

5-Fluorouracil	Coronary vasospasm Angina ST segment elevations Ventricular ectopy Arrhythmias	Myocardial ischemia	Prophylactic and PRN calcium channel blockers Serum cardiac enzymes pre- and post-drug
Taxanes (Paclitaxel)	Chest pain Hypotension Ventricular tachycardia	Atrioventricular conduction blocks Ventricular tachycardia Left bundle branch block Sinus bradycardia	Cardiac assessment ECG and echocardiogram baseline and postdrug

9. Assess the patient's activity and exercise levels and develop an appropriate plan.

▼ Cutaneous Toxicity

Chemotherapy can induce alterations of the integumentary system. These may be generalized or localized reactions and are often manifested on the skin, its appendages, and mucosal surfaces. Cutaneous reactions vary in site, onset, severity, and duration depending on the kind of cytotoxic agent used (Table 5-2). Cutaneous toxicity is generally transient because the skin regenerates its epidermal layer in 30 days. Unless the cutaneous reactions are severe, involving tissue necrosis, cutaneous toxicities eventually resolve. However, cutaneous reactions should be carefully evaluated because they can severely affect the patient's physical and mental health. Cutaneous toxicity can alter the skin's ability to protect the body against fluid loss, can alter temperature regulation, and can diminish sensations of pain and touch. Because most cutaneous manifestations are visible, they can have a tremendous impact on the patient's self-image and how others perceive him or her. Other than the use of cytotoxic agents, especially at high doses, potential causes for cutaneous symptoms are infection, cutaneous malignancy, metastatic spread, graft–host interaction, nutritional disorders, and other drugs, such as antibiotics and analgesics.

The chemotherapy cutaneous reactions include the following:

Alopecia
Acral erythema
Hyperpigmentation
Nail changes
Photosensitivity
Radiation enhancement and recall

Extravasation, hypersensitivity reactions, and mucositis, which are the acute and most serious of the cutaneous reactions, are discussed in another section.

ALOPECIA

Of all the complications of chemotherapy, the most devastating is hair loss. It is a visible and constant reminder of can-

Table 5-2. Cutaneous Toxicity Induced by Chemotherapeutic Agents

	Alopecia	Stomatitis	Pigmentation Disorders	Nail Disorders	Radiation Reactions
BCNU	2	2	3	3	3
Bleomycin	1	1	1	2	2
Busulfan	3	3	1	3	3
CCNU	3	2	3	3	3
Chlorambucil	3	3	3	3	3
Cisplatin	3	3	3	3	3
Cyclophosphamide	1	1	2	2	3
Cytarabine	3	2	3	3	3
Dacarbazine	3	3	3	3	2
Dactinomycin	1	1	2	3	1
Daunorubicin	1	1	2	2	3
Doxorubicin	1	1	1	2	1
Etoposide	2	2	3	3	2
5-Fluorouracil	1	1	1	2	2
Hexamethylmelamine	3	3	3	3	3
Hydroxyurea	2	3	2	2	2
Ifosfamide	1	3	3	3	3

(continued)

Table 5-2. Cutaneous Toxicity Induced by Chemotherapeutic Agents (*Continued*)

	Alopecia	Stomatitis	Pigmentation Disorders	Nail Disorders	Radiation Reactions
Mechlorethamine	2	3	3	3	3
Melphalan	3	3	3	3	3
6-Mercaptopurine	3	2	3	3	3
Methotrexate	2	1	2	3	1
Mithramycin	3	2	2	3	3
Mitomycin-C	3	2	3	3	3
Mitotane	3	3	3	3	3
Procarbazine	3	2	3	3	3
Streptozocin	3	3	3	3	3
6-Thioguanine	3	2	3	3	2
Thiotepa	2	3	3	3	3
Vinblastine	2	2	3	3	2
Vincristine	2	2	3	3	3
Vindesine	1	3	3	3	3

1, frequent; 2, occasional; 3, rare or nonexistent.
Modified from De Spain, J. D. (1992). Dermatologic toxicity. In: Perry, M. C. (Ed.), *The chemotherapy sourcebook* (pp. 531–547). Baltimore: Williams & Williams.

cer. The noticeable hair loss has a negative impact on one's body image. To a woman who has had a mastectomy or hysterectomy, alopecia represents an added threat to her femininity. To a young adolescent, the premature "baldness" can damage his or her relationships with peers. In addition to the scalp hair, the eyebrows, beard, pubic hair, and axillary hair can also be lost.

There are approximately 100,000 hair follicles in the body. These hair follicles undergo the phases of *anagen* (growth), *catagen* (transition), and *telogen* (dormancy). About 85% to 90% of hair follicles are in the anagen phase; the remainder are in the telogen phase or in a brief transitional state (Jacubovic & Ackerman, 1985). When a hair follicle enters the anagen phase, the upward growth of the new hair causes the dormant hair to shed. As a result of this growth and dormancy cycle, a normal person usually sheds 100 scalp hairs daily. The active hair bulbs duplicate every 12 to 24 hours, resulting in a daily growth of the hair shaft of 0.37 mm (Crounse & Van Scott, 1960). With high-dose chemotherapy, the hair follicles that are in the anagen phase atrophy, causing the hair to fall out spontaneously. Alopecia can also occur from the narrowing of the hair shaft, which causes defective and weak hair that is prone to breakage. This leads to thinning of the hair in various degrees and usually occurs with standard-dose chemotherapy.

The degree of alopecia may be minimal (less than 25% hair loss), moderate (25% to 50%), or severe (more than 50%). The degree depends on the drug or combination of drugs used, the dose, the serum half-life of the agent, and the duration of the infusion time. Hair loss is usually experienced within 2 weeks after chemotherapy administration, and hair regrowth may take 3 to 5 months after chemotherapy.

Management and Patient Education

1. Prepare the patient for the degree of possible hair loss and the time frame for regrowth.
2. Allow the patient to verbalize, acknowledge the meaning and impact of the hair loss on his or her body image and lifestyle, and plan ways to deal with the potential hair loss.
3. Do not recommend the use of a scalp tourniquet and hypothermia: these procedures may produce sanctuary sites or a refuge for circulating tumor cells.

4. Emphasize adequate nutrition. The use of vitamin E or gelatin supplements has not been proven to be of benefit.
5. Implement anticipatory interventions such as early referrals to a wig specialist. Wigs are tax-deductible and are covered by medical insurance. Encourage the patient to see a wig specialist during the early phase of chemotherapy so that the specialist can determine the natural color and style.
6. Refer the patient to the American Cancer Society's "Look Good, Feel Better" program and other support groups.
7. Assure the patient that alopecia is reversible and that regrowth will occur when chemotherapy is stopped. Review time frames. Provide emotional support, because the process can be slow and new growth may not be appreciable until after a few months.
8. Teach proper techniques for hair care, such as:
   a. Use mild shampoos; avoid perming, peroxide coloring, or chemical treatments.
   b. Minimize the use of heat, rollers, and vigorous brushing. Teach the patient to "finger-comb" the hair instead of using a hair brush.
   c. Wear attractive turbans, scarves, and hats.
   d. Consider cutting the hair to a shorter length.

ACRAL ERYTHEMA (HAND-FOOT SYNDROME)

The agent most implicated in this condition is high-dose cytarabine; other neoplastic agents can also produce this syndrome when given at high doses (methotrexate, 5-fluorouracil, hydroxyurea, capecitabine, and etoposide). The initial reactions are burning, swelling, tingling, and sharply demarcated erythema of the palm, the fingers, and the soles of the feet, which progress to blistering and desquamation of the affected areas. The scalp and chest can also be affected. Patients complain of tingling in the hands and feet progressing to flank pain when handling objects or walking.

Management and Patient Education

1. Frequently bathe hands and feet.
2. Administer pain medications as ordered.
3. Elevate affected extremities.
4. Provide heel cushions.

    5. Apply cold compresses and moisturize with lotion.
    6. Assist patients who have decreased mobility.

HYPERPIGMENTATION

The pathogenesis of altered pigmentation is poorly understood. It is believed to be due to a deviation in the amount and distribution of melanin and the direct stimulation of the melanocyte (Fitzpatrick & Hood, 1988). There is an increased incidence of hyperpigmentation in dark-skinned persons. It is usually manifested on the skin, but other areas, such as the nails, hair, and oral mucous membranes, have also been reported. Hyperpigmentation disappears with time, and the changes are rarely permanent. One of the cutaneous complications associated with 5-fluorouracil is serpiginous hyperpigmented streaks overlying the veins used for administration in the absence of the usual warning signs of phlebitis (Fig. 5-1). 5-fluorouracil is thought to produce endothelial fragility, which allows the drug to escape into the tissues, resulting in hyperpigmentation of the overlying skin (Hrushesky, 1980). A similar reaction of hyperpigmented linear streaks of the veins has also been reported with bleomycin (de Bast et al., 1971). Among African Americans, hyperpigmentation of the oral mucosa and the tongue has been noted after administration of doxorubicin, busulfan, and cyclophosphamide (Dunagin, 1982).

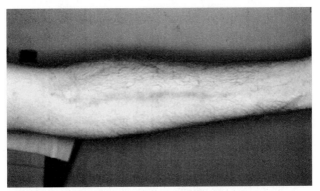

Fig. 5-1. Serpiginous hyperpigmented streaking noted from 5-fluorouracil infusion.

Management and Patient Education

1. Assess the patient's baseline skin condition and evaluate his or her skin care regimen.
2. Assure the patient that hyperpigmentation will resolve in time.
3. Ask the patient about concomitant medications that may influence skin reactions.
4. Instruct the patient to use sunscreen.
5. Monitor the infusion site when administering 5-fluorouracil; discontinue the infusion at the first sign of irritation and restart a new line.

NAIL CHANGES

Certain chemotherapeutic agents can cause alterations to the nails. Not as significant and distressing as the other cutaneous reactions, these changes include brittleness, banding, and hyperpigmentation of the matrix of the nails. They are temporary and resolve when chemotherapy is completed. Hyperpigmentation of the nail is due to the deposition of melanin in the nail plate. Blue discoloration of the nail plate has also been observed after the administration of 5-fluorouracil and doxorubicin. Transverse banding—multiple white horizontal lines along the fingernails—has also been reported. Another abnormality in the nail consists of thin transverse grooves across the nail plate, called *Beau's lines*. This is also seen in patients with myocardial infarction and may involve all 20 nails. *Onycholysis* (partial separation of the nail from the nail bed) has been noted in patients receiving 5-fluorouracil, doxorubicin, and bleomycin (De Spain, 1992).

Management and Patient Education

1. Assess the patient's nails before chemotherapy administration.
2. Advise the patient of potential changes in the nails and ask him or her to report any changes. These usually occur 5 to 10 weeks after chemotherapy.
3. Reassure the patient that the changes are usually temporary.
4. Cover nails with nail polish.
5. Encourage the patient to wear gloves if he or she is embarrassed about the appearance of the nails.
6. Teach the patient about good nail care:

a. Avoid cutting cuticles.
b. Apply oil to nails.
c. Do not cut the nails too close to the nail bed.

PHOTOSENSITIVITY

Photosensitivity is caused by cytotoxic agents that have radiosensitizing properties. The cutaneous reaction is thought to occur by means of a phototoxic mechanism involving UVB light (De Spain, 1992). Photosensitivity is manifested as an exaggerated sunburn accompanied by urticaria and stinging; it resolves with hyperpigmentation.

Management and Patient Education

1. Review medications that are associated with photosensitivity.
2. Instruct the patient to take the following precautions:
   a. Avoid exposure to direct, indirect, and artificial sunlight.
   b. Use protective sunblocks (SPF 30 or greater), applied at least 15–30 minutes before sun exposure.
   c. Wear protective clothing, wide-brimmed hats, and long-sleeved shirts.

RADIATION ENHANCEMENT AND RECALL

Cutaneous reactions may occur as a result of the synergistic effect of irradiation and cytotoxic agents on both normal and target cancer tissues. Enhancement reactions occur if chemotherapy is administered within a week of irradiation. Recall reactions may happen within weeks or months to even years after radiation; however, they appear more frequently with shorter time intervals and high-dose chemotherapy. These reactions can occur in the skin, lung, heart, and gastrointestinal tract. They are manifested by erythema, blisters, hyperpigmentation, edema, vesicle formation, exfoliation, and sometimes ulcers. The management of radiation recall and enhancement effects is similar.

Management and Patient Education

1. Consider longer intervals between the chemotherapy administration and the radiation therapy, if possible.
2. Perform a thorough skin assessment; note color, moisture, and turgor. Instruct the patient to report any changes in the skin.

3. Teach the patient to avoid trauma or irritation to the affected areas.
4. Instruct the patient on good skin care to maintain skin integrity:
   a. Wash the skin with mild soap (e.g., Dove, Ivory) or cleanser (Cetaphil) and tepid water.
   b. Use a soft cloth, avoid rubbing, and use a gentle patting motion to cleanse and dry the area.
   c. Use sunscreen (SPF 30 or greater).
   d. Wear loose and nonconstrictive clothing; avoid materials that might irritate the skin.
   e. Use mild detergents when laundering clothes.
   f. Avoid extremes in temperature.
   g. Do not use adhesives or occlusive dressings over affected skin. Expose the area to air.
   h. If shaving is necessary, use an electric razor.
   i. Do not use any skin care product unless it is prescribed by the nurse or doctor.
5. If the area gets infected, gentle débridement might be necessary. An antimicrobial ointment can be used to keep the area moist. Cover with a nonadherent dressing.

▼ Gastrointestinal Toxicity

Chemotherapy can profoundly affect the gastrointestinal (GI) tract. Ninety percent of the GI crypt epithelium is composed of undifferentiated cells and goblet cells found in the small intestines. These are mitotically active cells and as such are vulnerable to cytotoxic attack. Because the GI tract functions as the major site of nutritional intake, and because malnutrition, anorexia, and cachexia are associated with cancer, any further insult to the functioning of the GI tract can severely compromise the host.

The common chemotherapy-induced toxicities to the GI system are nausea and vomiting, anorexia, mucositis, constipation, and diarrhea.

NAUSEA AND VOMITING

Among all the symptoms that are dreaded by patients receiving chemotherapy, nausea and vomiting are considered to be at the top of the list. It is thought that 70% to 80% of patients receiving chemotherapy have some degree of nausea and vomiting. Nausea often precedes vomiting and is an unpleasant feeling of the need to vomit. It is a separate event from vomiting and may or may not result in vomiting. Retching, also known as dry heaves, is another phenomenon that may or may not accompany emesis. It is caused by the rhythmic contraction of the abdominal and respiratory muscles. Vomiting is the forceful expulsion of the gastric contents through the mouth. It is accompanied by weakness, pallor, tachycardia, decreased blood pressure, and increased respiration.

The exact mechanism of chemotherapy-induced emesis is not completely understood. It is postulated that emesis is induced by stimulation of the true vomiting center (TVC), the nucleus tractus solitarius, located in the general area of the lateral reticular formulation of the fourth ventricle. The physiologic stimulation of the TVC is mediated by neurotransmitters, including serotonin ($5-HT_3$), dopamine, norepinephrine, and histamine. The receptor sites for these transmitters are located in the chemoreceptor trigger zone (CTZ) and the GI tract. The TVC receives afferent impulses from four sources (Borison & Wang, 1953):

1. The CTZ, located in the area postrema in the brain stem, responds directly to chemical toxins (chemotherapy) in the blood and the cerebrospinal fluid.
2. The GI tract at the level of the small intestine is the primary location of the serotonin receptor, which when stimulated sends impulses by sympathetic and afferent pathways.
3. The higher cortical centers transmit psychogenic stimuli.
4. The vestibular apparatus of the middle ear (motion sickness) is also involved.

When impulses from any of these four trigger points exceed the threshold, vomiting occurs.

Patient characteristics and prognostic factors that affect the incidence of nausea and vomiting include:

- Age: Younger patients experience more nausea and vomiting than older patients.
- Gender: A higher incidence in women is believed to be due to the more highly emetogenic drugs given to women and lesser alcohol intake.
- Alcohol intake: High alcohol intake has a positive effect on control of emesis.
- History of motion sickness or severe emesis during

pregnancy: These patients are more susceptible to chemotherapy-induced nausea and vomiting.

- Anxiety, expectations of severe side effects, and previous chemotherapy experience are other predisposing factors.
- Food intake, change in taste sensations, and the amount of sleep before chemotherapy can affect the incidence of nausea and vomiting.

Patterns of chemotherapy-induced emesis are anticipatory, acute, delayed, and refractory.

Anticipatory Emesis

Anticipatory emesis is a conditioned or learned aversion to chemotherapy-related cues. Any stimulus (sight, smell, place) elicits a classic pavlovian reflex, even in the absence of cytotoxic drug administration. Approximately 10% to 44% of chemotherapy patients experience anticipatory nausea and vomiting (Morrow et al., 1991). The following risk factors are associated with anticipatory nausea and vomiting:

- Severe posttreatment side effects
- Age younger than 50 years
- History of motion sickness
- Anxiety and depression
- Tastes and odors
- Schedule and number of chemotherapy cycles

The best intervention for this type of emesis is prevention—that is, giving the patient the best antiemetic regimen during the initial drug cycle to avoid any untoward associations. Behavioral techniques such as guided imagery, relaxation, hypnosis, and distraction have also been proven to be beneficial. Antiemetics are ineffective for acute emesis.

Acute Emesis

Acute emesis is the most common and most studied emetic syndrome. It may happen minutes after drug exposure but usually occurs 2 to 6 hours after treatment. Most of the research in antiemetic therapy has been conducted to determine the best regimen for this type of emesis.

Delayed Emesis

The mechanism for delayed emesis is unclear. It persists for 1 to 4 days after chemotherapy administration. It is usually associated with high-dose regimens of cisplatin and combination regimens of cyclophosphamide and an anthracycline. Although it is not as distressing as acute emesis, it may severely affect the patient's food intake and prolong the hospital stay.

Refractory Emesis

Refractory emesis refers to emesis that does not respond to antiemetic therapy. Patients with this type of emesis usually respond if an anxiolytic agent is added to the regimen.

Management and Patient Education

PHARMACOLOGIC APPROACHES

The degree and incidence of emesis depend on the emetogenic potential of the drug, the dose, and the administration schedule. Recent advances in antiemetic therapy have provided regimens that have lessened the incidence and degree of nausea and vomiting, allowing better and more affordable control of treatment-related emesis. In 1999, the American Society of Clinical Oncology's panel of experts developed clinical practice guidelines for antiemetic therapy (Gralla et al., 1999). Tables 5-3 through 5-7 give the evidence-based recommendations of this group.

Serotonin receptor antagonists are an important class of antiemetic drugs that have provided effective emetic control with minimal side effects. These agents include dolasetron, granisetron, ondansetron, and tropisetron. All of these agents are equally effective and act in a similar fashion as antagonists of the 5-HT$_3$ receptor. They are preferable to metoclopramide because of the absence of central nervous system effects, extrapyramidal reactions, and sedation. This mild side effect profile is particularly attractive for younger patients. The side effects noted with the serotonin antagonists are slight headache, mild asymptomatic transaminase elevation, and constipation (most common adverse effect).

Corticosteroids are valuable and have a high therapeutic index, especially in acute emesis control. They are frequently prescribed with single-agent use in low-risk settings but are also effective when combined with serotonin receptor antagonists for patients receiving highly emetogenic chemotherapy.

Metoclopramide works as a serotonin antagonist but is also thought to have substantial activity by the dopamine receptor pathway, which explains the extrapyramidal reactions. It is less expensive than the serotonin antagonists but as effective at higher doses. Its side effects are acute dystonic reactions, akathisia, and sedation.

Table 5-3. Antiemetic Agents, Doses, and Administration Schedule

Antiemetic Agent (trade name)	Dose Range	Schedule (for acute chemotherapy-induced emesis, unless otherwise noted)
Agents With Highest Therapeutic Index		
Serotonin Receptor Antagonists		
Dolasetron (Anzemet)	100 mg or 1.8 mg/kg IV	One time, before chemotherapy
	100 mg PO	One time, before chemotherapy
Granisetron (Kytril)	1 mg or 0.01 mg/kg IV	One time, before chemotherapy
	2 mg PO	One time, before chemotherapy
Ondansetron (Zofran)	8 mg or 0.15 mg/kg IV	
	Oral doses vary (12–24 mg/d) (8 mg doses usually used in delayed or RT emesis)	One time, before chemotherapy (two to three times daily in delayed or RT emesis)
Tropisetron (Navoban)	5 mg IV	One time, before chemotherapy
	5 mg PO	One time, before chemotherapy
Corticosteroids		
Dexamethasone (Decadron)	20 mg IV	One time, before chemotherapy
Methylprednisolone (Medrol)	40–125 mg	One time, before chemotherapy
Agents of Lower Therapeutic Index		
Dopamine Receptor Antagonists		
Metoclopramide (Reglan)	2–3 mg/kg IV	Before chemotherapy and 2 hours after chemotherapy
	20 mg or 0.5 mg/kg PO for delayed or RT emesis	2–4 times a day for delayed emesis
Prochlorperazine (Compazine)	10 mg to 30 mg IV	Every 3–4 hours
	10 to 20 mg PO	Every 3–4 hours

RT, radiation therapy
Adapted from Gralla, R. J., Osoba, D., Kris, M. K., et al. (1999). Recommendations for the use of antiemetics: Evidence-based, clinical practice guidelines. *Journal of Clinical Oncology,* 17(9), 2971.

Table 5-4. High Emetic Risk: Chemotherapeutic Agents and Guidelines for Acute and Delayed Emesis

Acute Emetic Category	Chemotherapy Agent (trade name)	Guideline for Acute Emesis	Guideline for Delayed Emesis
High: cisplatin	Cisplatin (Platinol)	Pretreatment: 5-HT$_3$ antagonist plus a corticosteroid	Oral cortico-steroid plus oral metoclopramide (or plus an oral 5-HT$_3$ antago-nist) Dexamethasone 8 mg twice daily for 3–4 days, plus either Metoclopramide 30–40 mg, 2–4 times per day for 2–4 days, or
High: noncisplatin	Dacarbazine (DTIC-Dome)		5-HT$_3$ antago-nists at doses in Table 5-3, for 2–3 days (guide-line for all agents in this class, ex-cept cisplatin)
	Actinomycin-D (Cosmegen)		Dexamethasone 8 mg twice daily for 2–3 days, plus either
	Mechlorethamine (Mustargen) Streptozocin (Zanosar)		Metoclopramide 30–40 mg, 2–4 times per day for 2–3 days, or
	Hexamethyl-melamine (Hexalen) Carboplatin (Paraplatin) Cyclophospha-mide (Cytoxan) Lomustine (CeeNU) Carmustine		5-HT$_3$ antago-nists at doses in Table 5-3, for 2–3 days

(continued)

Table 5-4. High Emetic Risk: Chemotherapeutic Agents and Guidelines for Acute and Delayed Emesis *(Continued)*

Acute Emetic Category	Chemotherapy Agent (trade name)	Guideline for Acute Emesis	Guideline for Delayed Emesis
High: noncisplatin *(continued)*	(BiCNU) Daunorubicin (DaunoXome) Doxorubicin (Adriamycin) Epirubicin (Pharmorubicin) Idarubicin (Idamycin) Cytarabine (Cytosar) Ifosfamide (Ifex)		

Adapted from Gralla, R. J., Osoba, D., Kris, M. K., et al. (1999). Recommendations for the use of antiemetics: Evidence-based, clinical practice guidelines. *Journal of Clinical Oncology,* 17(9), 2971.

Table 5-5. Intermediate Emetic Risk: Chemotherapeutic Agents and Guidelines for Acute and Delayed Emesis

Acute Emetic Category	Chemotherapy Agent (trade name)	Guideline for Acute Emesis	Guideline for Delayed Emesis
Intermediate	Irinotecan (Camptosar) Mitoxantrone (Novantrone) Paclitaxel (Taxol) Docetaxel (Taxotere) Mitomycin (Mutamycin) Topotecan (Hycamtin) Gemcitabine (Gemzar) Etoposide (Vepesid) Teniposide (Vumon)	Pretreatment: a corticosteroid (such as dexamethasone 4–8 mg by mouth, given once before chemotherapy)	No regular preventive use of antiemetics for delayed emesis

Adapted from Gralla, R. J., Osoba, D., Kris, M. K., et al. (1999). Recommendations for the use of antiemetics: Evidence-based, clinical practice guidelines. *Journal of Clinical Oncology,* 17(9), 2971.
    Note: Individual patients may require treatment similar to that recommended for high-emetic-risk agents. Combinations of agents in this class are not well studied, but they may occasionally cause more emesis for some patients, requiring treatment similar to that recommended for high-emetic-risk agents.

Table 5-6. Low Emetic Risk: Chemotherapeutic Agents and Guidelines for Acute and Delayed Emesis

Chemotherapy Agent (trade name)	Guideline for Acute Emesis	Guideline for Delayed Emesis
Bleomycin (Blenoxane) Busulfan (Myleran) Chlorambucil (Leukeran) 2-chlorodeoxyadenosine (Leustatin) Fludarabine (Fludara) Fluorouracil (Efudex) Hydroxyurea (Hydrea) L-asparaginase (Elspar) Melphalan (Alkeran) Mercaptopurine (Purinethol) Methotrexate (Rheumatrex) Tamoxifen (Nolvadex) Thioguanine (Lanvis) Vinblastine (Velban) Vincristine (Oncovin) Vindesine (Eldisine) Vinorelbine (Navelbine)	No routine pretreatment antiemetics	No regular preventive use of antiemetics for delayed emesis

Adapted from Gralla, R. J., Osoba, D., Kris, M. K., et al. (1999). Recommendations for the use of antiemetics: Evidence-based, clinical practice guidelines. *Journal of Clinical Oncology, 17*(9), 2971.

NOTE: Individual patients may require treatment similar to that recommended for intermediate-emetic-risk agents. Combinations of agents in this class are not well studied, but they may occasionally cause more emesis for some patients, requiring treatment similar to that recommended for intermediate-emetic-risk agents.

The other antiemetic agents—phenothiazines (prochlorperazine, thiethylperazine), butyrophenones (haloperidol, droperidol), and cannabinoids (dronabinol, nabilone, levonantradol)—are considered to be substantially lower in efficacy. They have more side effects; phenothiazines cause orthostatic hypotension.

Adjunctive medications such as benzodiazepines (lorazepam) and antihistamines (diphenhydramine, hydroxyzine, benztropine) may be added to an antiemetic regimen but should not be used alone as antiemetic agents. Diphenhydramine is more commonly used to prevent extrapyramidal reactions.

NONPHARMACOLOGIC APPROACHES

1. Try the following dietary interventions
   a. Eat foods cold or at room temperature; smells from hot foods might induce nausea or vomiting.

Table 5-7. Summary of Guidelines

Anticipatory Emesis

Prevention: Use of the most active antiemetic regimens appropriate for the chemotherapy being given to prevent acute or delayed emesis is suggested. Such regimens must be used with the initial chemotherapy, rather than after assessment of the patient's emetic response to less effective treatment.

Treatment: If anticipatory emesis occurs, behavioral therapy with systematic desensitization is effective and is suggested.

Special Emetic Problems

Emesis in pediatric oncology: The combination of a 5-HT$_3$ antagonist plus a corticosteroid is suggested before chemotherapy in children receiving chemotherapy of high emetic risk.

High-dose chemotherapy: A 5-HT$_3$ antagonist plus a corticosteroid is suggested.

Vomiting and nausea despite optimal prophylaxis in current or prior cycles: It is suggested that clinicians (1) conduct a careful evaluation of risk, antiemetic, chemotherapy, tumor, and concurrent disease and medication factors; (2) ascertain that the best regimen is being given for the emetic setting; (3) consider adding an antianxiety agent to the regimen; and (4) consider substituting a dopamine receptor antagonist, such as high-dose metoclopramide, for the 5-HT$_3$ antagonist (or add the dopamine antagonist to the regimen).

Adapted from Gralla, R. J., Osoba, D., Kris, M. K., et al. (1999). Recommendations for the use of antiemetics: Evidence-based, clinical practice guidelines. *Journal of Clinical Oncology,* 17(9), 2971.

  b. Try eating frequent light meals throughout the day. Rinse the mouth to remove the unpleasant taste and smell of emesis.

  c. Avoid foods that are spicy, greasy, or sweet and have strong odors.

  d. Eat bland or sour foods.

  e. Drink clear, cold liquids such as apple juice, ginger tea, lemonade, Gatorade, or cola. Sip the liquids slowly.

  f. Avoid food intake 1 to 2 hours before and after chemotherapy.

2. Get enough rest in a quiet and comfortable environment.

3. Minimize stimuli that might precipitate an emetic response, such as strong and unpleasant odors or the sight and sounds of other patients vomiting.

4. Use behavioral techniques such as relaxation, guided imagery, hypnosis, or acupuncture.

5. Use distraction, such as listening to music, reading, watching favorite TV programs or movies, and having pleasant conversations.

6. Use strategies that have worked in dealing with past emetic episodes (chemotherapy-related or not).
7. Try the newly approved, over-the-counter, drug-free devices, such as the ReliefBand®. This device, worn like a wristband, is believed to relieve nausea and vomiting by delivering gentle electrical signals that stimulate the underside of the wrist, carrying impulses to the nervous system and affecting areas that produce nausea and vomiting.

ANOREXIA

Alterations in the cancer patient's nutritional status can be induced by chemotherapy. These symptoms of anorexia and cachexia can severely compromise the patient's nutritional status, which can be irreversible and fatal. Anorexia is the lack of desire to eat, accompanied by decreased food intake. It is multifactorial, caused by the abnormally increased synthesis of serotonins, which stimulates a feeling of satiety; alterations in taste and smell; cancer treatments; aversion to certain foods; and an inability to digest nutrients (Robuck & Fleetwood, 1992). In cancer, the tumor cells compete for nutrients with the normal cells. As the tumor grows, body mass decreases and the patient loses weight.

Management and Patient Education

1. Obtain the patient's baseline height and weight. Ask the patient for a history of weight loss. Observe the patient's weight before each chemotherapy treatment. Teach the patient to weigh himself or herself once a week and to report a weight loss of 3 lb or more each week.
2. Monitor protein and albumin levels.
3. Analyze dietary intake and instruct the patient to keep a 3-day journal of intake.
4. Assess how the patient's mood or relationship with others affects his or her intake. Investigate any social or psychological factors that may affect eating patterns.
5. Determine the patient's ability to prepare and obtain food. Refer him or her to available community resources such as Meals on Wheels.
6. Urge the patient to eat high-protein, high-calorie foods.
7. Encourage small, frequent meals in a pleasant atmosphere. Having a glass of wine or another alcoholic beverage before a meal can stimulate the appetite.

8. Instruct the patient to take antiemetics to minimize nausea and vomiting.
9. Administer appetite stimulants (megestrol acetate) as ordered.
10. Provide electrolyte, mineral, and other nutritional supplements if needed.
11. Assess the patient's need for enteral or total parenteral nutrition.

MUCOSITIS

Managing alterations of the mucous membranes that line the oral, GI, and female reproductive cavities is a major challenge for oncology nurses. This condition is generally called mucositis. *Stomatitis* refers specifically to inflammation of the oral lining of the mouth (lips, gums, gingiva, tongue, palate, floor of the mouth) or throat. Approximately 40% of cancer patients have this complication. It is a major concern because it can lead to life-threatening events such as sepsis, infection, and malnutrition that may not be reversed without aggressive measures. It also affects quality-of-life issues because it can affect the patient's appearance and ability to communicate.

Factors that affect the degree of stomatitis include the type of cancer, the patient's age and oral health, the type of drug, and concomitant therapy. Patients with hematologic malignancies are more prone to oral complications than those with solid tumors. These patients are functionally myelosuppressed because of their cancer. Because hematologic malignancies are more common in younger patients, it follows that stomatitis often occurs in patients younger than 20 years old. Patients receiving combination chemotherapy, radiation treatment, antimicrobials, and corticosteroids are at the greatest risk (Mitchell, 1992). Patients who drink alcohol and smoke tobacco are also at high risk.

Chemotherapy has direct and indirect effects on the oral mucosa. *Direct stomatoxicity* occurs because chemotherapy decreases the renewal rate of the basal layer of epithelial cells that line the oral cavity. The epithelium normally regenerates every 10 to 14 days. With the cytotoxic attack on normal and malignant cells, these rapidly dividing epithelial cells are susceptible. The result is a thinning of the epithelium, leading to localized or diffuse ulceration about 2 to 3 weeks after drug administration. Drugs that cause stomatitis are the antimetabolites (e.g., 5-fluorouracil, methotrexate) and the antitumor antibiotics (e.g., doxorubicin, dactinomycin). *Indirect stomatitis* is the result of the myelosuppressive effect of chemotherapy on the bone marrow. The onset of indirect stomatitis depends on the agent used. Most drugs exert their myelotoxic effect within 10 to 14 days after treatment. It is believed that because the renewal rates of the oral mucosal cells and the leukocytes are similar, stomatitis is observed near the drug nadir, with resolution after marrow recovery (Sonis & Clark, 1992).

Other alterations in the oral mucosa include xerostomia (dryness of the mouth because of decreased production of saliva), ageusia (absence of taste perception), dysgeusia (unusual taste perception), and hypogeusia (decrease in taste acuity).

Management and Patient Education

1. Perform oral assessment daily. Using an oral assessment guide (Table 5-8) allows the patient and nurse to observe and document oral status systematically before and during treatment. Teach the patient to do self-assessment.
2. Refer the patient for a dental consultation before chemotherapy starts.
3. Teach the patient a good daily oral hygiene regimen:
   a. Perform preventive mouth care every 4 hours while awake. If mild stomatitis occurs, do mouth care every 4 hours around the clock; in severe stomatitis, every 2 hours is recommended (Bruya et al., 1975).
   b. Brush the teeth gently with a soft toothbrush or toothettes after meals and at bedtime. Use waxed dental floss because it is easier on the gums.
   c. Avoid using commercial mouthwashes containing alcohol because they irritate and dry the tissues. Rinse the mouth with warm saline (1 teaspoon of salt to 1 glass of water) or with sodium bicarbonate rinses (1 teaspoon of sodium bicarbonate to 1 pint of warm water). Hydrogen peroxide mouthwash is not recommended because it disturbs the normal flora of the mouth (Daeffler, 1980) and causes overgrowth of fissures and white papillae of the tongue, leading to candidiasis (Segelman & Doku, 1977).
   d. Wear dentures only if necessary.

Table 5-8. The Oral Cavity Assessment Form

Category	Rating	1	2	3	4
Lips	1 2 3 4	Smooth, soft, pink, moist, and intact	Slightly dry, wrinkled, reddened areas	Dry, rough, swollen, inflammatory line of demarcation	Very dry, inflamed, cracked, blistered, ulcerated, and bleeding
Tongue	1 2 3 4	Smooth, firm, pink, moist, and intact	Papillae prominent particularly at base, dry, pink with reddened areas	Raised, red papillae all over tongue giving peppered appearance: (very dry and swollen), coating at base	Very dry, thick, grooved, and coated; tip very red and demarcated, sides blistered
Oral mucosa	1 2 3 4	Smooth, pink, moist, and intact	Pale, slightly dry, reddened areas or white pustules	Red, dry, inflamed, edematous, ulcerated	Very red, shiny, edematous with blisters and/or ulcerations
Teeth or dentures	1 2 3 4	Shiny, no debris, well fitting	Slightly dull with slight debris, slightly loose	Dull with debris on half of visible enamel; loose with areas of irritation	Very dull, covered with debris, unable to wear due to irritation
Saliva	1 2 3 4	Thin, watery, sufficient saliva quantity	Saliva amount increased	Saliva scant, mouth dry	Saliva thick, ropy, viscid, or mucid

Total score: Mild dysfunction: 6–10, Moderate dysfunction: 11–15, Severe dysfunction: 16–20.

Directions: 1. Determine rating for each category. 2. Add up ratings. 3. Institute care based on ratings total score.
Reprinted with permission from Beck, S. L., & Yasko, J. M. (1984). *Guidelines for oral care.* Newbury Park, CA: Sage.

110

4. Advise the patient to eat a high-protein diet and to drink as much as 3 L/day, if not contraindicated. Avoid hot, spicy foods or foods high in sugar. Avoid oral irritants such as alcohol and tobacco.

5. Treat oral infection early with antifungal or antiviral agents as ordered. Agents commonly used are nystatin as an oral tablet, a vaginal tablet, or an oral suspension ("swish and swallow") four times a day. Other recommended agents are clotrimazole troches, chlorhexidine, Neosporin ointment applied to perioral infections, sucralfate, and allopurinol mouthwash.

6. Administer local or systemic pain medications (or both) as ordered. These medications may include 2% viscous lidocaine (Xylocaine) administered half an hour before eating, dyclonine hydrochloride in a 0.5% to 1.0% solution as a topical anesthetic, or diphenhydramine hydrochloride (Benadryl) elixir.

7. Use a topical protective agent to promote healing, such as kaolin–pectin preparations, with a Maalox substrate. (Allow the antacid to settle, pour off the liquid portion, and use the pasty residue to swab the affected area.) Rinse with saline or water after 20 minutes.

8. If the patient has xerostomia, use saliva substitutes and sialagogues (agents that increase salivary flow). Other measures are sucking on hard, sugarless candy, chewing sugarless gum, and keeping the lips and oral cavity moist with petroleum jelly or butter.

9. Teach the patient to notify the nurse or physician if the temperature exceeds 38°C or if bleeding and poor pain control occur, which can compromise nutritional intake.

CONSTIPATION

The oncology patient is at risk for constipation. Although the associated discomfort and high incidence of constipation are widely recognized, it is often considered a trivial problem by health care providers. To the patient, this can be a distressing and important problem. Constipation is defined as a "chronic (longer than 6 weeks) gastrointestinal disorder consisting of hard stools, fewer than three stools per week, or the inability to expel stool, whether hard or soft" (Donnatelle, 1990). In the oncology patient, constipation is due to the malignant process itself or is iatrogenically induced. Agents that commonly produce constipation are the vinca alkaloids, opioids given for pain relief, and antiemetics, particularly the serotonin (5-HT$_3$) receptor antagonists.

Management and Patient Education

1. Assess the patient's bowel function and elimination pattern.
2. Review with the patient the signs and symptoms of constipation and when to report the symptoms.
3. Ask the patient about the use of concomitant medications that may cause constipation.
4. Help the patient establish a daily bowel regimen.
5. Encourage the patient to increase his or her intake of foods rich in fiber and bulk (raw fruits and vegetables, grains and cereals) and to drink 8 to 10 glasses of fluids daily. Warm fluids and prune juice are helpful.
6. Encourage physical activity as tolerated.
7. Advise the patient to take prescribed medications. Call if the problem continues for 2 days.

DIARRHEA

Diarrhea is more common than constipation and produces more deleterious effects. If not promptly managed, diarrhea can lead to serious problems such as dehydration, electrolyte imbalances, weakness, lethargy, and metabolic acidosis. Diarrhea is the passage of frequent and watery stools, in this context caused by the destruction of the GI epithelium by chemotherapeutic agents. Diarrhea is often associated with antimetabolite administration and is a dose-limiting factor for 5-fluorouracil and irinotecan. Other causes of diarrhea, such as infection, intestinal obstruction, laxative abuse, and hypocalcemia, should be ruled out before initiating treatment. Diarrhea is best managed by pharmacologic intervention with anticholinergic drugs (atropine sulfate, belladonna) and opiates (loperamide, diphenoxylate, codeine, paregoric). Octreotide, a stable analogue of somatostatin, has shown efficacy for its antisecretory effect in chemotherapy-induced diarrhea (Harris et al., 1995).

Management and Patient Education

1. Assess the patient for signs and symptoms of diarrhea and dehydration. Review these with the patient so the patient can monitor and self-report.

2. Assess bowel function and elimination pattern.
3. Monitor weight, intake and output, and electrolytes. Administer IV fluids or electrolytes as ordered.
4. Administer antidiarrheal medications as ordered. Explain medications to the patient.
5. Encourage the patient to eat a low-residue, high-protein, high-calorie diet, increase fluid intake, and avoid foods such as beans, peas, milk, and caffeine. Avoid spicy and fatty foods, alcohol, and tobacco.
6. Instruct the patient to practice good perianal hygiene after each episode of diarrhea.
7. Encourage rest and decreased activity.
8. Consider discontinuing the drug or modifying the dose if diarrhea persists.

▼ Hematologic Toxicity

MYELOSUPPRESSION

Myelosuppression is the most common dose-limiting side effect of chemotherapy. Few cytotoxic agents are not myelosuppressive. Although this condition is generally reversible, it can cause complications because of infection and bleeding complications. Myelosuppression or bone marrow depression occurs because the antineoplastic agents are not selective; they attack the cancer cells and the mitotic normal cells. Recent research in the use of hematopoietic growth factors (discussed in an earlier chapter on biotherapy) and a new generation of antibiotics have lessened the incidence of myelosuppression, especially in high-dose regimens and in intense multimodality therapy. The main manifestations of myelosuppression are anemia, neutropenia, and thrombocytopenia. A brief discussion of hematopoiesis will help the nurse understand how the different agents may cause this type of toxicity.

Hematopoiesis is regulated by endogenous glycoproteins called colony-stimulating factors. These substances are growth factors responsible for the production of precursor and progenitor cells of all the major cell lines. The bone marrow contains the pluripotent stem cells, the precursors to the main blood components, including erythrocytes, leukocytes, and platelets. The normal laboratory values for these components are listed in Table 5-9. Figure 5-2 shows how the multipotent progenitor cells become differentiated and com-

Table 5-9. Normal Values and Survival Time for Blood Components

Blood Component	Normal Value	Survival Time
Red blood cells (RBCs)		120 days
Hemoglobin (Hgb)	Male: 14–16 g/dL	
	Female: 12–14 g/dL	
Hematocrit (Hct)	Male: 42%–51%	
	Female: 37%–47%	
Platelets	145,000–364,000/mm³	5–10 days
White blood cells	5,000–10,000/mm³	6–8 h circulat-
(WBCs–granulocytes)		ing in blood,
Neutrophils	35%–73%	2–3 days in
Bands	0%–11%	tissues
Eosinophils	0%–5%	
Basophils	0%–2%	
Lymphocytes	15%–52%	100–300+ days
Monocytes	2%–14%	

Absolute neutrophil count (ANC) = (% neutrophils + % bands) ÷ 100 × WBC.

mitted to specific cell lines to form mature blood cells in the peripheral blood. Myelosuppression is caused by the destruction of these circulating progenitor cells, which depletes the number of circulating mature blood cells. This reduction causes the blood count to drop. The lowest level to which a blood cell count drops is called its *nadir*.

The degree of bone marrow depression is attributed to the following (Cawley, 1990; Gastineau & Hoagland, 1992):

- Kinetics of a particular cell line
- Patient characteristics
- Drug characteristics
- Concomitant therapy

As shown in Table 5-9, the half-lives of the various cell lines differ. Anemia has a later onset than neutropenia, irrespective of the drug administered, because the half-life of each cell line differs substantially.

Patient Characteristics

The patient's age, health status, and nutritional status influence the degree of myelosuppression. Older and debilitated patients are at greater risk from the myelotoxic effects of chemotherapy. Patients with a compromised organ such as

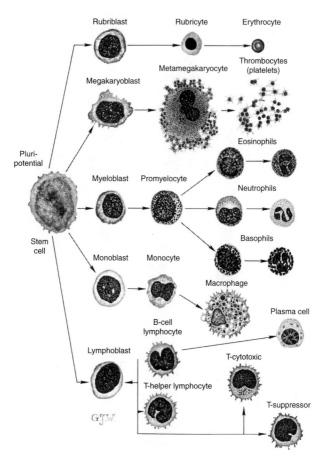

Fig. 5-2. Components of blood derived from a single stem cell. (Reprinted with permission from Belcher, A. E. [1992]. *Cancer nursing.* St. Louis: Mosby.)

the liver or kidney may tolerate chemotherapy poorly, because these organs play a key function in the metabolism and elimination of these drugs.

Drug Characteristics

The type, dose, schedule, and mode of administration of a drug help predict its myelosuppressive effects. Table 5-10 shows when myelosuppression occurs with some of the most

Table 5-10. Myelosuppressive Effects of Antineoplastic Agents

Drug	Neutropenia	WBC Nadir (days)	WBC Recovery (days)	Thrombocytopenia	Platelet
Altretamine	Mild to moderate	21–28	42	Mild to moderate	NA
Amsacrine	Moderate	11–14	17–25	Moderate	NA
Bleomycin	Rare	10	14	Rare	NA
Busulfan	Marked	11–30	25–54	Marked	NA
Carboplatin	Marked	21	28	Marked	NA
Carmustine	Marked	28–42	42–56	Marked	28–35
Chlorambucil	Moderate	21–28	42–56	Moderate	7–14
Cisplatin	Moderate	18–23	21–39	Moderate	14
Cladribine	Mild to moderate	11	42–56	Moderate	NA
Cyclophosphamide	Moderate	8–14	18–25	Mild	10–25
Cytarabine	Marked	12–14	22–24	Marked	22–24
Dacarbazine	Mild	21–28	28–35	Mild	14–28
Dactinomycin	Marked	14–21	22–25	Marked	10–14
Daunorubicin	Marked	10–14	21	Marked	10–14
Doxorubicin	Marked	10–14	21	Marked	NA
Etoposide	Moderate	7–14	16–20	Mild	9–16
Fludarabine	Moderate to severe	3–25		Moderate to severe	NA
5-Fluorouracil	Mild	7–14	20–30	Mild	7–17

Hydroxyurea	Marked	7	14–21	Moderate to severe	NA
Idarubicin	Moderate to severe	10–14	21–23	Platelet-sparing	NA
Ifosfamide	Moderate	10	18		28
Lomustine	Marked	40–50	60	Marked	28
Mechlorethamine	Moderate to marked	6–8	16–28	Moderate to marked	10–14
Melphalan	Moderate to marked	14–21	28–35	Moderate to marked	7–14
6-Mercaptopurine	Moderate to marked	7	14–21	Moderate to marked	10–14
Methotrexate	Moderate to marked	7–14	14–21	Moderate to marked	5–12
Mitomycin-C	Rare	28–42	42–70	Rare	NA
Mitoxantrone	Moderate	10–14	21	Marked	8–16
Pentostatin	Mild	10	14	Mild	NA
Plicamycin	Mild	14	21	Marked	NA
Procarbazine	Moderate	25–36	35–50+	Marked	21
Streptozocin	Mild	10–14	14–21	Mild	NA
Taxol	Marked	8–15	21	Marked	8–15
6-Thioguanine	Moderate to marked	14–28	28–35	Moderate to marked	14
Vinblastine	Marked	5–10	7–14	Marked	4–10
Vincristine	Mild	4–5	7–10	Mild	NA
Vindesine	Dose-related	3–6	7–10	Mild	7

Myelosuppressive course may vary with the dose, route, schedule of drug administration, and the patient's bone marrow reserve.

Adapted with permission from Goodman, M. (1992). *Cancer chemotherapy and care* (2nd ed.). Princeton: Bristol-Myers Oncology Division: Tanenbaum, L. (1994). *Cancer chemotherapy and biotherapy* (2nd ed.). Philadelphia: W. B. Saunders.

commonly used drugs. The phase specificity of a drug is related to the onset of myelosuppression. Thrombocytopenia and granulocytopenia are most noted with cell cycle–specific drugs, particularly those that are active in the S and M phases, such as 5-fluorouracil and the vinca alkaloids. Nadir recovery is quicker with these drugs. In contrast, the cell cycle–nonspecific drugs, such as the alkylating agents, have a delayed and prolonged effect. The use of high-dose or combination regimens can cause persistent nadirs because of the intense damage to the stem cell population. In terms of method of administration, the intra-arterial infusion of 5-fluorouracil is less myelosuppressive than systemic infusion.

Concomitant Therapy

The bone marrow is compromised when different treatment regimens are given sequentially or concomitantly. These treatments may be multimodal, such as chemotherapy, radiation therapy, and immunotherapy. These therapies as single interventions can also cause bone marrow depression. With radiation and chemotherapy, myelosuppression is more pronounced when they are given simultaneously or when chemotherapy is administered after radiation (von der Masse, 1994). Studies have shown that interferon potentiates the myelotoxic effects of chemotherapy (Gastineau & Hoagland, 1992). Also, non-neoplastic agents that the patient is taking may enhance myelosuppression.

ANEMIA

Anemia (decreased number of circulating red cells) is not as alarming as the changes induced in the other blood elements. It is usually slow in onset because of the long life span of the red cells (120 days) compared with that of the neutrophils (4 days) and the platelets (10 days). It is not a dose-limiting factor in chemotherapy and rarely occurs from chemotherapy alone. The signs and symptoms of anemia include a fall in the hematocrit and hemoglobin, fatigue, hypotension, shortness of breath, tachypnea, tachycardia, headaches, dizziness, and irritability.

Management and Patient Education

1. Obtain a baseline complete blood count and monitor the count during chemotherapy as indicated.

2. Assess the patient for signs and symptoms of anemia, and teach the patient to report these.
3. Assess the patient for other conditions that may cause anemia, such as bleeding.
4. If the hemoglobin falls below 8%, the hematocrit drops to 25%, or the patient becomes symptomatic, transfusion of packed cells might be indicated.
5. Administer oxygen when oxygen saturation is less than 90% or when the patient is symptomatic.
6. Evaluate dietary intake. Encourage the patient to eat foods that are rich in iron, vitamins, and minerals.
7. Suggest nutritional or iron and vitamin supplements if necessary.
8. Encourage the patient to modify and pace activities and to get enough rest and sleep.
9. Teach the patient the importance of exercise and ways of incorporating it into his or her daily activities.
10. Administer recombinant human erythropoietin (epoetin alfa) as ordered, and teach the patient how to inject the drug.
11. Instruct the patient's family to assist the patient in tasks and activities of daily living.

NEUTROPENIA

The white blood cell, the body's defense against infection, is vulnerable to the myelosuppressive effect of chemotherapy. The life span of a white cell is 6 to 8 hours in the blood and 2 to 3 days in the tissues. There are six types of white cells: neutrophils, eosinophils, basophils, monocytes, lymphocytes, and bands. The first three subtypes are called granulocytes because of their appearance. The neutrophils are considered the body's first line of defense because they neutralize and localize infective bacteria. The major indicator of bacterial infection is *neutropenia,* the reduction of the absolute neutrophil count to 1,500/mm^3 or less. The absolute neutrophil count is calculated by multiplying the total white cell count by the percentage of neutrophils and bands.

When there are not enough neutrophils and macrophages, which are responsible for ingesting and digesting bacteria (phagocytosis), the body is at risk for infection. Bacteria can invade the skin, respiratory tract, oral cavity, sinuses, and perianal area. In the cancer patient, infection can be life-threatening, especially when complications such as sepsis occur. Fever is the first and in some cases the only sign; therefore, other diagnostic tests such as chest x-rays and cultures are needed to confirm the diagnosis of infection. The white blood cell count nadir is reached in 7 to 14 days; recovery occurs in 14 to 28 days. Patients who have neutropenic fevers are usually given broad-spectrum antibiotics and colony-stimulating factors. The chemotherapy doses are either modified or discontinued if the problem persists.

Management and Patient Education

1. Obtain baseline data before chemotherapy; assess and monitor the complete blood count, particularly the absolute neutrophil count, during treatments and at ordered intervals.
2. Assess the patient for signs and symptoms of infection.
3. Teach the patient about neutropenia and when to report symptoms.
4. Administer prophylactic antibiotics and antipyretics as ordered.
5. Teach the patient about colony-stimulating factors such as granulocyte colony-stimulating factor, if ordered. Instruct the patient in self-administration.
6. Urge the patient to maintain a safe and clean environment:
   a. Avoid people who have colds or any communicable disease, such as chicken pox or pneumonia.
   b. Do not eat raw fruits and vegetables; do not handle fresh flowers and plants.
   c. Do not handle pet excreta because of the potential of contracting a fungal or bacterial infection.
   d. Avoid stagnant water, which might harbor bacteria.
7. Emphasize the importance of meticulous personal hygiene:
   a. Bathe daily, rinse the skin thoroughly, and pat dry.
   b. Perform oral care every 4 hours or more often.
   c. Cleanse the perianal area after each bowel movement.
   d. Empty the bladder every 4 hours.
   e. Do not use rectal suppositories, enemas, douches, and tampons.
   f. Keep nails clean and short; observe good handwashing technique.

8. Maintain adequate nutrition:
   a. Eat a high-protein, high-carbohydrate diet.
   b. Drink at least eight glasses of fluid daily.
   c. Avoid raw and uncooked meat, fruits, and vegetables.

THROMBOCYTOPENIA

The thrombocytes or platelets are critical for maintaining vascular integrity and hemostasis by aggregating to each other to form a clot. A reduction in the number of platelets to less than 50,000/mm^3 indicates thrombocytopenia, which may result in bleeding. The sites of bleeding are the skin, mucous membranes, the GI system, the genitourinary system, the respiratory system, and the intracranial area. The onset of thrombocytopenia is slower than that of leukopenia. Chemotherapy can depress the platelet count, and drugs containing acetylsalicylic acid (aspirin), other forms of salicylates, or nonsteroidal anti-inflammatory agents can potentiate existing thrombocytopenia.

Management and Patient Education

1. Monitor the platelet count closely.
2. Assess for superficial or internal manifestations of bleeding such as petechiae, epistaxis, easy bruising, prolonged bleeding time, "coffee-grounds" emesis, and hematuria.
3. Test the stool for occult blood and check the urine for heme.
4. Teach the patient to observe the following precautions:
   a. Maintain a safe environment to prevent falls or trauma.
   b. Use stool softeners to avoid straining, which can cause rectal tearing and bleeding. Avoid performing the Valsalva maneuver when moving or defecating. Eat a high-fiber diet and drink plenty of fluids to avoid constipation.
   c. Postpone or minimize, if appropriate, any invasive medical or surgical procedures (e.g., dental extractions, multiple venipunctures, injections).
   d. Do not use sharp instruments (scissors, razors, blades) for grooming. Use an electric razor.
   e. Avoid medications that might prolong or exacerbate bleeding, such as steroids and over-the-counter medications containing aspirin. If these medications are

needed, the patient should take antacids, H_2 blockers, or food concomitantly.

f. Use a soft toothbrush; avoid flossing.

g. Use a water-soluble lubricant for sexual intercourse. Avoid intercourse when platelet count is less than $50,000/mm^3$.

5. Administer platelet transfusions as ordered. Check institutional policy for transfusion parameters. Premedicate the patient and monitor for platelet reaction.

▼ Hepatotoxicity

Certain cytotoxic agents (Table 5-11) have been implicated in hepatotoxicity. These drugs cause damage to the liver in the following forms: veno-occlusive disease, chronic fibrosis, fatty changes, cholestasis, and hepatocellular dysfunction. The clinical picture involves elevated liver enzyme and bilirubin levels, right upper quadrant pain, hepatomegaly, jaundice, ascites, hyperpigmentation of the skin, lethargy, anorexia, and nausea. These changes are often reversible; clinicians may wish to modify the drug dose to prevent chronic hepatic injury.

Table 5-11. Hepatotoxic Agents

Drug	Effect
Carmustine	Elevated liver enzymes
Cytosine arabinoside	Elevated liver enzymes
L-Asparaginase	Fatty metamorphosis
Lomustine	Elevated liver enzymes
6-Mercaptopurine	Cholestasis, necrosis
Methotrexate	Fibrosis, cirrhosis
Plicamycin	Acute necrosis
Streptozocin	Elevated liver enzymes

MANAGEMENT AND PATIENT EDUCATION

1. Obtain baseline liver function tests before initiating treatment.

2. Monitor hepatic enzymes, serum glutamic oxaloacetic transaminase (SGOT) and serum glutamic pyruvate

transaminase (SGPT), lactate dehydrogenase, and bilirubin periodically.
3. Ask whether the patient is taking any medications (antimicrobials) that might cause abnormal liver function.
4. Review signs and symptoms of hepatotoxicity.
5. Consider dose modifications or intermittent dosing schedules, if practical, if liver function test results are abnormal.
6. Instruct the patient to avoid alcohol.

▼ Fatigue

During the past decade, increasing attention has been paid to cancer-related fatigue, which has a broad impact on the quality of life of the cancer patient and his or her family. Clinical studies affirm that its prevalence is as high as 99% (Blesch et al., 1991), as a result of either the disease process or the aggressive therapies used. Fatigue has been identified as a major dose-limiting factor in patients receiving chemotherapy, radiation, and alpha-interferon. Piper et al. (1987) defined fatigue as "a subjective feeling of tiredness that is influenced by circadian rhythm [and] that varies in unpleasantness, duration, and intensity." Their fatigue model (Fig. 5-3) explains how the objective and subjective manifestations of fatigue are influenced by environmental, social, physiologic, psychological, and personal factors.

The clinician can use both pharmacologic and nonpharmacologic fatigue management strategies, but patient preparation and education are key. As clinicians, we must educate ourselves about this problem so that we can demystify it to patients and teach them self-management techniques. The oncology nurse should try to understand the fatigue phenomenon from the patient's perspective, including the degree of distress that the patient experiences from fatigue. This knowledge will help the nurse plan strategies to help the patient handle fatigue.

MANAGEMENT AND PATIENT EDUCATION

1. Assure the patient that the fatigue is a side effect of the chemotherapy and does not indicate treatment failure.
2. Obtain a fatigue profile by asking about the patient's fatigue pattern, the onset of fatigue, the impact of fatigue

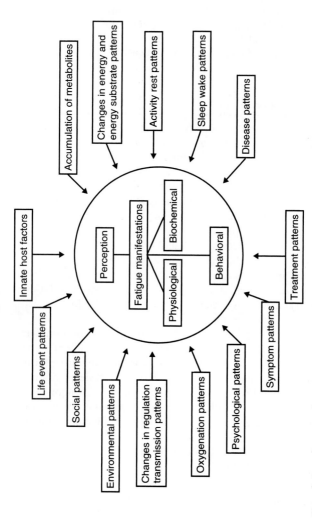

Fig. 5-3. Piper fatigue framework.

on his or her life and daily activities, and factors that might contribute to the degree of fatigue.

3. Help the patient set realistic goals for activity, rest, and sleep after evaluating his or her energy levels.

4. Advise the patient to get enough rest and sleep during the day.

5. Teach the patient the importance of maintaining good sleep hygiene:

   a. Go to bed at the same time each night.

   b. Create an environment conducive to sleep; turn off the TV and eliminate distracting noises. Avoid caffeine and alcohol at least 2 hours before going to bed.

6. Stress the importance of active exercise, 20 to 30 minutes a day.

7. Instruct the patient to pace activities according to his or her energy level.

8. Encourage the patient to seek assistance with activities of daily living; rest and do not do too much too soon.

9. Emphasize the importance of good nutrition, including moderate fluid intake, unless contraindicated, to eliminate cellular wastes.

10. Teach the patient relaxation techniques and other methods to conserve mental and emotional energy.

11. Administer packed red cells if ordered. Monitor the complete blood count and vital signs; assess for a hemolytic reaction.

12. Collaborate with the physician in the management of other potential causes of fatigue, such as dehydration, anemia, pain, and electrolyte imbalance.

13. Check the patient's medication profile for medications that might be contributing to fatigue, such as opioids and antiemetics.

14. Investigate the severity and chronicity of fatigue signs and symptoms, and make a psychiatric referral if there is a likelihood of clinical depression rather than fatigue.

▼ Nephrotoxicity

Some of the neoplastic agents known for their potential nephrotoxic effects are ifosfamide, cyclophosphamide, cisplatin, methotrexate, streptozocin, and the nitrosoureas (Table 5-12). Acute or chronic chemotherapy-induced nephrotoxicity may result from the direct effect of these drugs on the kid-

Table 5-12. Nephrotoxic Agents: Clinical Characteristics, Types of Nephrotoxicity, and Related Assessment and Intervention

Agent	Clinical Characteristics	Type of Nephrotoxicity	Assessment and Interventions
Carboplatin	Elevated creatinine studies (BUN, creatinine, serum creatine)		Creatinine studies: baseline and after drug administration IV hydration pre- and postdrug
Carmustine	Elevated creatinine studies	Inflammatory changes	Monitor creatinine studies
Cisplatin	Most common 10–20 days after administration: elevated clearance studies, hyperuricemia, elevated serum electrolytes	Proximal tubule damage Distal tubule damage	Creatinine studies baseline and postdrug Copious IV hydration pre- and postdrug Administration of mannitol, furosemide, or both pre-, intra-, and postdrug Monitor urine output
Cyclophosphamide	Elevated creatinine studies Hematuria	Bladder mucosa damage Hemorrhagic cystitis	Creatinine studies baseline and after drug administration IV hydration pre- and postdrug Fuorsemide pre-, intra-, and postdrug Monitor urine output Mesna pre- and intradrug administration (protective coating for bladder mucosa) Teach patient to void every 2 hours to excrete drug metabolites Dipstick all urine for hematuria; if present, increase IV hydration rate to flush drug metabolites
Ifosfamide	Elevated creatinine studies Hematuria	Proximal tubular damage Impaired tubular re-	Creatinine studies baseline and postdrug IV hydration pre- and postdrug

Drug			Nursing interventions
		absorption Bladder mucosa damage Hemorrhagic cystitis	Monitor urine output Dipstick urine for hematuria; if present, increase IV hydration to flush metabolites Mesna administration (protective coating for bladder mucosa) Teach patient to void every 2 hours
Lomustine	Onset most common months to years after therapy	Tubular atrophy Glomerular sclerosis Renal tubule damage Renal tubule obstruction	
Methotrexate	Elevated creatinine studies Azotemia Electrolyte abnormalities Acidosis Oliguria		Creatinine studies baseline and postdrug IV hydration pre- and postdrug Monitor urine output Sodium bicarbonate pre-, intra-, and postdrug Maintain urine pH above 7 because drug precipitates in acidic urine; if pH is less than 7, give sodium bicarbonate dose to maintain alkaline urine above 7. Citrovorum administration postdrug to prevent lysis of normal cells Obtain and monitor serum drug levels after administration
Mithramycin	Elevated creatinine studies Azotemia Electrolyte abnormalities Hemolytic uremic syndrome	Irreversible renal tubule damage Renal failure Renal tubular necrosis	Creatinine studies baseline and postdrug IV hydration postdrug Monitor urine output

(continued)

127

Table 5-12. Nephrotoxic Agents: Clinical Characteristics, Types of Nephrotoxicity, and Related Assessment and Intervention (*Continued*)

Agent	Clinical Characteristics	Type of Nephrotoxicity	Assessment and Interventions
Mitomycin-C	Hemolytic uremic syndrome Thrombocytopenia Azotemia	Dose is cumulative Renal tubule damage Glomerulus damage	Monitor serum creatinine Monitor platelet count Transfuse with platelets as necessary
Thioguanine	Elevated creatinine studies Azotemia	Renal parenchyma damage Kidney occlusion	Monitor BUN and creatinine during routine visits

ney or the glomerular distal tubule pathway. The renal alterations are manifested by hemorrhagic cystitis, oliguria, dysuria, an increased creatinine level, suprapubic discomfort, and low back pain. Hyperuricemia is associated with the use of high-dose methotrexate, and delayed renal failure may occur months to years after carmustine therapy.

MANAGEMENT AND PATIENT EDUCATION

1. Monitor renal function by checking serum creatinine, electrolytes, and creatinine clearance values before treatment.
2. Ensure adequate hydration before and after treatment by giving fluids intravenously and orally.
3. Maintain adequate diuresis (100 mL/hour for 2 to 4 hours before treatment and for 4 to 6 hours after treatment). Administer mannitol if indicated.
4. Alkalinization of the urine to a pH of more than 7 is important to prevent precipitate formation with high-dose methotrexate administration. If oral sodium bicarbonate or citrovorum rescue (leucovorin) is ordered, make sure the patient knows the importance of taking these medications as scheduled.
5. Encourage the patient to drink enough fluids before and after treatment.
6. Give uroprotectants such as mesna or allopurinol to enhance uric acid excretion, if ordered.
7. Teach the patient to void frequently, especially at bedtime, to prevent urinary stasis.
8. Instruct the patient to avoid foods that may irritate the bladder, such as coffee, tea, alcohol, and spices.
9. Teach the patient signs and symptoms of renal toxicity, their management, and when to report them.

▼ Neurotoxicity

One must understand the nervous system, the agents associated with neurologic symptoms, and the presenting signs and symptoms of neurologic syndromes to diagnose chemotherapy-induced neurotoxicity. The nervous system regulates and maintains body function through stimuli reception and response. The components of the nervous system are the peripheral nervous system, the central nervous system (CNS), and the autonomic nervous system. Toxicity affecting these different components has separate symptoms. Toxicity to the peripheral nervous system, which comprises the sensory and motor nerves, results in paresthesias, numbness, and tingling of the hands and feet. The CNS, composed of the brain and spinal cord, is responsible for the neurologic functions of mental status, level of consciousness, sensory and motor functions, cerebellar function, and cranial nerve function. The toxic manifestations are confusion, dizziness, and unsteady gait. Toxicity to the autonomic nervous system results in constipation, urinary retention, impotence, and postural hypotension.

Another component of the nervous system that is important to understand is the blood–brain barrier. The blood–brain barrier determines whether a cytotoxic agent can reach the nervous system. It blocks some agents from entering the system at a cellular level. Penetration of the CNS is different from that of the peripheral nervous system. Subsequently, the chemotherapeutic agents that can penetrate to the peripheral nervous system cause neurologic changes involving sensation and pain, whereas agents that can penetrate the blood–brain barrier to the CNS cause alterations in cranial nerve, mental, cerebellar, motor, and sensory function.

The varied factors known to cause neurologic symptoms in oncology patients, combined with the neurotoxic effects of many antineoplastic agents, often make it difficult to discern the cause of chemotherapy-induced neurotoxicity. The risk factors speculated to predispose patients receiving potentially neurotoxic agents to toxicity are:

- Intrathecal administration
- Concomitant cranial irradiation
- Impaired renal function
- Concomitant use of aminoglycosides
- High-dose therapy
- Cumulative vinca alkaloid doses
- Increasing age
- Previous neurotoxic sensitivity

Before the administration of a potentially neurotoxic agent, the patient should be evaluated for the presence of risk factors, should undergo a neurologic examination, and should have renal function studies performed. The exact incidence of chemotherapy-related neurotoxicity is not known, although the frequency is increasing, especially with high-dose regimens (Kaplan & Wiernik, 1982).

Table 5-13 lists the most common neurotoxicities associated with specific antineoplastic agents, signs and symptoms, and interventions. The chemotherapy-induced neurotoxic reactions include the following:

- Cerebellar toxicity
- Cranial neuropathy
- Encephalopathy
- Peripheral neuropathy
- Autonomic neuropathy

▼ Pulmonary Toxicity

Chemotherapy-induced pulmonary toxicity is not well understood. It is believed that the cause is direct damage to the lung parenchyma and the altered proliferation and migration of pneumocytes. The damage caused by the cytotoxic agents causes destruction of the alveolar and interstitial epithelium, making capillary exchange of oxygen and carbon dioxide difficult. Alveolitis, interstitial pneumonitis, and fibrosis can occur, all of which reduce the functional residual capacity and elasticity of the lungs. These effects are significant because they are the precursors to life-threatening respiratory failure.

Awareness of the risk factors associated with pulmonary toxicity is important in identifying patients predisposed to pulmonary damage. These risk factors include the use of pulmonary-toxic drugs, pre-existing lung disease, age older than 60 years, renal dysfunction, high-dose oxygen therapy, history of smoking, and concomitant radiation therapy to the chest. Pulmonary toxicity may develop within days of therapy or may have a chronic onset after months or years of therapy.

The two cytotoxic agents that commonly cause pulmonary damage are bleomycin and busulfan. The pulmonary damage caused by bleomycin is dose-related; patients who receive a cumulative dose of greater than 450 units show a higher incidence of toxicity than those who receive a lower cumulative dose. In busulfan therapy, the busulfan lung syndrome (discussed in the busulfan drug monograph) can occur and has a poor prognosis.

Dyspnea is the cardinal symptom of chemotherapy-induced pulmonary toxicity. Other signs and symptoms are fever, fatigue, dry cough, tachypnea, and rales. Chest pain is unusual but may occur with paclitaxel and docetaxel admin-

Table 5-13. Neurotoxic Agents

Toxicity	Agents	Characteristics	Interventions
Autonomic nervous system	Arabinoside Cytosine (IT) Methotrexate (IT) Vincristine Vinblastine	Bladder atony Abdominal pain, tenderness Bladder incontinence Bowel incontinence Constipation Paralytic ileus	PO hydration Prophylactic stool softener High-fiber diet Avoid constipating foods Ambulate (if able to) Bladder/bowel training for incontinence or urinary retention Reduce or hold future doses for paralytic ileus
CNS: cerebellar	Cytosine arabinoside 5-Fluorouracil	Ataxia Tremor Decreased coordination Nystagmus Diplopia Dysarthria Slurred speech	Discontinue therapy Speech, occupational, and physical therapy consultation Institute safety precautions Assistive devices
CNS: cranial neuropathy— cranial nerve II	Carboplatin Cisplatin	Impaired visual acuity	Test visual acuity Assess visual fields Inspect optic discs

Problem	Drugs	Signs and Symptoms	Interventions
CNS: cranial neuropathy—cranial nerve III, IV, VI	Carboplatin Cisplatin Cyclophosphamide	Impaired extraocular movements Papilledema, nystagmus	Test pupillary reaction to light Assess extraocular movement for nystagmus, diplopia Test visual acuity Assess visual fields Check optic discs
CNS: cranial neuropathy—cranial nerve VII	Vincristine	Jaw pain Facial nerve palsy	Assess for diminished contraction of masseter muscles and jaw pain Give soft foods and pain medication for jaw pain
CNS: cranial neuropathy—cranial nerve VIII	Cisplatin	Impaired hearing	Audiogram, whisper test, Weber and Rinne tests
CNS: cranial neuropathy—cranial nerve IX, X	Vincristine Vinblastine	Hoarse or absent voice	Listen to quality of voice Minimize use of laryngeal nerve
CNS: encephalopathy	Carmustine Cyclophosphamide Cystosine arabinoside Ifosfamide L-Asparaginase Methotrexate Procarbazine Thiotepa	Confusion Hallucinations Altered consciousness Seizures Lethargy Altered cognitive function Agitation	Discontinue drug Assess level of consciousness Institute seizure precautions Neuropsychiatric consult Teach memory improvement strategies Instruct family or significant other to supervise patient activity and institute safety precautions
CNS: peripheral neuropathy: motor	Paclitaxel Vinblastine Vincristine	Muscle weakness Foot drop	Assess muscle strength in major muscle groups Active or passive range-of-motion exercises TID-QID

(continued)

133

Table 5-13. Neurotoxic Agents (Continued)

Toxicity	Agents	Characteristics	Interventions
CNS: peripheral neuropathy: sensory	Carboplatin	Diminished or absent sensation	Assess deep tendon reflexes
	Cisplatin	Jaw pain	Assess sensation discrimination
	Cytosine arabinoside	Diminished or absent deep tendon reflexes	Soft foods and pain medication PRN for jaw pain
	Etoposide	Neuropathic pain	Pain medication for neuropathic pain
	Paclitaxel		Avoid extreme temperatures and temperature changes
	Vinblastine	Paresthesias of fingers and toes	Assistive devices as necessary
	Vincristine	Loss of proprioception	

Table 5-14. Pulmonary Toxic Agents

Agent	Toxicity	Interventions
Bleomycin	Pulmonary capillary and cellular destruction	Pulmonary assessment Pulmonary function tests (PFTs) pre- and postdrug Avoid high fractions of inspired oxygen
Busulfan	Progressive pulmonary fibrosis	Pulmonary assessment Pending pulmonary assessment:
	Precursors to fibrosis: atypical alevolar and interstitial epithelium changes Pulmonary edema Insterstitial pneumonitis	PFTs, chest x-ray Restrict fluids with pulmonary edema Provide supportive therapy as necessary
Carmustine	Pulmonary parenchyma changes	Same as above
Cyclophosphamide	Pulmonary edema Aveolitis Interstitial pneumonitis	Same as above
Cytosine arabinoside	Pulmonary edema Respiratory distress Respiratory failure	Same as above
Lomustine	Pulmonary fibrosis	
Melphalan	Progressive bronchopulmonary tissue changes Interstitial pneumonitis Pulmonary fibrosis	Same as above
Methotrexate	Pulmonary edema Interstitial pneumonitis Eosinophilia Irreversible interstitial fibrosis	Same as above
Mitomycin	Pulmonary parenchyma damage and atypical changes in interstitial lung tissues	Same as above
Procarbazine	Hypersensitivity Pneumonitis	Same as above
Teniposide	Bronchospasm	

Note: The characteristics of pulmonary toxicity are the same for all of the drugs in this table and include dyspnea, dry cough, tachypnea, fever, and rales.

istration. The best intervention for pulmonary alterations is prevention (Table 5-14).

MANAGEMENT AND PATIENT EDUCATION

1. Obtain a baseline assessment of pulmonary function, including a chest x-ray, pulmonary function tests, and arterial blood gas analysis.
2. Observe the patient's respiratory rate and breathing patterns, and note any changes with position and exertion.
3. Ask the patient whether he or she has problems performing activities of daily living.
4. Review with the patient the signs and symptoms of pulmonary toxicity and measures for coping with these problems.
5. Instruct the patient to avoid smoking and exposure to irritants such as noxious gases and aerosol sprays.
6. Teach the patient to breathe properly and to alternate periods of activity and rest.
7. If the patient is undergoing therapy and develops severe pulmonary complications, consider discontinuing the drug.
8. Monitor the dose given for bleomycin therapy; the recommended maximum is 400 to 500 units.
9. Consider the use of steroid prophylaxis for patients who develop capillary leak syndrome.
10. Avoid using high fractions of inspired oxygen to prevent further lung damage.
11. Provide supportive therapy, such as loop diuretics to decrease pulmonary congestion or vasodilators or bronchodilators (theophylline) as needed.
12. Restrict fluid intake.
13. Position patient for comfort.

▼ Sexuality and Fertility Effects of Chemotherapy

Because of the growing number of cancer survivors, the effect of chemotherapy on male and female sexuality and fertility has become an issue. The damaging systemic effects caused by the lysis of rapidly dividing cells such as those that compose the bone marrow, the hair follicles, and the digestive tract cause pallor, alopecia, and GI-related weight loss, which alter the patient's appearance, body image, and sexual desire (Smith & Babaian, 1992). The implications of altered sexual desire are significant, because desire is the initial phase of the sexual response cycle (Hughes, 1995). Lack of desire causes dysfunction and impairs sexual health (Hughes, 1996).

The chemotherapy-induced sexuality and fertility reactions include gonadal dysfunction (perimenopause, premature menopause), infertility, testicular dysfunction (azospermia, oligospermia), and teratogenicity or mutagenicity.

GONADAL DYSFUNCTION

Perimenopause is caused by failing or dysfunctional ovaries, and premature menopause by failed ovaries (Chapman, 1992). Perimenopause and premature menopause are indicated by elevated levels of follicle-stimulating hormone and luteinizing hormone, irregular or absent menses, and menopausal symptoms (Chapman, 1992; Lamb, 1995). Menopausal symptoms include decreased sexual desire, amenorrhea, vaginal atrophy, dryness, stenosis, hot flashes, itching, irritation, dyspareunia, and sterility (Aikin, 1995; Smith, 1994). These effects not only impair libido but also prevent women from participating in sexual activity.

INFERTILITY

Chemotherapy-associated infertility occurs in women from direct injury to the ova or from granulosa follicular cell suppression, damage, or death (Chapman, 1992). The length of time the patient will remain infertile is not understood: some women regain ovarian function on completing treatment, some do so with time, and others never do so (Chapman, 1992; Lamb, 1995).

In men, chemotherapy-associated infertility results from lysis of spermatocytes and damage to the Sertoli cells and the seminiferous tubules. Because the process of spermatogenesis begins at 13 years of age, male patients older than age 13 should be given the option of banking sperm.

TESTICULAR DYSFUNCTION

Testicular dysfunction induced by chemotherapy is caused by altered sexual desire, suppression of testicular function, or suppression of spermatogenesis (Kaempfer, 1981). Because spermatocytes are rapidly dividing cells, chemotherapy quickly suppresses spermatogenesis. Azoospermia (absence of sperm in the semen) is induced by the suppression of spermatogenesis. Oligospermia is a low sperm count induced by impaired spermatogenesis after chemotherapy. Depending on the drug used and the duration of treatment, some recovery of spermatogenesis after completion of therapy is believed to be possible (Smith & Babaian, 1992).

TERATOGENICITY AND MUTAGENICITY

The possible restoration of spermatogenesis or ovarian function after therapy has led to the question of reproduction after receiving chemotherapy. Reproduction after therapy remains controversial because these agents, in the laboratory setting, have demonstrated the potential to cause mutagenicity (the potential to cause genetic mutation) and teratogenicity (the potential to cause abnormal structure development in an embryo, which may result in a deformed fetus).

Health care providers need to be aware of which drugs have the potential to impair sexual and reproductive health. Table 5-15 lists the agents associated with these sexuality and fertility reactions.

MANAGEMENT AND PATIENT EDUCATION

1. Assess previous sexual history.
2. Advise the patient of the physical, sexual, and reproductive changes that may occur after therapy. Inform the patient of the potential for sterility.
3. Encourage the patient to ask questions and discuss concerns.
4. Encourage the patient to discuss future plans for pregnancy.
5. Educate male patients about sperm banking and female patients about *in vitro* fertilization.
6. Provide information about contraception. Stress the importance of avoiding pregnancy during therapy.
7. Instruct the patient to use water-soluble lubricating agents if vaginal dryness occurs during intercourse.
8. Advise the patient to plan intercourse for times of higher energy.

9. Give the patient the American Cancer Society's booklet *Sexuality and Cancer*.
10. Teach patient techniques for "setting the mood," such as romantic, candlelight dinners, massage, sensual clothing, and so on.
11. Address activities and prosthetic devices that promote a positive body image, such as good hygiene or the use of wigs and perfumes.

Table 5-15. Effects of Chemotherapeutic Agents on Sexual Function

Class/Drug	Effects on Sexual Function
Alkylating Agents	
Busulfan	Gonadal function
	Fertility
Chlorambucil	Gonadal function
	Fertility
	Mutagenic
Cyclophosphamide	Gonadal function
	Fertility
	Sterility
	Teratogenic
Melphalan	Gonadal function
	Fertility
Nitrogen mustard	Testicular function
	Fertility
	Teratogenic
	Mutagenic
Thiotepa	Teratogenic
Nitrosoureas	
Lomustine	Gonadal function
Antitumor Antibiotics	
Bleomycin	Mutagenic
Dactinomycin	Mutagenic
Daunorubicin	Mutagenic
	Teratogenic
Doxorubicin	Gonadal function
	Fertility
	Teratogenic

(continued)

Table 5-15. Effects of Chemotherapeutic Agents on Sexual Function *(Continued)*

Class/Drug	Effects on Sexual Function
Antitumor Antibiotics	
(continued)	
Mithramycin	Azoospermia
Mitomycin	Mutagenic
Antimetabolites	
Cytosine arabinoside	Gonadal function
	Fertility
	Teratogenic
5-Fluorouracil	Gonadal function
	Fertility
	Teratogenic
Methotrexate	Gonadal function
	Fertility
	Teratogenic
	Mutagenic
Procarbazine	Gonadal function
	Fertility
	Mutagenic
	Erectile dysfunction
Vinca Alkaloids	
Vinblastine	Gonadal function
	Fertility
	Teratogenic
Vincristine	Possible erectile dysfunction and retrograde ejaculation

Data from MSKCC (1996), Glasel (1994), Chapman (1992), and Kaempfer, S. (1981). The effects of chemotherapy on reproduction: A review of the literature. *Oncology Nursing Forum, 8,* 11–17.

6

Management of Hypersensitivity Reactions and Extravasation

▼ Hypersensitivity Reactions

Hypersensitivity reactions (HSRs) are common in patients receiving chemotherapy. These reactions, which may be local or systemic, are believed to be immunologically mediated (Weiss, 1992a; 1992b); however, there are other mechanisms that may explain their occurrence (Table 6-1). An HSR can involve any of the four types of reactions defined by Gell and Coombs (1975; Table 6-2).

When a patient develops an HSR to a chemotherapeutic agent, most likely the drug will be stopped. The decision to use it again depends on the severity of the reaction, the treatment plan, and the availability of alternative agents.

Although it may be difficult to pinpoint the cause of the HSR, it is important to understand the reaction and its relation to the drug administered, as well as to distinguish the reaction from an immunologically mediated response. It can be difficult for the clinician to ascertain a true HSR, because some reactions mimic immunologic reactivity by direct release of mediators. Other drugs being administered concurrently, the drug formulation, and the diluents used can be contributing factors; these factors should be ruled out before diagnosing an HSR. Drugs such as cytarabine preserved in

Table 6-1. Cancer Chemotherapeutic Agents Causing Hypersensitivity Reactions

Drug	Type of Reaction	Frequency	Probable Mechanism of Reaction
Anthracycline antibiotics	I	Varies depending on anthracycline ($< 1\%$–15%)	Unknown (nonspecific release)
L-Asparaginase	I	10%–20%	IgE; IgG, complement?
Bleomycin	I	Case reports	Unknown
Chlorambucil	I	Case reports	Unknown
Cisplatin	I	Intravesically: up to 20% Intravenously: $< 5\%$	IgE; nonspecific release?
Cisplatin analogues	I	Up to 10%	Unknown
Cyclophosphamide	I	Case reports	Unknown
Cytarabine	I	Case reports	IgE
Dacarbazine	I	Case reports	Unknown
Etoposide	I	Case reports	Unknown
5-Fluorouracil	I	Case reports	Unknown
Ifosfamide	I	Case reports	Unknown
Mechlorethamine:			
Topical	IV	10%–20%	T-cell sensitization
Intravenous	I	Case reports	Unknown
Melphalan:			
Intravenous	I	2%–5%	Unknown
Methotrexate	I	Case reports	Unknown
	III	Case reports	Immune complexes?
	II	Case reports	IgG
Mitomycin	I or III?	Case reports	Unknown
Mitoxantrone	I	Case reports	Unknown
Paclitaxel	I	Up to 10%	Nonspecific release of vasoactive substances?
Procarbazine	I	Up to 15%	Unknown
	III	Case reports	Immune complexes?
Teniposide	I	5%–15% (depending on cancer being treated)	Nonspecific release?
Trimetrexate	I	Case reports	Unknown
Vinca alkaloids	I	Case reports	Unknown

Table 6-2. Types of Hypersensitivity Reactions (Gell and Coombs Classification)

Type	Major Signs and Symptoms	Mechanisms
I	Urticaria, angioedema, rash, bronchospasm, abdominal cramping, extreme pain, agitation and anxiety, hypotension	Antigen interaction with IgE bound to mast cell membrane causes degranulation. Drug binding to mast cell surface causes degranulation. Activation of classic or alternative complement pathway produces anaphylatoxins. Neurogenic release of vasoactive complement.
II	Hemolytic anemia	Antibody reacts with cell-bound antigen and activates complement.
III	Deposition of immune complexes in tissues, resulting in various forms of tissue injury	Antigen–antibody complexes form intravascularly and deposit in or on tissues.
IV	Contact dermatitis, granuloma formation, homograft rejection	Sensitized T lymphocytes react with antigen to release lymphokines.

benzyl alcohol have been reported to produce HSRs (Wilson et al., 1986).

Clinicians who administer these agents should know the clinical manifestations of an HSR so they can anticipate the symptoms and manage them quickly, whether they relate to a localized reaction or to a severe anaphylaxis reaction, which can be very alarming to the patient. The clinical manifestations are as follows:

- Urticaria
- Lightheadedness or dizziness
- Generalized or localized itching
- Abdominal cramping
- Nausea
- Restlessness
- Periorbital or facial edema
- Shortness of breath with or without wheezing
- Hypotension
- Chills
- Chest tightness

NURSING MANAGEMENT

1. Obtain the patient's allergy profile.
2. Inform the patient of the potential for an HSR. Instruct the patient to notify the nurse if he or she experiences any of the HSR symptoms.
3. Perform a scratch test or a skin test or administer a test dose for drugs with known hypersensitivity potential, such as bleomycin.
4. Administer premedications as ordered.
5. Have emergency equipment and medications ready (Table 6-3).
6. Obtain a physician's orders for emergency medications before initiating the drug (Brown & Hogan, 1990).
7. Obtain baseline vital signs and monitor the patient closely during treatment.
8. Ensure that a physician is in attendance during the first 15 minutes of the initial drug dosing.
9. If an HSR occurs, stop the drug. Maintain an IV line for emergency drugs and stay with the patient.
10. If a localized HSR occurs:
    a. Monitor and evaluate symptoms (urticaria, localized erythema, wheals).
    b. Administer diphenhydramine, corticosteroids, or both in accordance with the physician's order.
    c. Monitor vital signs every 15 minutes for the first hour.
    d. Avoid using the drug; if the clinician wants to use it again, the patient should be premedicated with antihistamines, corticosteroids, or both.

Table 6-3. Emergency Medications and Equipment for Potential Hypersensitivity Reactions

Drugs	Equipment
Epinephrine 1:1000 for SC injection	IV solutions and administration sets
Epinephrine 1:10,000 for IV injection	Oxygen and setup
Diphenhydramine (Benadryl) 25–50 mg for IV injection	Suction setup
Solu-Medrol® 30–60 mg Solu-Cortef® 100–500 mg Dexamethasone 10–20 mg	Crash cart

    e. If the reaction is an anthracycline flare, stop the drug and flush the vein with saline. If the flare reaction resolves, continue the infusion slowly. Monitor for repeated flare reactions; it may be necessary to change the infusion site if this happens.

11. If a generalized HSR occurs (usually within the first 15 minutes of the drug infusion):

    a. Stay with the patient; reassure the patient and family.

    b. Discontinue the infusion immediately.

    c. Maintain an IV infusion of normal saline solution.

    d. Administer emergency drugs as ordered.

    e. Maintain a patent airway and be ready to give cardiopulmonary resuscitation if necessary.

    f. Notify the physician.

    g. Monitor vital signs as needed.

    h. Document the occurrence, the measures undertaken, and the patient's responses.

    i. Tell the patient to inform the clinician, on subsequent dosing, about the history of HSRs and measures undertaken that were effective.

12. If the clinician deems it necessary to use the drug again, the following precautions should be undertaken:

    a. Physician-guided desensitization

    b. Premedication with antihistamines, corticosteroids, or both

    c. A longer infusion time

    d. Increased volume of the solution used for dilution

    e. Substitution of a similar drug, such as *Erwinia* L-asparaginase instead of the *Escherichia coli* form (Weiss, 1992).

▼ Extravasation

Extravasation is the accidental infiltration of chemotherapeutic drugs into subcutaneous tissues. An unfortunate side effect of chemotherapy administration, it is not unusual in cancer patients because their thin, fragile, and mobile veins have experienced multiple punctures. The degree of extravasation varies from mild erythema to severe tissue damage with involvement of deeper structures such as tendons and joints (Fig. 6-1).

    There are two categories of extravasation injury: those in-

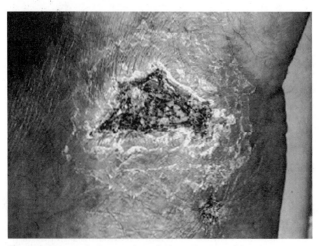

Fig. 6–1. Progressive necrosis and ulceration noted in an extravasation.

volving agents that do not bind to tissue nucleic acids, and those that do. Examples of nonbinding agents are hyperalimentation solutions, sodium bicarbonate, norepinephrine, and certain chemotherapeutic drugs such as vinblastine, vincristine, nitrogen mustard, carmustine, and 5-fluorouracil. The second category of agents, those that bind to nucleic acids, can cause destructive and prolonged tissue injuries. It is believed that anthracyclines such as doxorubicin form free radicals that bind to DNA. These free radicals are toxic to the tissues and especially impede wound healing. The DNA–doxorubicin complex is retained and recirculates in the tissues, which sets up a pattern of continuous tissue damage (Rudolph & Larson, 1987).

It is important to distinguish between an extravasation event, an irritation of the vein, and a flare reaction. The definitions are as follows:

Extravasation: An infiltration or leakage of a vesicant agent into the tissue surrounding the administration site that may result in local tissue damage. Symptoms usually occur 6 to 12 hours after the event; the patient may complain of itching but not pain. Blood return is usually absent or sluggish.

Irritation: A local inflammatory reaction to an irritant drug that does not lead to tissue damage.

Flare reaction: A raised, red streak along the course of the vein. The onset is within minutes of drug infusion and the reaction disappears within 30 to 90 minutes after the infusion. It is usually seen with daunorubicin and doxorubicin. The patient may experience pain. Blood return is usually present.

The following factors affect the severity of the extravasation injury:

- Vesicant potential of the drug
- Volume of extravasated drug
- Dose of the drug
- Site of infiltration
- Length of exposure
- Immediate measures undertaken to manage the extravasation

The administration of vesicants (Table 6-4) by a skilled and knowledgeable professional gives the patient the best protection from extravasation. The nurse needs to know the vesicant properties of the drug, the acute and delayed signs and symptoms for which to monitor, the special techniques used in vesicant administration, and the immediate measures to take in case of extravasation (Table 6-5).

CARE OF THE PATIENT RECEIVING VESICANT CHEMOTHERAPY

Before vesicant administration, the nurse should:

1. Be knowledgeable about the vesicants to be administered and the institutional policies relating to vesicant administration.

Table 6-4. Chemotherapeutic Agents with Vesicant Properties

Cisplatin	Mechlorethamine
Dactinomycin	Mitomycin-C
Daunorubicin	Mitoxantrone
Doxorubicin hydrochloride	Paclitaxel
Epirubicin	Vinblastine
5-Fluorouracil	Vincristine
Idarubicin	Vindesine
	Vinorelbine

Table 6-5. Vesicants and Irritants

Chemotherapeutic Agents	Antidote	Antidote Preparation	Local Care	Comments
Cisplatin	Isotonic sodium thiosulfate	Prepare 1/6 molar solution: a. If 10% Na thio-sulfate solution, mix 4 mL with 6 mL sterile water for injection. b. If 25% Na thio-sulfate solution, mix 1:6 mL with 8.4 mL sterile water.	1. Inject 1–4 mL through existing IV line. 2. Remove needle. 3. Inject SC.	1. Vesicant potential seen when more than 20 mL of 0.5 mg/mL concentration extravasated. If less than this, drug is an irritant; no treatment recommended. 2. Time is essential in treating extravasation. 3. Heat and cold not proved effective. Although clinically accepted, reports of the benefits are scant.
Dactinomycin	None		1. Apply ice. 2. Elevate × 48 h.	1. Little information. 2. In mouse experiments, some benefit from topical dimethyl sulfoxide (DMSO).
Daunorubicin	None			
Doxorubicin	None		Apply cold pad with circulating ice water, ice	1. Exatravasations of less than 1–2 mL often heal spontaneously. If

Drug	Antidote	Preparation	Treatment	Comments
		pack, or cryogel pack for 15–20 min at least four times per day for the first 24–48 h.		greater than 3 mL, ulceration often rsults. 2. Protect from sunlight and heat. 3. Some studies suggest benefit of 99% DMSO 1–2 mL applied to site every 6 hours. Other studies show delayed healing with DMSO.
Epirubicin Idarubicin (Idamycin)	None			1. Antidote and local care measures unknown. 2. Cold, DMSO, and corticosteroids ineffective in experiments with mice.
5-Fluorouracil	None			Rare weak vesicant. Few documented cases of small ulcerations and pulp necrosis seen with extravasation.
Mechlorethamine	Isotonic sodium thiosulfate	Prepare 1/6 molar solution a. If 10% Na thiosulfate solution, mix 4 mL with 6 mL sterile water for injection.	1. Immediately inject Na thiosulfate through IV cannula, 2 mL for every mg extravasated. 2. Remove needle. 3. Inject antidote into subcutaneous tissue.	1. Na thiosulfate neutralizes nitrogen mustard, which is then excreted by the kidneys. 2. Time is essential in treating extravasation. 3. Heat and cold not proved effective. Although clinically

(continued)

Table 6-5. *Vesicants and Irritants (Continued)*

Chemotherapeutic Agents	Antidote	Antidote Preparation	Local Care	Comments
		b. If 25% Na thio-sulfate solution, mix 1.6 mL with 8.4 mL sterile water.		accepted, reports of the benefits are scant.
Mitomycin	None			1. Protect from sunlight. 2. Delayed skin reactions have occurred in areas far from original IV site. 3. Some research studies show benefit with use of 99% DMSO, 1–2 mL applied to site every 6 h for 14 d. More studies needed.
Mitoxantrone	Unknown			1. Antidote or local care measures unknown. 2. Ulceration: none unless concentrated dose infiltrates.
Paclitaxel (Taxol)	Hyaluronidase (Wydase) Ice	Mix 300 units of hyaluronidase with 3 mL saline.	1. Inject hyaluronidase into IV line, 1 mL for each 1 mL infiltrated. 2. If IV removed, inject SC.	1. Recent documentation of vesicant potential. 2. Paclitaxel has rare vesicant potential (probably due to dilution

Drug				
Vinblastine	Same as above, excpet for ice	Same as above	3. Apply ice pack for 15–20 min at least 4 times per day for the first 24 h.	in 500 mL diluent). 3. If infiltrated, is considered intermediate vesicant. 4. Ice and hyaluronidase were effective in decreasing local tissue damage in a mouse model.
			Same as 1 and 2 above.	Apply heat for 15–20 min at least four times per day for the first 24–48 hrs.
Vincristine	Hyaluronidase	Mix 150 units hyaluronidase with 1–3 mL saline.	1. Inject hyaluronidase into IV line, 1 mL for each 1 mL infiltrated. 2. If IV removed, inject SC. 3. Apply warm pack for 15–20 min at least four times per day for the first 24–48 h and elevate.	1. Same as above. 2. Hyaluronidase should be stored in a refrigerator. 3. These two methods of treatment are very effective for rapid absorption of drug.
Vindesine	Same as above	Same as above	Same as above	Same as above
Vinorelbine	Same as above	Same as above	Same as above	1. Same treatment as for vincristine and vinblastine. 2. Moderate vesicant. 3. Studies in mice found warmth and hydrocortisone to be ineffective. Warmth still recommended in humans.

(continued)

Table 6-5. Vesicants and Irritants *(Continued)*

Chemotherapeutic Agents	Antidote	Antidote Preparation	Local Care	Comments
				4. Manufacturer recommends administering drug over 6–10 min into side port of free-flowing IV line closest to the IV bag, followed by flush of 75–125 mL IV solution to reduce incidence of phlebitis and severe back pain. In clinical studies, the incidence of venous irritation and severe back pain with varying infusion times were 6% and 9%, respectively, when infused over 1–2 min; 11% and 3% when infused 6–10 min; and 20% and 1% when infused over 20–30 min.
Irritants				
Bleomycin				May cause irritation to tissue; little information known.
Ifosfamide Carboplatin				May cause phlebitis; antidote or local care measures unknown.
Carmustine				May cause phlebitis; antidote and local care measures unknown.

Dacarbazine		1. May cause phlebitis. 2. Protect from sunlight.
Doxorubicin liposome		1. May produce redness and tissue edema. 2. Low ulceration potential. 3. If ulceration begins or pain, redness, or swelling persists, treat like doxorubicin.
Etoposide	Mix 150 units hyaluronidase, 1 mL with 1–3 mL saline.	1. Inject hyaluronidase into IV line for each 1 mL infiltrated. 2. If IV removed, inject SC. 3. Apply warm pack.	1. Treatment necessary only if large amount of concentrated solution extravasates. In this case treat like vincristine or vinblastine. 2. May cause phlebitis, urticaria, and redness.
Hyaluronidase		
Menogaril		1. May cause phlebitis, venous edema, and induration. 2. Increased incidence if concentrations greater than 1 mg/mL infiltrate or administration occurs in more than 2 h.
Teniposide	Same as etoposide	Same as etoposide	Same as etoposide
	Same as etoposide		

Adapted with permission from Oncology Nursing Society. (1996). *Cancer chemotherapy guidelines and recommendations for practice.* Pittsburgh: Oncology Nursing Press.

2. Assess the patient's risk factors for chemotherapy extravasation:
   a. Poor venous condition secondary to the disease process, age, venous sclerosis, lymphedema, or superior vena cava syndrome
   b. Altered mental status and drugs that may produce sedation
   c. Peripheral neuropathy

3. Inform the patient about the signs and symptoms (immediate and delayed), and instruct the patient to report them immediately. Immediate signs and symptoms include pain and burning at the administration site and redness or swelling at the site of the injection. Delayed signs and symptoms include pain, skin discoloration, and change in skin integrity.

4. Select the optimal site for peripheral placement. Do not use an old IV line (inserted more than 24 hours earlier) because of questionable integrity. Avoid sites such as the inner wrist, the dorsum of the hand, and the antecubital fossa because of the underlying tendons and blood vessels. Use larger veins located between the wrist and the elbow joint.

5. Use a 20- to 23-gauge (for adults) and a 23- to 25-gauge (for children) butterfly needle or flexible catheter.

6. Verify for adequate blood return before proceeding with the treatment. For peripheral lines, ensure the patency of the vein by feeling for a bruit along the venous track with a 10-mL normal saline IV push. Do not pinch the IV tubing to check patency.

7. Confirm the CVAD placement before accessing for the first time.

8. Anchor the needle (peripheral or implanted port) securely to prevent dislodgement and to allow direct visualization of the insertion site.

9. Use a transparent, occlusive dressing for better visualization of the insertion site.

10. Assess blood return continuously by drawing back after every 1 to 2 mL of the drug is administered.

TECHNIQUES FOR VESICANT ADMINISTRATION

Side Arm Technique

1. Ensure the proper venous access site.

2. Use at least a 20-gauge needle to access the vein.
3. Secure the cannula but do not obstruct the entrance site.
4. Check for blood return.
5. Test the vein with 50 to 100 mL of IV solution to ensure an adequate and swift flow of the infusion. The solution should be additive-free.
6. With a continuously flowing IV line, slowly inject the vesicant into the IV line.
7. Do not allow the vesicant to backflow.
8. Do not pinch off tubing except to check the blood return.
9. Assess for blood return after every 1 to 2 mL of injection.
10. Flush the needle with saline at the completion of administration.

Two-Syringe Technique

This technique is recommended for children.

1. Select an appropriate vein.
2. Begin a new IV line using a 23- to 25-gauge scalp vein needle.
3. Flush the line with 8 to 10 mL of normal saline. Assess for a brisk, full blood return and any evidence of infiltration. Check for swelling, redness, or pain at the site and lack of blood return.
4. Once access is ensured, switch to the syringe containing the vesicant.
5. Inject the drug slowly.
6. Assess for blood return every 1 to 2 mL of infusion.

Continuous Infusion

If a vesicant is administered as a continuous infusion, it should always be given through a central line. Vesicants may be given as continuous infusions using a central venous device (implanted port, Hickman or Broviac catheter). The following guidelines should be used for continuous infusion:

1. Confirm line placement before initiating treatment.
2. Inspect needle site every 2 hours for signs of infiltration or dislodgement.
3. Infuse the drug using an infusion pump especially for 24-hour infusions.
4. Teach the patient to observe for signs and symptoms of

dislodgement, leakage, and edema around the insertion site.

5. For continuous infusion of a vesicant at home, choose a Broviac or Hickman catheter instead of an implanted port to avoid needle displacement.

MANAGEMENT OF SUSPECTED OR ACTUAL EXTRAVASATION

Extravasation can occur with peripheral or central venous access administration of vesicant agents. Peripheral extravasation has been reported in 0.1% to 6.0% of patients (Dorr, 1990). With central venous access devices, the most common cause of extravasation is needle dislodgement.

Management of extravasation includes both pharmacologic and nonpharmacologic measures. There has not been a completed randomized trial in humans on the management of extravasation from cytotoxic agents because of the ethical issues surrounding the trying of different treatment options that may or may not be beneficial to the patient. Therefore, the basis for these measures is empirical evidence taken from cumulative clinical case reports and uncontrolled studies.

Pharmacologic management involves the use of antidotes for many of the vesicant drugs. The drugs most commonly used are

1. *Corticosteroids:* Corticosteroids are useful in the treatment of anthracycline extravasations because of their positive effect on the inflammatory process. However, histology studies have shown that inflammation is not a major component of tissue necrosis. Further, animal studies have shown that hydrocortisone increases the skin toxicity of vinca alkaloids and that high doses of steroids injected intradermally may even be harmful.

2. *Dimethyl sulfoxide (DMSO):* Case reports show that this drug, applied topically, is effective and well tolerated in the treatment of extravasation. Because DMSO has potent free radical–scavenging properties, it is postulated that it acts on the local tissue damage that is produced by hydroxyl radical formation.

3. *Sodium bicarbonate:* The use of sodium bicarbonate is discouraged because of extravasation of sodium bicarbonate itself. Experimental evidence has also shown

that this agent can increase the cellular uptake of anthracyclines in the tissues.

4. *Hyaluronidase:* This enzyme degrades hyaluronic acid,
   thus promoting the absorption of injected substances.
   Hyaluronidase is effective in the management of vinca
   alkaloid extravasations but detrimental for doxorubicin
   infiltrations. It is also effective in epipodophyllotoxin
   extravasations (e.g., etoposide).

5. *Sodium thiosulfate (sodium hyposulfite):* Clinical studies
   have advocated the use of this antidote in extravasations of dacarbazine and concentrated cisplatin (more
   than 0.4 mg/mL).

6. *Beta-adrenergic compounds* such as propranolol and iso-
   prenaline and antioxidants such as acetylcysteine, beta-
   carotene, and retinol are being tested in animal models.

Nonpharmacologic management involves the use of cold or
warm compresses on the administration site. Heat produces
vasodilation and promotes the removal of the extravasated
drugs. Warm compresses are useful for vinca alkaloid extravasations. Topical cooling has been shown to be a better
choice than hyperthermia, except in vinca infiltrations. Cold
causes vasoconstriction, which decreases the absorption of
the extravasated agent into the tissues, thus localizing the tissue injury. Proponents also believe that cold disrupts the
metabolic activities of the cells, thus lessening the destructive
effects of the white blood cells during the inflammatory
process. Cold or warm compresses are applied for 15 minutes
to the affected site three or four times a day for 24 to 48 hours.

Peripheral Extravasation

1. Stop administration of vesicant and IV infusion.
2. Disconnect the IV line and try to aspirate the residual
   drug with a syringe. Do not apply pressure to the site.
   Cover lightly with a sterile occlusive dressing.
3. Apply cold or warm compresses as recommended.
4. Notify the physician.
5. Administer the necessary antidote as ordered.
   a. If the antidote is administered intravenously, instill the
      appropriate amount and discontinue the IV catheter.
   b. If the antidote is administered subcutaneously, dis-
      continue the IV catheter. Using a 25-gauge needle,
      inject the antidote into the subcutaneous tissue.
6. Instruct the patient to rest and elevate the arm for 48

hours. For a child, immobilize the affected extremity with a sling or an arm board.

7. Photograph the extravasation site if necessary.
8. Assess the need for a plastic surgery consultation.
9. Document:
   a. The patient's name and the date and the time of the incident
   b. Needle type and gauge
   c. Administration site, location, and appearance
   d. Names and sequence of drugs given before extravasation
   e. Name of vesicant drug and the approximate amount and volume that infiltrated
   f. Patient symptoms and assessment
   g. Interventions undertaken and patient's response
   h. Time physician was notified and name of physician
   i. Patient teaching and plans for follow-up
   j. Nurse's signature

Central Venous Access Device Extravasation

1. Immediately discontinue chemotherapy and IV infusion if the patient reports pain or there is redness or swelling at the central access site, or if there is a change in the IV flow.
2. Ascertain that the needle is not dislodged if the patient has an implanted port.
3. Aspirate the vesicant drug from the port pocket or at the exit site of the tunneled catheter. If the cause of the extravasation is a dislodged needle, attempt to aspirate the pooled drug from the subcutaneous tissue.
4. Administer the appropriate antidote and proceed with nursing measures as noted in the peripheral extravasation guidelines.

PATIENT EDUCATION IN VESICANT ADMINISTRATION

1. Review possible side effects of vesicant or irritant administration.
2. Emphasize the importance of prompt reporting of immediate and delayed symptoms of reaction.
3. Provide written materials related to drugs and self-care of the extravasation site if a suspected or actual extravasation has occurred:
   a. Do not use lotions or creams other than as instructed.

b. Do not wear constrictive clothing or apply excessive pressure on the affected area.

c. Avoid direct exposure of the area to sunlight.

d. Notify the physician or nurse of pain; a temperature of 101°F or higher; signs of skin breakdown such as erythema, induration, blistering, ulceration, or necrosis; or decreased mobility of the affected extremity.

4. Discuss follow-up plans and continued assessment over the telephone. (See an example of an extravasation follow-up record, Fig. 6-2.)

MEMORIAL SLOAN-KETTERING
CANCER CENTER
DIVISION OF NURSING

FLOWSHEET FOR SUSPECTED/ACTUAL
CHEMOTHERAPY EXTRAVASATION

Date: _____   Date extravasation occurred: _____   addressograph stamp

DESCRIPTION OF EXTRAVASATION   INITIAL EVALUATION (DAY 0)
Name and volume of drug given: _____
IV site location: (indicate on diagram and describe):
_____
Needle type and gauge: _____
IV site appearance: _____
Patient complaints: _____
Physician notified (name): _____
R.N. (name): _____

rt. lt.   rt. lt.
Anterior   Posterior

INITIAL INTERVENTIONS   ADDITIONAL INTERVENTIONS   PATIENT TEACHING

Date   Date   Date
____ Antidote admin.*   ____ Dermatology Consult*   ____ Extravasation
(specify) ____   ____ Plastic Surg. Consult*   fact card given and
____ Cold compresses   ____ Wound Care (describe)   reviewed
____ Warm compresses   ____   ____ Follow-up
____ 1% Hydrocortisone   ____   schedule reviewed
cream applied   ____ Follow-up photo
____ Baseline photo

FOLLOW-UP FLOW CHART*** Patient phone #: _____

	Day 1	Day 3	Day 5	Day 7	Day 14	Day 21**	Day 28**	Day 35**	Day 42**
Date									
Call/Visit									
Skin color									
Skin temp.									
Skin integrity									
Edema									
Mobility									
Pain									
Fever									
RN initial****									

*   Requires M.D. order
**   May omit if no signs of extravasation
***   Refer to Grading Scale on reverse side
****   Full signature required on reverse side   forward

Fig. 6-2. Flow sheet for chemotherapy extravasation. (Reprinted with permission from Memorial Sloan-Kettering Cancer Center, New York, NY.)

| GRADE | 0 | I | GRADING SCALE | | |
			II	III	IV
COLOR	normal	pink	red	blanched center surrounded by red	blackened
INTEGRITY	unbroken	blistered	superficial skin loss	tissue loss exposing subcutaneous tissue	tissue loss exposing muscle/bone with a deep crater or necrosis
SKIN TEMP.	normal	warm	hot		
EDEMA	absent	nonpitting	pitting		
MOBILITY	full	slightly limited	very limited	immobile	
PAIN	rate on 0–10 scale		0= no pain	10= worst pain	
FEVER	normal	elevated (record 24 hour temp. max)			

INITIAL	SIGNATURE/TITLE	INITIAL	SIGNATURE/TITLE

Fig. 6-2. (*Continued*)

7

Patient Education

Patient education is an important component of care. An increasing number of cancer patients are undergoing multiple treatment modalities, and they need knowledge and skills to cope with them. It is estimated that more than 30% of Americans will be faced with a diagnosis of cancer, presenting a challenge to health care providers in terms of sheer numbers.

Recent changes in health care and the health care system have also underscored the importance of patient education. Among these changes are the emphasis on health promotion, patients' rights, and cost containment (with the resulting move toward home health care). Standards by the Joint Commission on Accreditation of Health Care Organizations (JCAHO) mandate that hospitals operationalize policies to ensure "the right of the patient, in collaboration with his/her physician, to make decisions involving his/her health care . . . and the right of the patient to the information necessary to enable him/her to make treatment decisions that reflect his/her wishes" (JCAHO, 1998). This expanded role can give the patient a sense of control and build self-esteem. Because of the emphasis on cost containment, lengths of stay have been shortened, reducing the amount of time available for patient education. The rapid growth of technology and the availablity of medical devices for the administration of various conventional chemotherapeutic drugs and immunological agents have shifted clinical care to the outpatient and home settings. Patients and caregivers need to be taught about equipment such as venous access devices and ambulatory infusion pumps, to name just a few. This expectation for more active participation puts added demands and reponsibilities on the patient and his or her family.

The major areas of education that a cancer patient needs are treatment options, side effects of the treatment modalities, management of side effects, coping mechanisms and support systems, treatment devices, self-care activities, and management at home. Patients who are educated in these areas are more likely to cooperate with the treatment regimen, suffer fewer side effects, and experience less anxiety and stress (Adams, 1992).

All of these areas involve the three domains of learning: cognitive, affective, and psychomotor. The cognitive domain comprises behaviors that deal with the recall or recognition of knowledge and the development of intellectual skills, such as being able to identify the common side effects of a chemotherapeutic agent. Affective learning relates to the patient's attitudes, feelings, and coping mechanisms, such as being able to deal with the side effects of anticancer agents and the changes in appearance and lifestyle. The psychomotor domain relates to behaviors that affect the performance of skills, such as caring for a venous access device or troubleshooting a problem with an ambulatory infusion pump.

▼ The Dot.com: The Role of the Internet in Patient Education

The Internet has revolutionized patient education. With the growing number of computers at home, at work, in the community, and in schools, the Internet provides a steady and convenient way to obtain information. Some patients may seek medical information online because they do not receive it from their health care provider. However, there is growing concern over the quality of the information available on the Internet, and patients may need help evaluating the information they find. The nurse should ask the patient specific questions about what information he or she is seeking online. Does that information match what was already given? What needs reinforcement? How can the online information add to the patient's understanding of the treatment plan? The nurse can play a pivotal role in providing education and helping patients evaluate the information they find on their own.

▼ Nursing Process in Patient Education

Patient education requires time, energy, and resources. The nursing process—assessment, planning, implementation, evaluation, and documentation—is a useful framework for the patient education process, whether the nurse is teaching one patient or is designing a patient education program for an entire hospital.

ASSESSMENT AND PLANNING

A complete assessment is crucial to successful patient education. It should include the multidimensional aspects of the learner (physiologic, social, psychological, cultural, environmental, and spiritual dimensions), because these variables can enhance or limit learning. Patient responses during the initial assessment are good indicators as to what type of teaching the patient will need. Because of economic constraints and shorter hospital stays, the nurse should start patient education on admission or during the first office encounter.

After making an initial assessment of the patient's learning needs, the nurse must clarify and validate these with the patient. Glaring differences often exist between what the educator perceives the learner needs and what the learner believes he or she needs.

Timing is important. The least appropriate time to engage the patient in a learning activity is at the time of diagnosis. The patient's anxiety level is exceedingly high, and this can cloud comprehension. The educator should not present a barrage of information that the patient cannot process; rather, this time is better spent listening to the patient's fears and uncertainties. Education can be delayed until the patient's cognitive and emotional comprehension is better.

Ongoing assessments should also be done during subsequent visits or hospital admissions, and by telephone calls when the patient is discharged.

The teaching process is a partnership between the patient and the nurse, but usually a caregiver (a family member or significant other) is also involved and should not be overlooked. Many family members faced with the caregiver role experience high levels of stress and feel overwhelmed. They suffer from loss of sleep and often get sick or injured themselves; they may even reach a breaking point as a result of the heavy demands. They too can benefit from a carefully designed education program.

IMPLEMENTATION

Nurses can choose from a wide variety of media to deliver the right information in the right way. Whatever the method, it should be appropriate, accurate, and accessible to the user. The nurse must match the method to the patient and should use creative flair in getting the message across, especially when there is limited time for patient education. Because patients are going home more quickly, it is best to combine different methods so that patients can learn in an interesting environment, which will enhance the learning process.

Printed Materials

The most common form of educational intervention is the use of printed materials. Health care workers depend greatly on printed materials to impart valuable information to patients, especially when inpatient stays are shorter and patients are expected to care for themselves at home.

Research has suggested that written materials combined with other teaching methods produce more positive outcomes than when used alone. There is an abundant supply of excellent printed materials dealing with cancer-related topics. Most can be obtained at minimal or no cost from the American Cancer Society and the National Cancer Institute. Appendix A lists the major publications available from the National Cancer Institute in English and Spanish. Pharmaceutical and biomedical companies are also rich sources of written materials, as are health care organizations, private foundations, and community outreach programs.

In hospitals, patient education materials are developed and tailored to specific patient needs to supplement what is available from outside sources. Helpful strategies in preparing appropriate written materials are:

- Know the target audience; keep them in mind when preparing the materials.
- Focus on "need-to-know" information.
- Break complex information into small chunks.
- Because verbal instructions are more understandable,

supplement printed materials with simple audiovisual materials. Use examples.

- Pretest the materials on a sample audience before final publication to assess the relevancy and appropriateness of the content. Edit as needed.

Appendix B shows samples of written fact cards and instructional materials developed for patients. These typical handouts provide a ready, easy, and consistent method of presenting the necessary information. When patients go home, these handouts can be read at a later time.

The Readability and Literacy Issue: Can Patients Understand Patient Education Materials

Readability and literacy levels are important considerations when preparing patient education materials: written materials can benefit patients only if the patients understand what they read. One study showed that approximately 20% of American adults read at or below the fourth-grade level (Meade et al., 1992). Another study (Cooley et al., 1995) found that a patient's reported grade level does not accurately denote his or her actual reading ability. That study recommended screening a patient's reading ability initially so that appropriate patient education materials can be given. Literacy can be determined by using the Wide-Range Achievement Test to assess grade level and the Cloze Method to determine reading comprehension. The grade level should be indicated on printed materials so the nurse can select appropriate publications.

Two scales are widely used to assess the readability of materials: the FRY scale and the SMOG scale. The former is considered a better tool for readability, but the latter is more commonly used because it requires less time and is easier to use (Doak et al., 1985). To calculate the SMOG reading grade level:

1. Count all the three-syllable words in 10 consecutive sentences.
2. Apply the following scale to determine the grade level: grade 4, 0 to 2; grade 5, 3 to 6; grade 6, 7 to 12; grade 7, 13 to 20; grade 8, 21 to 30; grade 9, 31 to 42; grade 10, 43 to 56; grade 11, 57 to 72; grade 12, 73 to 90.

Audiovisual Materials

Videotapes are effective, but producing them requires time and money, which may be in short supply in this era of cost cutting. Videos ensure consistent teaching and can portray live situations with which patients can identify. They are particularly effective with the affective and psychomotor domains of learning, and can reach patients with a broad range of literacy levels. Patients can fast-forward past the information that is not needed and rewind to a segment that needs clarification or reinforcement.

Patients prefer an interactive approach and multimedia learning. A study by Garvey and Kramer (1983) showed that a combination of approaches reduced nursing teaching hours by 50% without compromising quality. Nurses are therefore challenged to develop creative, innovative, and flexible educational opportunities to convey important messages to patients and their caregivers.

The Adult Learner

When teaching adults, the nurse should incorporate the principles of adult learning. Adult patients learn differently from children: they are not passive learners, and they need a different environment to be fully engaged in the learning process. Malcolm Knowles, the father of *androgogy* (adult learning), outlined four assumptions about adult learning (Knowles, 1975) that are essential to keep in mind:

- Self-concept moves from dependency toward self-direction. The adult sees himself or herself as capable of managing his or her own decisions and taking responsibility for consequences.
- A reservoir of life experiences is a valuable resource for learning.
- Readiness to learn is strongly influenced by developmental tasks and social roles.
- The adult's time perspective is different. The adult learner needs immediate application of knowledge; learning is problem-centered rather than subject-centered.

Adults will learn when they believe that knowledge and skill are of value. Some helpful strategies are:

- Set the tone for success. Convey the desired result to the learner.
- Ensure consistency of information.
- Vary the presentation; keep the learner actively involved.
- Do not inundate the patient with details or too many printed materials.

- Assess the patient's baseline knowledge of the subject matter before preparing an educational package.
- Keep information as streamlined as possible; add more if needed.
- Provide ample opportunities for feedback by asking questions or asking for return demonstration of skills. Give feedback promptly and often.
- Keep educational sessions short; timing is important.
- Provide a quiet and nonthreatening environment where the patient can remain focused and his or her attention span can be sustained (the same applies to children).
- Recognize the patient's need for reinforcement of teaching.
- Connect new knowledge and skills with those from past experiences.

The Child Learner

Teaching children requires strategies and styles very different from those involved in teaching adults. The information provided to children should be appropriate for their developmental stage, cognitive abilities, previous experiences, and support system. A child's readiness to learn should also be considered. Although the common mistakes made in teaching adults are similar to those made in teaching children, there are added pitfalls to avoid when dealing with children.

Parents have a more difficult time accepting the diagnosis and consequences of cancer than a child. Parents should be encouraged to communicate information to the child at an understandable level. A protective instinct often causes parents to exclude the child from discussions or avoid answering questions. When the child senses this "conspiracy of silence," he or she will turn to outside resources, mostly peers, to discuss concerns. Often, parents fail to realize that children are masters at perceiving what adults are reluctant to share with them. When the anxiety level is high in the family, excluding the child increases the child's anxiety level through fear of the unknown and creates a sense of isolation and loss of parental support.

Some helpful hints for teaching children are:
- Keep sessions brief; children have a short attention span.
- Offer a supportive and nurturing environment.
- Use play to get the message across.

- Use language appropriate for the child's cognitive and developmental age.
- Allow active participation; children love interactive, "high-tech" and "high-touch" media.

The Elderly Learner

It is estimated that 12% of the U.S. population is composed of people older than 65 years. More than 50% of this aging population are people diagnosed with cancer. This trend is predicted to double to nearly 50 million by the year 2030 (Boyle et al., 1992; Derby, 1991; Newell et al., 1989). Many oncology patients are elderly, and geriatric patients have special learning needs. As part of the aging process, cognitive ability and psychomotor skills decline. Concomitant illnesses and the multiple medications associated with these diseases can slow cognitive and psychomotor abilities. The elderly person may also have a lack of support from family.

Some helpful hints for teaching older patients are (Bernardini, 1985):

- Keep sessions brief; sessions may need to be repeated.
- Use larger print and easy-to-read fonts for printed material.
- Do not "overdesign" visuals; keep them simple and conservative.
- If the patient needs glasses or hearing aids, make sure that he or she uses them.
- Speak slowly in front of the patient and in a lower tone.
- Allow sufficient time for the patient to assimilate and understand the information. Elicit feedback by asking simple questions or having the patient give return demonstrations.
- Give praise.
- Ensure that the patient has adequate support and resources available.

Cultural Diversity

Minorities account for one third of the U.S. population. Most recently, ethnicity has become a major consideration for the effective delivery of patient care. Health behaviors are culturally patterned, so the nurse providing patient education needs to be aware of the patient's health beliefs and incorporate them into teaching. A cultural assessment should be done to determine the patient's belief systems, values, and practices, because these may influence intervention strategies. Other relevant information includes the patient's family network, patterns of decision making, and communication styles.

A shortcoming of many health education programs is that they do not include information about ethnic differences. Health care professionals often talk about "difficult" or "noncompliant" patients, but the problem may actually be due to miscommunication, misunderstandings, or cultural stereotyping.

For patients who do not speak English, written materials and audiovisual tools can be translated to suit the patient population. Interpreters are valuable but are lacking in many institutions.

Cross-cultural programs are being implemented to raise the level of awareness and explore culturally appropriate strategies, but as a whole, the health care profession is poorly equipped to handle today's culturally diverse patient population. To provide quality care to everyone in our pluralistic society, health care professionals need to reexamine their assumptions and perceptions about patients from different ethnic groups.

EVALUATION

Patient education is not just the giving of information; the end point is a behavioral change on the part of the patient. The nurse can gauge the effectiveness of educational interventions by evaluating the progress made toward the outcomes set at the onset of the teaching process. Goal setting is essential because goals provide the basis for the expected behavioral change. Goals are mutually defined by the teacher and the learner and involve a contractual relationship, with time frames, between the two parties. They establish priorities and set attainable and specific expectations. Evaluation allows the teacher to determine what works for the patient and to modify the original strategy.

Significant others should be encouraged to participate in goal setting, because this participation signals "buy-in." This support is crucial, especially for a patient who is anxious because of the physical and emotional impact of the disease. The family's input is also a valuable tool in evaluating the patient's progress toward the goals.

DOCUMENTATION

Documentation of patient education is a critical element of the teaching process. Documenting the information given, the tools used, and significant changes in the patient's behaviors provides a useful point of reference for other members of the health team. A good documentation system shows accountability for clinical practice, ensures quality and continuity of care, ensures compliance with regulatory standards, and provides an evaluation of the outcomes of the teaching process.

The system recommended is the integrated method, which involves many disciplines. Each person caring for the patient contributes to the process with each patient encounter. Historically, nurses do most of the teaching and therefore are expected to do most of the charting. People from other disciplines may sometimes fail to document the teaching given or may duplicate the nurse's efforts. Integrated charting solves some of these problems. It is efficient and clinically effective. This system also helps acknowledge each person's contribution to the teaching process. To avoid the tedious paper trail of the patient's medical record, the charting system should be set up to follow the patient as he or she moves through the different patient care settings (e.g., inpatient, outpatient, emergency room, or home care). This sharing of information across the settings prevents the information gaps created when the information is not accessible and the frustration felt by patients when they must repeatedly answer the same set of questions regarding their history.

Figure 7-1 shows an example of a chemotherapy patient education documentation form. This flowsheet format outlines the necessary elements of an educational program for a patient receiving chemotherapy. It is started on admission. The variables that may affect the patient's ability to learn are identified, and the expected outcomes are enumerated. The program content is comprehensive and includes information about chemotherapy, side effects, self-care measures, and indications for calling the physician. This information is reinforced during the teaching sessions. The nurse who participates in the educational plan charts the progress of the patient and significant other so that other caregivers can continue the teaching process. The teaching aids are listed to ensure continuity and consistency of information. When the patient is dis-

PATIENT IDENTIFICATION

MEMORIAL SLOAN-KETTERING CANCER CENTER
PATIENT EDUCATION DOCUMENTATION FORM

DATE	LEARNING NEEDS ASSESSMENT
	Check any of the following that impact teaching/ learning:
INITIALS	— Physical disability — Religion — Cognitive changes — Culture — Emotional issues — Language — Lack of agreement with learning objectives

Date and initial all entries.
Document all comments on the reverse side; indicate by circling your initials in the appropriate column.

Taught to: ____ patient ____ other ________

EXPECTED OUTCOMES	Teaching Sessions 1		2		3		Outcome Achieved	
THE PATIENT / FAMILY IS ABLE TO:	Date	Initials	Date	Initials	Date	Initials	Date	Initials
1. Describe how chemotherapy works.								
2. Name the chemotherapy agents the patient is receiving and the side effects as listed on the Chemotherapy Fact Card. Specify: 1.								
2.								
3.								
4.								
3. List procedures to be performed at home before treatment: (circle) drink fluids : quantity ______ collect urine take medications: specify ______ change diet: specify______ other: ______								
4. Describe procedures/routines for chemotherapy treatment. (circle) ambulatory routine inpatient same day								
5. List self-care measures to minimize side effects: (circle) a. po fluids b. antiemetics c. relaxation techniques d. laxatives/stimulants e. antidiarrheal agents f. increased activity g. dietary changes - specify: h. avoiding contact with known sources of infection i. oral care - specify: j. wigs/scarves k. G-CSF stop date: l. other:								
6. List indications for calling MD _ >100.5°F temp (38°C) _ bleeding _ inability to take po fluids _ intractable vomiting _ >4 loose BM/day _ mouth sores — Other______								
7. State telephone number and describe how to contact MD during regular and weekend hours.								
8. State how to access appropriate resources (e.g., Look Good...Feel Better).								

CHEMOTHERAPY - ACTION AND SIDE EFFECTS

Revised January 1995
MRC approved 1/26/95

SEE BACK FOR COMMENTS/NOTES/SIGNATURE/RESOURCES
56-11496

B58

Fig. 7-1. Example of a patient education documentation form for chemotherapy. (Reprinted with permission from Memorial Sloan-Kettering Cancer Center, New York, NY.)

charged, the form becomes a part of the medical record and can be used during subsequent visits to the hospital.

▼ Home Care

Providing care at home has become a major health care trend. In the past 10 years, the home health care industry has experienced tremendous growth driven by three factors: cost containment, new technology, and patient choice.

INITIALS	SIGNATURE / TITLE	INITIALS	SIGNATURE / TITLE

EDUCATIONAL MATERIALS/METHODS

Hematology
___ Blood Counts and Infections
___ Facts About Blood and Blood Counts
___ Guidelines for Patients with a Low Platelet Count
Information
___ Hair Loss Following Chemotherapy
Nutrition
___ Nutrition: A Guide for Patients with Cancer
Pharmacology
___ Chemotherapy and You
___ Common Medicines Containing Aspirin and Ibuprofen
___ Fact card _____

___ Fact card _____

___ Fact card _____
___ Special Measures for Patients Receiving Chemotherapy

Procedures
___ Collection of Urine for Creatinine Clearance
___ Basic Mouth Care Guidelines
___ Mouth Care Guidelines for Patients Who May Develop
         Mouth Sores
___ Oral Care Guidelines for Patients Receiving Cancer
         Therapies
___ Prevention of Constipation
___ Other_____

___ Other_____

___ Other_____
Other
___ Other_____

___ Other_____

___ Other_____

DATE	COMMENTS / NOTES

Fig. 7-1. (*Continued*)

Escalating health care costs, which have outpaced the inflation rate, have prompted the government and third-party payers to examine where health care dollars are going and for what services they are paying. Prospective payment systems have caused hospitals to cut the length of stay, so patients are being discharged "sicker and quicker." This phenomenon has increased the population base for the home health care business.

Advances in technology such as venous access devices and user-friendly ambulatory infusion pumps now allow chemotherapeutic agents and supportive therapies to be administered at home. In addition, many antineoplastics are now available in oral form and can be taken on an outpatient basis.

The third reason for the expansion of home health care is that it offers an improved quality of life for the patient and family. More and more patients choose to be treated at home. Home care allows the patient active participation in and more control over the treatment regimen. There is also a wide perception in the lay public that hospitals are not pleasant and safe places, especially in this current era of downsizing. Traveling to a health care facility causes fatigue, and patients feel much more comfortable in their homes under the watchful eye of a significant other. For the family, there is less disruption when they can take care of the patient at home.

Nurses must enhance their telephone triage skills so that they can monitor patient compliance and help patients manage symptoms at home, thus making them more active participants in their care.

Cancer patients may have traditional home care needs or high-technology home care needs. The latter include chemotherapy and biotherapy treatments, pain management, antibiotic therapy, hydration needs, and nutritional support.

The standards of care for home care are the same as those in other settings. However, the methods of attaining these standards may be different because of the location and resources available. Therefore, it is important to establish criteria for what type of patients and services are appropriate for home care. These selection criteria should include patient characteristics such as physical stability, motivation and ability for self-care, support system, coping skills, ability and willingness to participate in care, and living environment. The nurse should be aware of the dual role of recipient and provider that the patient assumes in the home care setting; this can be overwhelming to the patient and the significant other. Therefore, a well-designed educational program is important to help the patient and family make the transition to these roles.

If a home care agency is used, standards of care must be shared and clarified with the agency to ensure continuity and safe care. This can be accomplished early during discharge planning, when the patient is still in the hospital.

The educational needs of patients receiving chemotherapy at home include the drugs, management of side effects and toxicities, care of infusion devices (including troubleshooting), and handling and safe disposal of equipment and drugs. The necessary materials should be provided, such as a chemotherapy spill kit. Patients should also be taught about reporting untoward reactions; they should have telephone access and should know how to access medical care when needed. Patients should be encouraged to keep diaries of relevant occurrences at home and their responses to self-care measures. Written instructions are useful references for the patient and family.

The home has become a reasonable setting for chemotherapy and other therapies in oncology because of economic, technological, and quality-of-life issues. Given these changes, it is important that the various efforts be coordinated beyond the hospital to the outpatient setting, including home health agencies and community resources, to ensure continuity and quality care. Appendix C lists organizations and agencies that provide assistance to cancer patients and their families.

Bibliography

CHAPTER 1: OVERVIEW OF CHEMOTHERAPY

Alberts, B., Bray, D. Lewis, J., Raff, M., Roberts, K., & Watson, D. (1994). *Molecular biology of the cell* (3rd ed.). New York: Garland Publishing.

Association of Pediatric Oncology Nurses. (1990). *Cancer chemotherapy*. Richmond, Va.: Author.

Bakemeier, R., & Quazi, R. (1993). Basic concepts of cancer chemotherapy and principles of medical oncology. In P. Rubin (Ed.), *Clinical oncology* (pp. 98–110, 864–870). Philadelphia: W. B. Saunders.

Balmer, C., & Valley, A. W. (1997). Basic principles of cancer treatment and cancer chemotherapy. In J. T. DiPiro, R. L. Talbert, G. C. Yee, G. R. Matzke, B. G. Wells, & L. M. Posey (Eds.), *Pharmacotherapy: A pathophysiologic approach* (3rd ed. pp. 2403–2465). Stamford, CT: Appleton & Lange

DeVita, V. T, Hellman, S., & Rosenberg, S. A. (1997). *Cancer: Principles and practice of oncology* (5th ed.). Philadelphia: Lippincott-Raven.

Fischer, D. S., Knobf, M. T., & Durivage, H. J. The cancer chemotherapy handbook (4th ed). St. Louis: Mosby.

Groenwald, S., Frogge, M., Goodman, M., & Yarbro, C. (1995). *Comprehensive cancer nursing review* (2nd ed., pp. 118–125). Boston: Jones and Bartlett.

Guy, J. L., & Ingram, B. A. (1996). Medical oncology: The agents. In R. McCorkle, M. Grant, M. Frank-Stromborg, & S. B. Baird (Eds.), *Cancer nursing: A comprehensive textbook* (2nd ed., pp. 359–394). Philadelphia: W. B. Saunders.

Haskell, C. M. (1995). Antineoplastic agents. In C. M. Haskell (Ed.), *Cancer treatment* (4th ed., pp. 78–165). Philadelphia: W. B. Saunders.

Pfeifer, K. (1994). Pathophysiology. In S. Otto (Ed.), *Oncology nursing* (pp. 3–12). St. Louis: Mosby–Year Book.

Tenenbaum, L. (1994). *Cancer chemotherapy and biotherapy: A reference guide* (2nd ed.). Philadelphia: W. B. Saunders.

Widnell, C., & Pfenninger, K. (1990). *Essential cell biology.* Baltimore: Williams and Wilkins.

Yarbro, J. (1992). The scientific basis of cancer chemotherapy. In M. C. Perry (Ed.), *The chemotherapy source book* (pp. 2–14). Baltimore: Williams & Wilkins.

CHAPTER 2: BIOLOGIC RESPONSE MODIFIERS

Aggarwal, B. B., & Gutterman, J. U. (Eds.). (1992). *Human cytokines: Handbook for basic and clinical research.* Cambridge, MA: Blackwell Scientific.

Amgen. (1994). *Epogen (epoetin alfa)* [Package insert]. Thousand Oaks, Calif.: Author.

Amgen. (1998). *Neupogen (filgrastim)* [Package insert]. Thousand Oaks, Calif.: Author.

Baggiolini, M., Imboden, P., & Detmers, P. (1992). Neutrophil activation and the effects of interleukin-8/neutrophil-activating peptide 1 (IL-8/NAP). *Cytokines, 4*(1), 1–17.

Baquiran, D. C., Dantis, L., & McKerrow, J. (1996). Monoclonal antibodies: Innovations in diagnosis and therapy. *Seminars in Oncology Nursing, 12*(2), 130–141.

Bodey, B., Siegel, S. E., & Kaiser, H. E. (1996). Human cancer detection and immunotherapy with conjugated and non-conjugated monoclonal antibodies. *Anticancer Research, 16,* 661–670.

Brunda, M. J. (1994). Interleukin-12. *Journal of Leukocyte Biology, 52,* 280–288.

Chapman, P. B., Scheinberg, D. A., DiMaggio, J. J., & Houghton, A. N. (1991). Unconjugated monoclonal antibodies as anticancer agents. *Immunology and Allergy Clinics of North America, 11,* 257–273.

Chiron. (1998). *Proleukin (aldesleukin)* [Package insert]. Emeryville, CA: Author.

Conrad, K. J., & Horrell, C. J. (1995). *Biotherapy: Recommendations for nursing course content and clinical practicum.* Pittsburgh, PA: Oncology Nursing Press.

Cytogen (1993). *OncoScint (satumomab pendetide)* [Package insert]. Princeton, NJ: Author.

De La Pena, L., Tomaszewski, J. G., Bernato, D. L., Kryk, J. A., Molenda, J., & Gantz, S. (1996*a*). Interleukins. *Cancer Nursing, 19,* 60–73.

De La Pena, L., Wooley, M., Tomaszewski, J. G., Gantz, S., Bernato, D. L., DiLorenzo, K., Molenda, J., & Kryk, J. A. (1996*b*). Hematopoietic growth factors. *Cancer Nursing, 19,* 135–151.

Ding, A. H., & Porteu, F. (1992). Regulation of tumor necrosis factor receptors on phagocytes. *Proceedings of the Society for Experimental Biology and Medicine, 200,* 458–465.

Dranoff, G., Crawford, A. D., Sadelain, M., Ream, B., Rashid, A., Bronson, R. T., Dickersin, G. R., Bachurski, C. J., Merk, E. L., Whitsett, J. A., & Mulligan, R. C. (1994). Involvement of granulocyte-macrophage colony-stimulating factor in pulmonary homeostasis. *Science, 264,* 713–716.

Dudjak, L. A., & Fleck, A. E. (1991). BRMS: New drug therapy comes of age. *Registered Nurse, 54*(10) 42–47.

Durum, S. K., & Oppenheim, J. J. (1993). Proinflammatory cytokines and immunity. In W. E. Paul (Ed.), *Fundamental immunology* (3rd ed., pp. 801–835) New York: Raven.

Eckardt, K. V., Pugh, C. W., Meier, M., Tan, C. C., Ratcliffe, P. J., & Kurtz, A. (1994). Production of erythropoietin by liver cells in vivo and in vitro. *Annals of the New York Academy of Sciences, 718*(50), 50–60.

Engelking, C., & Wujcik, D. (1994). Biologic response modifiers (BRMs). In L. Tenenbaum (Ed.), *Cancer chemotherapy and biotherapy: A reference guide* (2nd ed., pp. 151–179). Philadelphia: W. B. Saunders.

Farrell, M. M. (1996). Biotherapy and the oncology nurse. *Seminars in Oncology Nursing, 12*(2), 82–88.

Frendl, G. (1992). Interleukin 3: From colony-stimulating factor to pluripotent immunoregulatory cytokine. *International Journal of Immunopharmacology, 14,* 421–430.

Gabrilove, J. L., & Golde, D. W. (1997). Hematopoietic growth factors. In V. T. Devita, S. Hellman & S. A. Rosenberg (Eds.), *Cancer: Principles & practice of oncology* (4th ed., pp. 2275–2291). Philadelphia: Lippincott.

Gantz, S., Tomaszewski, J. G., DeLaPena, L., Molenda, J., Bernato, D. L., & Kryk, J. (1995). Biotherapy module III: Interferons. *Cancer Nursing, 18,* 479–491.

Gdicke, E., & Riethmller, G. (1995). Prevention of manifest metastasis with monoclonal antibodies: A novel approach to immunotherapy of solid tumours. *European Journal of Cancer, 31A*(7/8), 1326–1330.

Genetic Institute. (1997). *Neumega (Oprelvekin).* [Package insert]. Cambridge, MA: Author.

Groenwald, S. L., Frogge, M. H., Goodman, M., & Yarbro, C. H. (1995). *Comprehensive cancer nursing review* (2nd ed.). Boston: Jones & Barlett.

Hansen, R. M., & Borden, E. C. (1992). Current status of interferons in the treatment of cancer. *Oncology, 6,* 19–24.

Holter, W. (1992). Regulation of interleukin 4 production and of interleukin 4-producing cells. *International Archives of Allergy Immunology, 98,* 273–278.

Hood, L. E., & Abernathy, E. A. (1996). Biotherapy. In R. McCorkle, M. Grant, M. Frank-Stromborg & S. B. Baird (Eds.), *Cancer nursing: A comprehensive textbook* (2nd ed., pp. 434–457). Philadelphia: W. B. Saunders.

Hoover, H. C., & Hanna, M. G. (1991). Immunotherapy by active specific immunization: Clinical applications. In V. T. Devita, S. Hellman & S. A. Rosenberg (Eds.), *Biologic therapy of cancer* (pp. 670–682). Philadelphia: J. B. Lippincott.

Howard, M. C., Miyajima, A., & Coffman, R. (1993). T-cell derived cytokines and their receptors. In W. E. Paul (Ed.), *Fundamental immunology* (3rd ed., pp. 763–800) New York: Raven.

Hwu, P. (1995). The gene therapy of cancer. *PPO Updates: Principles & Practice of Oncology, 9*(4), 1–11.

Immunex. (1998). *Leukine (sargramostim)* [Package insert]. Seattle, WA: Author.

Jorde, L. B. (1994). Genes and genetic disease. In K. L. McCance & S. E. Huether (Eds.), *Pathophysiology: The biologic basis for disease in adults and children* (2nd ed., pp. 126–165). St. Louis, Mo.: Mosby–Year Book.

Jurcic, J. G., Scheinberg, D. A., & Houghton, A. N. (1997). Monoclonal antibody therapy of cancer. In H. M. Pinedo, D. L. Longo & B. A. Chabner (Eds.), *Cancer chemotherapy and biological response modifiers* Annual 16, (pp. 168–188). Amsterdam: Elsevier Science BV.

Keith, J. F. (1990). Overview of the immune system. In J. Koeller & J. Tami (Eds.), *Concepts in immunology and immunotherapeutics* (pp. 6–36). Bethesda, MD: American Society of Hospital Pharmacists.

Kohler, G., & Milstein, C. (1975). Continuous culture of fused cells secreting antibody of predefined specificity. *Nature, 256*, 495–597.

Komschlies, K. L., Gregorio, T. A., Gruys, M. E., Buck, T. O., Faltyneck, C. R., & Wiltrout, R. H. (1994). Administration of recombinant human IL-7 to mice alters the composition of B-lineage cells and T cell subsets, enhances T cell function, and induces regression of established metastases. *Journal of Immunology, 152*, 5776–5784.

Kosits, C., & Callahan, H. (2000). Rituximab: A new monoclonal antibody therapy for non-Hodgkin's lymphoma. *Oncology Nursing Forum, 27*(1), 51–9.

Koury, S. T., Bondurant, M. C., Semenza, G. L., & Koury, M. J. (1993). The use of in situ hybridization to study erythropoietin gene expression in murine kidney and liver. *Microscopy Research and Technique, 25*(1), 29–39.

Kwok, K. (1990). Monoclonal antibodies. In J. Koeller & J. Tami (Eds.), *Concepts in immunology and immunotherapeutics* (pp. 348–409). Bethesda, Md.: American Society of Hospital Pharmacists.

Livingston, P. (1991). Active specific immunotherapy in the treatment of patients with cancer. *Immunology and Allergy Clinics of North America, 11*, 401–419.

Lotze, M. T. (1991). Interleukin-2: Basic principles. In V. T. DeVita, S. Hellman, & S. A. Rosenberg (Eds.), *Biologic therapy of cancer* (pp. 159–177). Philadelphia: Lippincott.

Lotze, M. T., & Rosenberg, S. A. (1991). Interleukin-2: Clinical applications. In V. T. DeVita, S. Hellman, & S. A. Rosenberg (Eds.), *Biologic therapy of cancer* (pp. 178–196) Philadelphia: Lippincott.

Mayer, D. K. (1990). Biotherapy: Recent advances and nursing implications. *Nursing Clinics of North America, 25,* 291–308.

McCance, K. L., Roberts, L. K., & Mooney, K. H. (1994). Tumor metastasis in adults and cancer in children. In K. L. McCance & S. E. Huether (Eds.), *Pathophysiology: The biologic basis for disease in adults and children* (2nd ed., pp. 366–392). St. Louis, Mo.: Mosby–Year-Book.

Mukaida, N., Harada, A., Yasumoto, K., & Matsuschima, K. (1992). Properties of pro-inflammatory cell type-specific leukocyte chemotactic cytokines, interleukin 8 (IL-8) and monocyte chemotactic and activating factor (MCAF). *Microbiology and Immunology, 36,* 773–789.

O'Garra, A., Macatonia, S. E., Hsieh, C. S., & Murphy, K. M. (1993). Regulatory role of IL4 and other cytokines in T helper cell development in an alpha beta TCR transgenic mouse system. *Research Immunology, 144,* 620–625.

Old, L. J. (1996). Immunotherapy for cancer. *Scientific American, 275*(3), 136–143.

Olsson, T. (1992). Cytokines in neuroinflammatory disease: Role of myelin autoreactive T cell production of interferon gamma. *Journal of Neuroimmunobiology, 40,* 211–218.

Ortho Biotech. (1998). *Procrit (epoetin alfa)* [Package insert]. Raritan, NJ: Author.

Ortho Biotech. (1995). *Orthoclone (muromonab-CD3)* [Package insert]. Raritan, NJ: Author.

Parkinson, D. R. (1996). Immune therapies for cancer. In M. C. Brain, P. P. Carbone, J. G. Kelton, & J. H. Schiller (Eds.), *Current therapy in hematology-oncology* (5th ed., pp. 34–39). St. Louis, MO: Mosby-Year Book.

Peschon, J. J., Morrissey, P. J., Grabstein, K. H., Ramsdell, F. J., Maraskousky, E., Gliniak, B. C., Park, L. S., Ziegler, S. F., Williams, D. E., & Ware, C. B. (1994). Early lymphocyte expansion is severely impaired in interleukin-7 receptor-deficient mice. *Journal of Experimental Medicine, 180,* 1955–1960.

Pitler, L. R. (1996). Hematopoietic growth factors in clinical practice. *Seminars in Oncology Nursing, 12*(2), 115–129.

Post-White, J. (1996a). The immune system. *Seminars in Oncology Nursing, 12*(2), 89–96.

Post-White, J. (1996b). Principles of immunology. In R. McCorkle, M. Grant, M. Frank-Stromborg, & S. B. Baird (Eds.), *Cancer nursing: A comprehensive textbook* (2nd ed., pp. 171–189). Philadelphia: W. B. Saunders.

Rieger, P. T., & Haeuber, D. (1995). A new approach to managing chemo-related anemia: Nursing implications of epoetin alfa. *Oncology Nursing Forum, 22,* 71–81.

Rosenberg, S. A. (1992). Gene therapy of cancer. In V. T. DeVita, S. Hellman, & S. A. Rosenberg (Eds.), *Important advances in oncology* (pp. 293–324). Philadelphia: Lippincott.

Rosenberg, S. A. (1993*a*). Adoptive immunotherapy for cancer. *Scientific American Medicine* [Special Issue], 94–101.

Rosenberg, S. A. (1993*b*). Principles and applications of biologic therapy. In V. T. Devita, S. Hellman, & S. A. Rosenberg (Eds.), *Cancer principles & practice of oncology* (4th ed., pp. 17–38). Philadelphia: Lippincott.

Rote, N. S. (1994). Immunity. In K. L. McCance & S. E. Huether (Eds.), *Pathophysiology: The biologic basis for disease in adults and children* (2nd ed., pp. 205–233). St. Louis, Mo.: Mosby–Year Book.

Rust, D. M., Wood, L. S., & Battiato, L. A. (1999). Oprelvekin: An alternative treatment for thrombocytopenia *Clinical Journal of Oncology Nursing, 3*(2), 57–62.

Sandstom, S. K. (1996). Nursing management of patients receiving biological therapy. *Seminars in Oncology Nursing, 12*(2), 152–162.

Scheinberg, D. A., & Chapman, P. B. (1995). Therapeutic applications of monoclonal antibodies for human disease. In J. R. Birch & E. S. Lennox (Eds.), *Monoclonal antibodies: Principles and applications* (pp. 45–105). New York: Wiley-Liss.

Schindler, L. W. (1988). *Understanding the immune system* (NIH Publication No. 88–529). Washington, DC: U. S. Department of Health and Human Services.

Schirrmacher, V. (1995). Tumor vaccine design: Concepts, mechanisms, and efficacy testing. *International Archives of Allergy Immunology, 108*, 340–344.

Seragen, Inc. (1999). *Denileukin diftitox (Ontak).* [Package insert]. Hopkinton MA: Author.

Skalla, K. (1996). The interferons. *Seminars in Oncology Nursing, 12*(2), 97–105.

Tomaszewski, J. G., De La Pena, L., Gantz, S. B., Beranto, D. L., Woolery-Antill, M., DiLorenzo, K., Molenda, J., & Folts, S. (1995*a*). The immune system and cancer. *Cancer Nursing, 18*, 313–330.

Tomaszewski, J. G., De La Pena, L., Molena, J., Gantz, S., Bernato D. L., & Folts, S. (1995*b*). Overview of biotherapy. *Cancer Nursing, 18*, 397–414.

Trinchieri, G., Wysocka, M., D'Andrea, A., Rengaraju, M., Aste-Amezaga, M., Kubin, M., Valiante, N. M., & Chehimi, J. (1992). Natural killer cell stimulatory factor (NKSF) or interlukin-12 is a key regulatory of immune response and inflammation. *Progress in Growth Factor Research, 4*, 355–368.

Upeslacis, J., Hinman, L., & Oronsky, A. (1995). Modification of antibodies by chemical methods. In J. R. Birch & E. S. Lennox (Eds.), *Monoclonal antibodies: Principles and applications* (pp. 187–230). New York: Wiley-Liss.

Urabe, A. (1994). Interferons for the treatment of hematological malignancies. *Oncology, 51,* 137–141.

Waddelow, T. (1990). Cellular and tissue components of the immune system. In J. Koeller & J. Tami (Eds.), *Concepts in immunology and immunotherapeutics* (pp. 40–73). Bethesda, Md.: American Society of Hospital Pharmacists.

Ward, E. S., & Bebbington, C. R. (1995). Genetic manipulations and expression of antibodies. In J. R. Birch & E. S. Lennox (Eds.), *Monoclonal antibodies: Principles and applications* (pp. 137–185). New York: Wiley-Liss.

Wujcik, D. (1993). An odyssey into biologic therapy. *Oncology Nursing Forum, 20,* 879–887.

Zurawsky, G., & deVries, J. (1994). Interleukin 13, an interleukin 4-like cytokine that acts on monocytes and B cells, but not on T cells. *Immunology Today, 15*(1), 19–26.

CHAPTER 3: CLINICAL TRIALS

Freireich, E. J., Gehan, E. A., & Rall, D. P. (1996). Quantitative comparison of toxicity of anticancer agents in mouse, rat, hamster, dog, monkey, and man. *Cancer Chemotherapy Reports, 50,* 219.

Galassi, A. (1992). The next generation: New chemotherapy agents for the 1990s. *Seminars in Oncology Nursing, 8,* 83–94.

Giacalone, S. B. (1997). Cancer clinical trials. In S. E. Otto (Ed)., *Oncology Nursing* (3rd ed., pp. 641–665). St. Louis, MO: Mosby.

Gross, J. (1989). Cancer drug development. In L. Tenenbaum (Ed.), *Cancer chemotherapy: A reference guide* (pp. 99–109). Philadelphia: W. B. Saunders.

National Commission for the Protection of Human Subjects of Biomedical and Behavioral Research. (1991, April 18). *The Belmont Report: Ethical principles and guidelines for the protection of human subjects of research.* Washington, DC: OPRR Reports.

National Cancer Institute. (1998). *Taking part in clinical trials: What cancer patients need to know* (NIH Publication No. 98–4250). Bethesda, MD: Author.

Nightingale, S. L., & Bagley, G. P. (1994). FDA sanctions for practitioners for violations of clinical trial regulations and other misconduct. *Federation Bulletin, 81,* 7–13.

Protection of Human Subjects (rev. 1991, June 18). (Rev. ed., Title 45, Code of Federal Regulations, Part 46).

Simon, R., & Friedman, M. (1992). The design of clinical trials. In M. C. Perry (Ed.), *The chemotherapy source book* (pp. 130–143). Baltimore: Williams & Wilkins.

Varrichio, C. E., & Vassak, P. F. (1989). Informed consent: An overview. *Seminars in Oncology Nursing, 2* (5), 95–98.

Zubrod, C. G. (1984). Origins and development of chemotherapy research at the National Cancer Institute. *Cancer Treatment Reports, 68,* 9–19.

CHAPTER 4: PREPARATION, ADMINISTRATION, AND HANDLING OF CHEMOTHERAPY

Alexander, J. (1991). Chemotherapy: Uses and safety considerations. *Dermatology Nursing, 3* (2), 107–109.

Almadrones, L., Campanc, P., & Dantis, E. (1995). Arterial, peritoneal, and intraventricular devices. *Seminars in Oncology Nursing, 3,* 194–202.

American Society of Hospital Pharmacists. (1990). Technical assistance bulletin on handling cytotoxic and hazardous drugs. *American Journal of Hospital Pharmacy, 47,* 1033–1049.

American Society of Hospital Pharmacists. (1993). Technical assistance bulletin on handling cytotoxic and hazardous drugs. *Practice Standards of ASHP, 1993–1994.* Bethesda, MD: Author.

American Society of Hospital Pharmacists. (1994). ASHP outlines procedures for handling cytotoxic drugs. *Hospital Employee Health, 13*(14), 44–46.

American Society of Hospital Pharmacists Council on Professional Affairs. (1992). Draft guidelines on preventable medication errors. *American Journal of Hospital Pharmacy, 49,* 640–648.

Attilio, R. (1996). Caring enough to understand: The road to oncology medication error prevention. *Hospital Pharmacy, 31,* 17–26.

Bonawitz, S., Hammell, E., & Kirkpatrick, J. (1991). Prevention of central venous catheter sepsis: A prospective randomized trial. *American Surgery, 57,* 618–623.

Bowles, C., & McKinnon, B. (1993). Selecting infusion devices. *American Journal of Hospital Pharmacy, 50,* 228–230.

Camp-Sorrell, D. (1992). Implantable ports: Everything you always wanted to know. *Journal of Intravenous Nursing, 15,* 262–273.

Camp-Sorrell, D. (1996). *Access device guidelines: Recommendations for nursing practice and education.* Pittsburgh: Oncology Nursing Society.

Carmignani, S., & Raymond, G. (1997). Safe handling of cytotoxic drugs in the physician's office: A procedure manual model. *Oncology Nursing Forum, 24*(Suppl. 1), 41–48.

Chisholm, L. G., Berman, A. R., de Carvalho, M., & Gorrell, C. G. (1993). Cancer chemotherapy: Alternative administration routes. *Cancer Nursing, 16,* 249–251.

Cohen, M. R. (2000). ISMP Medication safety alert! Educating the healthcare community about safe medication practices. 5 Issue 5

Cozzi, E., Hagle, M., Lachute McGregor, M., & Woodhouse, D. (1984). Nursing management of patients receiving hepatic arterial chemotherapy through an implanted infusion pump. *Cancer Nursing,* June, 229–234.

Dearborn, P., DeMuth, J., Requarth, A., & Ward, S. (1997). Nurse and patient satisfaction with three types of venous access devices. *Oncology Nursing Forum, 24*(Suppl. 1), 34–40.

Dunne, C. (1989). Safe handling of antineoplastic agents. *Cancer Nursing, 12*(2), 120–127.

Ensminger, W., Niederhuber, J., Dakhil, S., Thrall, J., & Wheeler, R. (1981). Totally implanted drug delivery system for hepatic arterial chemotherapy. *Cancer Treatment Reports, 65* (5–6), 393–400.

Fisher, D., Alfano, S., Knobf, M., Donvan, C., & Beauliue, N. (1996). Improving the cancer chemotherapy use process. *Journal of Clinical Oncology, 14,* 3148–3155.

Gibbs, J. (1991). Handling cytotoxic drugs. *Nursing Times, 87*(11), 54–55.

Goodwin, M., & Carlson, I. (1993). The peripherally inserted central catheter: A retrospective look at three years of insertions. *Journal of Intravenous Nursing, 16*(2), 92–103.

Graham, A., & Holohan, T. (1994). External and implantable infusion pumps. *Health Technology Review, 7,* 1–29.

Graseby Medical PIC. (1991). *Graseby Medical MS 16/26* [Product literature]. Millerville, MD: Author.

Gualtieri, F. (1992). Safe use of syringe pumps: A word of caution. *Journal of Pediatric Nursing, 7,* 256–257.

Gullo, S. (1988). Safe handling of antineoplastic drugs: Translating the recommendations into practice. *Oncology Nursing Forum, 15,* 595–601.

Gullo, S. (1993). Implanted ports, technologic advances and nursing care issues. *Nursing Clinics of North America, 28*(4), 859–870.

Hadaway, L. (1995). Comparison of vascular access devices. *Seminars in Oncology Nursing, 11*(3), 154–166.

Hall, P., Cederman, B., & Swedenborg, J. (1989). Implantable catheter systems for long-term intravenous chemotherapy. *Journal of Surgical Oncology, 41,* 39–47.

Hoff, S. (1987). Concepts in intraperitoneal chemotherapy. *Seminars in Oncology Nursing, 3,* 112–117.

Ingle, R. (1995). Rare complications of vascular access devices. *Seminars in Oncology Nursing, 11*(3), 184–193.

Ingram, J., Weitzman, S., Greenberg, M., Parkin, P., & Filler, R. (1991). Complications of indwelling venous access lines in the pediatric hematologic patient: A prospective comparison of external venous catheters and subcutaneous ports. *American Journal of Pediatric Hematology/Oncology, 13*(2), 130–136.

Johnson, G. (1993). Nursing care of patients with implanted pumps. *Nursing Clinics of North America, 28*(4), 873–83.

Keegan-Wells, D., & Stewart, J. (1992). The use of venous access devices in pediatric oncology. *Nursing, 9*(4), 159–169.

Koeppen, M., & Caspers, S. (1994). Problems identified with home infusion pumps. *Journal of Intravenous Nursing, 17*, 151–156.

Kwan, J. (1991). High-technology infusion devices. *American Journal of Hospital Pharmacy, 48*, S36–S51.

Laidlaw, J., Connor, T. & Theiss, J. (1984). Permeability of latex gloves and polyvinyl chloride gloves to 20 antineoplastic drugs. *American Journal of Hospital Pharmacy, 41*(12), 2618–2623.

Legislative Network for Nurses. (2000). Reducing medication errors. *17*(4), 25.

Lucas, A. (1991). A critical review of venous access devices: The nursing perspective. *Current Issues in Cancer Nursing Practice*, September, 1–10.

Markman, M. (1991). Intraperitoneal chemotherapy. *Seminars in Oncology, 18*, 248–254.

Memorial Sloan Kettering Cancer Center. (1996). *Nurse reference manual*. New York: Author.

Mioduszewski, J., & Zarko, A. (1987). Ambulatory infusion pumps: A practical view at an alternative approach. *Seminars in Oncology Nursing, 3*, 106–111.

Moosa, H., Julian, T., Rosenfeld, C., & Shadduck, R. (1991). Complications of indwelling central venous catheters in bone marrow transplant recipients. *Surgery Gynecology & Obstetrics, 172*, 275–279.

Muller, R. Common errors in prescribing, dispensing, and administering cancer chemotherapy. *Strategies for reducing chemotherapy-related medication errors [course outline]*. 22nd Annual Congress of the Oncology Nursing Society, New Orleans, 1997.

Oncology Nursing Society. (1998). *Cancer chemotherapy guidelines and recommendations for practice*. Pittsburgh, PA: Oncology Nursing Press.

Rapsilber, L., & Camp-Sorrell, D. (1995). Ambulatory infusion pumps: Application to oncology. *Seminars in Oncology Nursing, 3*, 213–220.

Rich, D. (1992). Evaluation of a disposable elastomeric infusion device in the home environment. *American Journal of Hospital Pharmacy, 49*, 1712–1716.

Rogers, B. (1999). Preventing and detecting chemotherapy drug errors. *Oncology Nursing Updates, 6*(1), 1–12.

Rumsey, K., & Richardson, D. (1995). Management of infection and occlusion associated with vascular access devices. *Seminars in Oncology Nursing, 11* (3), 174–183.

Ryder, M. (1993). Peripherally inserted central venous catheters. *Nursing Clinics of North America, 28*(4), 937–964.

Smetzer, J. (1998). Lesson from Colorado: Beyond blaming individuals. *Nursing Management, 29*, 49–51.

Starnes Doane, L. (1993). Administering intraperitoneal chemotherapy using a peritoneal port. *Nursing Clinics of North America, 28*(4), 885–897.

Swenson, K., & Erikson, J. (1986). Nursing management of intraperitoneal chemotherapy. *Oncology Nursing Forum, 13*(5), 33–39.

Wickham, R., Purl, S., & Welker, D. (1992). Long-term central venous catheters: Issues for care. *Seminars in Oncology Nursing, 8*(2), 133–147.

Winslow, M., Trammell, L., & Camp-Sorrell, D. (1995). Selection of vascular access devices and nursing care. *Seminars in Oncology Nursing, 11*(3), 167–173.

CHAPTER 5: MANAGEMENT OF TOXIC EFFECTS OF CHEMOTHERAPY

Aikin, J. (1995). Menopausal symptoms resulting from breast cancer therapies. *Innovations in Breast Cancer Care, 1*, 2–5, 21.

Allen, A. (1992). The cardiotoxicity of chemotherapeutic drugs. In M. Perry, *The chemotherapy source book* (pp. 583–597). Baltimore: Williams & Wilkins.

Anastasia, P., & Blevins, M. (1997). Outpatient chemotherapy: Telephone triage for symptom management. *Oncology Nursing Forum, 24*(Suppl. 1), 13–22.

Armstrong, T., Rust, D., & Kohts, J. (1997). Neurologic, pulmonary, and cutaneous toxicities of high-dose chemotherapy. *Oncology Nursing Forum, 24*(Suppl. 1), 23–39.

Beck, S., & Yasko, J. (1993). *Guidelines for oral care* (2nd ed.). Crystal Lake, Ill.: Sage Products Inc.

Blesch, K. S., Paice, J. A., & Wickham, R. (1991). Correlates of fatigue in people with breast or lung cancer. *Oncology Nursing Forum, 18*, 81–87.

Borison, H. L., & Wang, S. C. (1953). Physiology and pharmacology of vomiting. *Pharmacological Reviews, 5*, 193–230.

Brillet, G., Deray, G., Jacquiard, C., Mignot, L., Burker, D., Meillet, D., & Jacobs, C., (1994). Long-term effects of cisplatin in man. *American Journal of Nephrology, 14*(2), 81–84.

Bruya, M. A., Madeira, N. P., & Powell, N. (1975). Stomatitis after chemotherapy. *American Journal of Nursing, 75*, 1349–1352.

Callaway, M., Tyrrell, C., Williams, M., & Marshall, A. (1994). Chemotherapy-induced myocardial fibrosis. *Clinical Oncology, 6*(1), 55–56.

Cameron, J. (1993). Iphosphamide neurotoxicity. *Cancer Nursing, 16*, 40–46.

Cawley, M. M. (1990). Recent advances in chemotherapy: Administration and nursing implications. *Nursing Clinics of North America, 25*, 377–392.

Chang, A., Kuebler, J., Pandya, K., Israel, R., Marshall, B., & Tormey, D. (1986). Pulmonary toxicity induced by mitomycin C is highly responsive to glucocorticoids. *Cancer, 57,* 2285–2290.

Chapman, R. (1992). Gonadal toxicity and teratogenicity. In M. Perry, *The chemotherapy source book* (pp. 710–755). Baltimore: Williams & Wilkins.

Crounse, R. G., & Van Scott, E. J. (1960). Changes in scalp hair roots as a measure of toxicity from cancer chemotherapeutic drugs. *Journal of Investigative Dermatology, 35,* 83–90.

Daeffler, R. (1980). Oral hygiene measures for patients with cancer. *Cancer Nursing, 3*(Part 1), 347–356.

de Bast, C., Morianne, N., & Wanet, J. (1971). Bleomycin in mycosis fungoides and reticulum cell lymphoma. *Archives of Dermatology, 104,* 508–512.

De Forni, M., & Armand, J. (1994). Cardiotoxicity of chemotherapy. *Current Opinion in Oncology, 6,* 340–344.

De Spain, J. D. (1992). Dermatologic toxicity. In M. C. Perry, *The chemotherapy source book* (pp. 531–547). Baltimore: Williams & Wilkins.

Dirix, L., Schrijvers, D., Druwe, P., Van den Brande, J., Verhoeven, D., & Van Oosterm, S. (1994). Pulmonary toxicity and bleomycin. *Lancet, 344*(8914), 56.

Doll, D., Weiss, R., & Issell, B. (1985). Mitomycin: Ten years after approval for marketing. *Journal of Clinical Oncology, 3,* 276–286.

Donnatelle, E. (1990). Constipation: Pathophysiology and treatment. *American Family Physician, 42,* 1335–1432.

Dorr, R. T., & Von Hoff (1994). *Cancer-chemotherapy handbook* (2nd ed.). East Norwalk, Conn.: Appleton & Lange.

Dunagin, W. G. (1982). Clinical toxicity of chemotherapeutic agents: Dermatologic toxicity. *Seminars in Oncology, 9,* 14–22.

Engelking, C., & Wujcik, D. (1994). Biologic response modifiers (BRMs). In L. Tenenbaum (Ed.), *Cancer chemotherapy and biotherapy: A reference guide* (2nd ed.). Philadelphia: W. B. Saunders.

Ewer, M. S., & Benjamin, R. S. (1996). Cardiotoxicity of chemotherapeutic drugs. In M. C. Perry, *The chemotherapy source book* (2nd ed., pp. 649–663). Baltimore: Williams & Wilkins.

Frankel, J., Kool, G., & deKraker, J., (1995). Acute renal failure in high-dose carboplatin chemotherapy. *Medical and Pediatric Onocology, 24*(6), 473–474.

Fitzpatrick, J. E., & Hood, A. F. (1988). Histopathologic reactions to chemotherapeutic agents. *Advances in Dermatology, 3,* 161–184.

Gastineau, D. A., & Hoagland, H. C. (1992). Hematologic effects of chemotherapy. *Seminars in Oncology, 19,* 543–550.

Gilbert, M., & Yasko, J. (1994). Neurotoxicities. In J. Kirkwood, M. Lotze, & J. Yasko (Eds), *Current Cancer Therapeutics* (pp. 284–287). Philadelphia: Churchill Livingstone.

Glasel, M. (1994). Effects on reproduction/sexual function. In L. Tenebaum, *Cancer chemotherapy and biotherapy: A reference guide* (pp. 273–283). Philadelphia: W. B. Saunders.

Glasel, M. (1996). Cancer chemotherapy agents' effects on gonadal function, fertility, and sexuality. In *New York Memorial Sloan Kettering Cancer Center, Nurse reference manual.* New York: Author.

Gralla, R. J., Osoba, D., Kris, M. K., et al. (1999). Recommendations for the use of antiemetics: Evidence-based, clinical practice guidelines. *Journal of Clinical Oncology, 17*(9), 2971.

Harmon, W., Cohen, H., Schneeberger, W., & Grupe, E. (1979). Chronic renal failure in children treated with methyl CCN4. *New England Journal of Medicine, 300,* 1200–1203.

Harris, A. G., O'Dorisio, E. A., Woltering, L. B., et al. (1955). Consensus statement: Octreotide dose titration in secretory diarrhea. *Digestive Diseases and Sciences, 40,* 1464–1473.

Ho, P., Zimmerman, K., Wexler, L., Blaney, S., Jarosinski, P., Izraeli, S., & Basil, F., (1995). A prospective evaluation of ifosfamide-related nephrotoxicity in children and young adults. *Cancer, 76*(12), 2557–2564.

Hrushesky, W. J. (1980). Unusual pigmentary changes associated with 5-fluorouracil therapy. *Cutis, 26,* 181–182.

Hughes, M. (1995). Sexuality changes in the cancer patient. *Nursing Intervention in Oncology, 8,* 15–18.

Hughes, M. (1996). Sexuality issues: Keeping your cool. *Oncology Nursing Forum, 23*(10), 1597–1600.

Jakubovic, H. R., & Ackerman, A. B. (1985). Structure and function of skin: Development, morphology, and physiology. In S. L. Moschella & H. J. Hurley (Eds.), *Dermatology* (2nd ed., pp. 1–74). Philadelphia: W. B. Saunders.

Kaempfer, S. (1981). The effects of chemotherapy on reproduction: A review of the literature. *Oncology Nursing Forum, 8*(1), 11–17.

Kalaycioglu, M., Kavuru, M., Tuason, L., & Bolwell, B. (1995). Empiric prednisone therapy for pulmonary toxic reaction after high-dose chemotherapy containing carmustine (BCNU). *Chest, 107*(2), 482–487.

Kaplan, R., & Wiernik, P. (1982). Neurotoxicity of antineoplastic drugs. *Seminars in Oncology, 9,* 103–130.

Kaszyk, L. (1986). Cardiac toxicity associated with cancer therapy. *Oncology Nursing Forum, 13*(4), 81–88.

Kintzel, P., & Dorr, R. (1995). Anticancer drug renal toxicity & elimination: Dosing guidelines for altered renal function. *Cancer Treatment Reviews, 21*(1), 33–64

Koeppel, K. (1995). Sperm banking and patients with cancer. *Cancer Nursing, 18*(4), 306–312.

Kreisman, H., & Wolkove, N. (1992). Pulmonary toxicity of antineoplastic therapy. In M. C. Perry, *The chemotherapy source book* (pp. 598–619). Baltimore: Williams & Wilkins.

Lamb, M. (1995). Effects of cancer on the sexuality and fertility of women. *Seminars in Oncology Nursing, 11*(2), 120–127.

Lipshultz, S., Sanders, S., Gorin, A., Krischer, J., Sallan, S., & Colan, S. (1994). Monitoring for anthracycline cytoxicity. *Pediatrics, 93*(3), 433–437.

Lowenthal, R. M., & Eaton, K. (1996). Toxicity of chemotherapy. *Hematology Oncology Clinics of North America, 10,* 967–990.

Lundquist, D., & Holmes, W. (1993). Documentation of neurotoxicity resulting from high-dose cytosine arabinoside. *Oncology Nursing Forum, 20,* 1409–1413.

Lydon, A. (1986). Nephrotoxicity of cancer treatment. *Oncology Nursing Forum 13*(2), 68–77.

Meehan, J., & Johnson, B. (1992). The neurotoxicity of antineoplastic agents. *Current Issues in Cancer Nursing Practice,* (update) *1*(8), 1–11.

Memorial Sloan-Kettering Cancer Center. (1982). *Methotrexate learning module.* New York: Author.

Mills, B., & Roberts, R. (1979). Cyclophosphamide-induced cardiomyopathy. A report of two cases and review of the English literature. *Cancer, 43,* 2223–2226.

Mitchell, E. P. (1992). Gastrointestinal toxicity of chemotherapeutic agents. *Seminars in Oncology, 19,* 566–579.

Morrow, G. R., Lindke, J., & Black, P. M. (1991). Predicting development of anticipatory nausea in cancer patients: Prospective examination of eight clinical characteristics. *Journal of Pain and Symptom Management, 6,* 2155.

Muggia, F., Louie, A., & Sikic, B. (1983). Pulmonary toxicity of antitumor agents. *Cancer Treatment Reviews, 10,* 221–243.

Nail, L. (1997). Fatigue. In S. L. Groenwald, M. H. Frogge, M. Goodman, & C. H. Yarbro (Eds)., *Cancer nursing: Principles and practice* (4th ed., pp. 640–654). Boston: Jones & Bartlett.

National Institutes of Health. (1989). *Consensus development conference statement on oral complications of cancer therapies: Diagnosis, prevention and treatment.* Bethesda, MD.

O'Driscoll, B., Kalra, S., Gattamaneni, H., & Woodcock, A. (1995). Late carmustine lung fibrosis. Age at treatment may influence severity and survival. *Chest, 107*(5), 1355.

Ofman, U., & Auchincloss, S. (1992). Sexual dysfunction in cancer patients. *Current Opinion in Oncology, 4,* 605–613.

Patchell, R., White, C., Clark, A., Beschorner, W., & Santos, G. (1985). Neurologic complications of bone marrow transplantation. *Neurology, 35,* 300–306.

Piper, B. F., Lindsey, A. M., & Dodd, M. J. (1987). Fatigue mechanisms in cancer patients: Developing nursing theory. *Oncology Nursing Forum, 14,* 13–19.

Robuck, J. T., & Fleetwood, J. B. (1992). Nutritional support of the patient with cancer. *Focus on Critical Care, 19,* 129–138.

Sasson, Z., Morgan, C., Wang, B., Thomas, G., Mackenzie, B., & Platts, M. (1994). 5-fluorouracil-related toxic myocarditis: Case reports and pathological confirmation. *Canadian Journal of Cardiology, 10*(8), 861–864.

Schover, L. (1994). Sexuality and body image in younger women with breast cancer. *Monographs/National Cancer Institute, 16,* 177–182.

Segelman, A. E., & Doku, H. C. (1977). Treatment of the oral complications of leukemia. *Journal of Oral Surgery, 35,* 469–477.

Shearer, P., Katz, J., Bozeman, P., Jenkin, J., Laver, J., Krance, R., Hurwitz, C., Mahmoud, H., & Mirro, J. (1994). Pulmonary insufficiency complicating therapy with high-dose cytosine arabinoside in five pediatric patients with relapsed acute myelogenous leukemia. *Cancer, 74*(7), 1953–1958.

Silver, H., Morton, D. (1979). CCN4 nephrotoxicity following sustained remission in oat cell carcinoma. *Cancer Treatment Reports, 63,* 226–227.

Singal, P., Siveski-Ilishovic, N., Hill, M., Thomas, T., & Li, T. (1995). Combination therapy with probucol prevents Adriamycin-induced cardiomyopathy. *Journal of Molecular and Cellular Cardiology, 27*(4), 1055–1063.

Smith, D., & Babaian, J. (1992). The effects of treatment for cancer on male fertility and sexuality. *Cancer Nursing, 15*(4), 271–275.

Sonis, S., & Clark, J. (1992). Prevention and management of oral mucositis induced by antineoplastic therapy. *Oncology, 5,* 11–21.

Tomaszewski, J. G., De La Pena, L., Molena, J., Molena, J., Gantz, S., Bernato, D. L., & Folts, S. (1995). Overview of biotherapy. *Cancer Nursing, 18,* 397–414.

von der Masse, H. (1994). Complications of combined radiotherapy and chemotherapy. *Seminars in Radiation Oncology, 4*(2), 81–94.

Weidmann, B., Teipel, A., & Niederle, N. (1994). The syndrome of 5-fluorouracil cardiotoxicity: An elusive cardiopathy. *Cancer, 73*(7), 2001–2202.

Weiss, R., & Muggia, F. (1980). Cytotoxic drug-induced pulmonary disease update 1980. *American Journal of Medicine, 68,* 259–266.

Weiss, R., Poster, D., & Penta, J. (1981). The nitrosoureas and pulmonary toxicity. *Cancer Treatment Reviews, 8*(2), 111–125.

Weiss, R., & Thrush, D. (1982). A review of pulmonary toxicity of cancer chemotherapy agents. *Oncology Nursing Forum, 9*(1), 16–21.

Wickham, R. (1986). Pulmonary toxicity secondary to cancer treatment. *Oncology Nursing Forum, 13*(5), 69–79.

Wilkes, G., Ingwersenm, K., & Burke, M. (1994). *Oncology nursing drug reference.* London: Jones & Bartlett.

Winningham, M., Nail, L., Burke, M., et al. (1994). Fatigue and the cancer experience: The state of the knowledge. *Oncology Nursing Forum, 21,* 23–26.

Wujcik, D. (1992). Current research in side effects of high-dose chemotherapy. *Seminars in Oncology Nursing, 8*(2), 102–112.

CHAPTER 6: MANAGEMENT OF HYPERSENSITIVITY REACTIONS AND EXTRAVASATION

Bertelli, G. (1994). Prevention and management of extravasation of cytotoxic drugs. *Drug Safety, 12*(4), 245–255.

Boyle, D. M., & Engelking, C. (1995). Vesicant extravasation: Myths and realities. *Oncology Nursing Forum, 22,* 55–67.

Brown, J., & Hogan, C. (1990). Chemotherapy. In S. Groenwald, M. Frogge & M. Goodman (Eds.), *Cancer nursing, principles and practice* (pp. 230–284). Boston: Jones & Bartlett.

Dorr, R. T. (1990). Antidotes to vesicant chemotherapy extravasation. *Blood Reviews, 4*(1), 41–60.

Gell, P. H. G., & Coombs, R. R. A. (1975). *Clinical aspects of immunology.* Oxford: Blackwell Scientific.

Goodman, M. (1991). Delivery of cancer chemotherapy. In S. B. Baird, R. McCorkle, & M. Grant (Eds.), *Cancer nursing: A comprehensive textbook* (pp. 291–320). Philadelphia: W. B. Saunders.

McCaffrey, D. & Engelking, C. (1990). Ten fallacies associated with the nature and management of chemotherpy extravasation. *Progresssions: Development in Ostomy and Wound Care, 2*(4), 3–10.

Oncology Nursing Society. (1998). *Cancer chemotherapy guidelines: Recommendations for the management of extravasation, hypersensitivity and anaphylaxis.* Pittsburgh: Author.

Rudolph, R., & Larson, D. L. (1987). Etiology and treatment of chemotherapeutic agent extravasation injuries: A review. *Journal of Clinical Oncology, 5,* 1116–1126.

Weiss, R. B. (1992*a*). Hypersensitivity reactions. In M. C. Perry, *The chemotherapy source book* (pp. 553–569). Baltimore: Williams & Wilkins.

Weiss, R. B. (1992*b*). Hypersensitivity reactions. *Seminars in Oncology, 19,* 458–477.

Wilson, J. P., Solimando, D. A., & Edwards, M. S. (1986). Parenteral benzyl alcohol-induced hypersensitivity reaction. *Drug Intelligence and Clinical Pharmacy, 20,* 689–691.

CHAPTER 7: PATIENT EDUCATION

Adams, M. (1992). Information and education across the phases of cancer care. *Seminars in Oncology Nursing, 7,* 105–111.

Bernardini, L. (1985). Effective communication as an intervention for sensory deprivation in the elderly client. *Topics in Clinical Nursing, 6,* 72–81.

Boyle, D. M., Engelking, C., Blesch, K. S., Dodge, J., Sarna, L., & Weinrich, S. (1992). Oncology Nursing Society position paper on cancer and aging: The mandate for oncology nursing. *Oncology Nursing Forum, 19,* 913–933.

Cassileth, B. R., Zupkis, R. V., Sutton-Smith., & March, V. (1980). Information and participation preferences among cancer patients. *Annals of Internal Medicine, 92,* 832–836.

Cooley, M., Moriarty, H., & Berger, M. (1995). Patient literacy and the readability of written cancer education materials. *Oncology Nursing Forum, 22*(9), 1345–1351.

Derby, S. E. (1991). Ageism in cancer care of the elderly. *Oncology Nursing Forum, 18,* 921–926.

Doak, C. C., Doak, L. G., & Root, J. H. (1985). *Teaching patients with low literacy skills.* Philadelphia: J. B. Lippincott.

Frank-Stromborg, M. (1985). Evaluating patient education material. *Oncology Nursing Forum, 12,* 65.

Garvey, E., & Kramer, R. (1983). Improving cancer patients' adjustment to infusion chemotherapy: Evaluation of a patient education pprogram. *Cancer Nursing, 6,* 373–378.

Joint Commission on Accreditation of Healthcare Organizations. (1998). Patient and family education. *1998 accreditation manual for hospitals, Vol 1.* Oak Brook, IL: Author.

Knowles, M. (1975). *The modern practice of adult education.* New York: Associated Press.

Meade, C. D., Diekman, J., & Thornhill, D. G. (1992). Readability of American Cancer Society patient education literature. *Oncology Nursing Forum, 19,* 51–55.

Newell, G. R., Spitz, M. R., & Sider, J. G. (1989). Cancer and age. *Seminars in Oncology, 16*(1), 3–9.

Shanabrook, L. (1999). Evaluating health-related Web sites for use by patients. *Chemotherapy, 10*(2), 1–3.

Stephens, S. T. (1992). Patient education materials: Are they readable? *Oncology Nursing Forum, 19,* 83–85.

Welch-McCaffrey, E. (1985): Evolving patient education needs in cancer. *Oncology Nursing Forum, 12,* 65.

II.

Chemotherapeutic Agents, Biologic Response Modifiers, and Chemoprotectants

▼ FDA Pregnancy Categories

The Food and Drug Administration has established five categories to indicate the potential for a systemically absorbed drug to cause birth defects. The key differentiation among the categories rests upon the degree (reliability) of documentation and the risk–benefit ratio.

Category A: Adequate studies in pregnant women have not demonstrated a risk to the fetus in the first trimester of pregnancy, and there is no evidence of risk in later trimesters.

Category B: Animal studies have not demonstrated a risk to the fetus but there are no adequate studies in pregnant women.
or
Animal studies have shown an adverse effect, but adequate studies in pregnant women have not demonstrated a risk to the fetus during the first trimester of pregnancy, and there is no evidence of risk in later trimesters.

Category C: Animal studies have shown an adverse effect on the fetus but there are no adequate studies in humans; the benefits from the use of the drug in pregnant women may be acceptable despite its potential risks.
or
There are no animal reproduction studies and no adequate studies in humans.

Category D: There is evidence of human fetal risk, but the potential benefits from the use of the drug in pregnant women may be acceptable despite its potential risks.

Category X: Studies in animals or humans demonstrate fetal abnormalities or adverse reaction; reports indicate evidence of fetal risk. The risk of use in a pregnant woman clearly outweighs any possible benefit.

Regardless of the designated Pregnancy Category or presumed safety, *no* drug should be administered during pregnancy unless it is clearly needed.

◆ Aldesleukin

(al-des-**loo**'-ken) Proleukin, Pregnancy Category C
interleukin-2

Mechanism of Action

Inhibits tumor growth; exerts immunologic effects by activating the cellular immunity to increase lymphocytes, eosinophils, platelets, and cytokines, including tumor necrosis factor, interleukin-1, and gamma interferon.

Indications

Metastatic renal cell carcinoma in adults.

Metabolism/Excretion

Metabolized in the kidney; excreted in the urine. Serum half-life: 13 minutes after IV administration. Eliminated in 85 minutes.

Dosage Range

◆ **Adult:** 600,000 IU/kg (0.037 mg/kg) given every 8 hours by a 15-minute IV infusion for a total of 14 doses. After 9 days of rest, repeat the schedule for another 14 doses, for a maximum of 28 doses per cycle. Doses may be held for toxicities. Retreatment may be given if response to treatment is noted after 4 weeks. The patient should have a rest period of at least 7 weeks from the date of discharge before retreatment.

◆ **Pediatric:** Safety and efficacy not established.

Drug Preparation/Stability

Supplied in powder for injection: single-use, preservative-free vials contain 22 million IU (1.3 mg) of aldesleukin. Reconstitute with 1.2 mL sterile water for injection. When reconstituted, each milliliter contains 18 million IU (1.1 mg) of aldesleukin. Do not reconstitute with bacteriostatic water or sodium chloride. Store powder and reconstituted solution in the refrigerator at 2° to 8°C (36° to 46°F). Do not shake or freeze. Discard unused portions. Administer reconstituted solution within 48 hours.

Drug Administration

IV

Drug Interaction

◆ Interactions possible with concomitant administration of psychotropic drugs.

◆ Increased toxicity noted with nephrotoxic (aminoglycosides, indomethacin), myelotoxic (chemotherapy), cardiotoxic (doxorubicin), or hepatotoxic drugs (methotrexate, asparaginase).

◆ Decreased effectiveness with concomitant administration of glucocorticoids.

◆ Increased hypotensive effects with concomitant administration of antihypertensives.

Side Effects and Toxicities

◆ **Constitutional:** Fever, chills, pain, fatigue, weakness, malaise, weight gain, weight loss, headache

◆ **CNS:** Mental status changes, dizziness, sensory dysfunction

◆ **GI:** Nausea, vomiting, diarrhea, stomatitis, anorexia, GI bleeding, dyspepsia, constipation

◆ **GU:** Oliguria, anuria, BUN and serum creatinine elevation, proteinuria, hematuria

◆ **Hematologic:** Elevated bilirubin, transaminase, and alkaline phosphatase, anemia, thrombocytopenia, leukopenia, coagulation disorders, leukocytosis, eosinophilia; hypomagnesemia, acidosis, hypocalcemia, hypophosphatemia, hypokalemia, hyperuricemia, hypoalbuminemia, hypoproteinemia

◆ **Integumentary:** Pruritus, erythema, rash, dry skin, exfoliative dermatitis

◆ **Musculoskeletal:** Arthralgia, myalgia

◆ **Pulmonary and cardiovascular:** Congestion, dyspnea, pulmonary edema, respiratory failure, tachypnea, pleural effusion, wheezing; hypotension, sinus tachycardia, arrhythmias, bradycardia

◆ **Other:** Jaundice, edema, infection

Special Considerations

◆ Contraindicated in patients with known allergy to aldesleukin or any component of the product; abnormal thallium stress test or pulmonary function test results; or organ allografts. Contraindicated in patients who have experienced the following toxicities during a previous treatment: sustained ventricular tachycardia (more than five beats); cardiac rhythm disturbances not controlled by or unresponsive to management; recurrent chest pain with ECG changes, consistent with angina or myocardial infarction; intubation required for more than 72 hours; pericardial tamponade; renal dysfunction requiring dialysis for more than 72 hours; coma or toxic psychosis lasting more than 48 hours; repetitive or difficult-to-control seizures; bowel ischemia or perforation; or GI bleeding requiring surgery.

◆ Patients should have normal cardiac, pulmonary, hepatic, and CNS function before start of treatment.

◆ Assess for capillary leak syndrome, characterized by hypotension, hypoperfusion, edema, and effusions. Frequently monitor blood pressure, pulse, mental status, weight, and urine output. May need to administer dopamine (1 to 5 mcg/kg/min) to patients with capillary leak syndrome.

◆ Obtain laboratory tests (CBC with differential, blood chemistries, including renal and liver function tests) before and daily during therapy. Obtain a baseline chest x-ray, pulmonary function test with arterial blood gases, and stress thallium study. Repeat studies during therapy when clinically indicated.

◆ If adverse events occur that require dosage modifications, withhold treatment rather than decreasing dosage.

◆ Altretamine

(al-**treh**'-tah-meen)   Hexalen   Pregnancy Category D

Mechanism of Action

Unknown

Indications

◆ Palliative treatment for recurrent or persistent ovarian cancer after first-line therapy with cisplatin or alkylating agent; use as a single agent

◆ Lymphoma, lung cancer

Metabolism/Excretion

Undergoes rapid and extensive metabolism in the liver and is excreted by the kidneys. Half-life: 0.5 to 3.0 hours.

Dosage Range

◆ **Adult:** Given for 14 or 21 days in a 28-day cycle at a dosage of 260 mg/m^2 per day. Therapy may be temporarily discontinued (for more than 14 days) and subsequently restarted at 200 mg/kg per day for any of the following: GI intolerance unresponsive to symptomatic measures; WBC count <2000/mm^3 or granulocyte count <1000/mm^3; platelet count <75,000/mm^3; progressive toxicity.

◆ **Pediatric:** Safety and efficacy not established.

Drug Preparation/Stability

Available in 50- and 100-mg capsules. No stability data available.

Drug Administration

Give the total daily dose in four divided PO doses after meals and at bedtime.

Drug Interaction

Concurrent therapy with monoamine oxidase inhibitors may cause severe orthostatic hypotension.

Side Effects and Toxicities

◆ **CNS:** Peripheral neuropathy, mood disorders, disorders of consciousness, ataxia, vertigo

◆ **GI:** Nausea and vomiting

◆ **GU:** Elevated serum creatinine and BUN levels

◆ **Hematologic:** Leukopenia, thrombocytopenia, anemia

Special Considerations

◆ Do not give to patients with known hypersensitivity to the drug, severe bone marrow depression, or severe neurologic toxicity.

◆ If patients who have been heavily treated with cisplatin or alkylating agents and have cisplatin-induced toxicity are given altretamine, monitor their neurologic function before each course of treatment.

◆ Obtain peripheral blood counts before initiation of treatment.

◆ Administer antiemetics to patients receiving high-dose courses. For nausea and vomiting not controlled by antiemetics, the dose should be reduced or discontinued according to the patient's tolerance.

◆ Amifostine

(a-mee-**phos**'-tin)   Ethyol   Pregnancy Category C

Mechanism of Action

Amifostine is dephosphorylated at the tissue site by alkaline phosphatase to form free thiol. Once inside the cell, the free thiol binds with and neutralizes the reactive species of cisplatin. It also acts as a potent scavenger of oxygen free radicals. This action is important because free radicals can damage cell membranes, DNA, and other important cell components, which will lead to cell death.

Indications

Used to reduce the cumulative renal toxicity associated with cisplatin-based therapies in advanced ovarian cancer or non-small cell lung cancer. It is also indicated to alleviate moderate xerostomia associated with radiation therapy.

Metabolism/Excretion

Rapidly cleared from the plasma. Elimination half-life: about 88 minutes. Excreted by the renal system.

Dosage Range

◆ **With cisplatin therapy:** 910 mg/m^2 given as a 15-minute infusion once a day 30 minutes before the cisplatin-based treatment.

◆ **For moderate xerostomia:** 200 mg/m^2 given as a 3-minute IV infusion starting 15 to 30 minutes before standard fraction radiation therapy.

◆ Use in children, elderly patients, and patients with pre-existing cardiovascular or cerebrovascular conditions has not been evaluated.

Drug Preparation/Stability

Supplied as a sterile lyophilized powder in 10-mL single-use vials. Each vial contains 500 mg of the drug and 500 mg of mannitol. When stored in the refrigerator at 2° to 8°C, the unused vial is chemically and physically stable for 15 months. Reconstitute the drug with 9.5 mL of sterile 0.9% sodium chloride solution, resulting in a formulation containing 50 mg of amifostine and 50 mg of mannitol/mL. The reconstituted solution can be further diluted with sterile sodium chloride solution for dosage adjustment and should be adjusted to equal a 50-mL solution. Reconstituted amifostine is stable for 5 hours at room temperature (15° to 25°C) or for up to 24 hours under refrigeration (2° to 8°C).

Drug Administration

♦ **Before cisplatin treatment:** give as a 15-minute IV infusion 30 minutes before chemotherapy. The patient should be adequately hydrated and maintained in a supine position. Monitor blood pressure every 5 minutes during the infusion.

♦ **Before radiation:** give as a 3-minute IV infusion. Patients should be well hydrated before the infusion. Give antiemetics before and in conjunction with the drug. Monitor blood pressure before and after the infusion.

Drug Interaction

None known. Use caution in patients taking antihypertensive drugs or other drugs that could potentiate hypotension. Contraindicated in patients sensitive to mannitol or aminothiol compounds.

Side Effects and Toxicities

♦ **Cardiac:** Transient reduction in systolic blood pressure

♦ **GI:** Nausea and vomiting, which can be severe. Can be relieved with an antiemetic regimen containing dexamethasone (20 mg) and a serotonin 5-HT3 receptor antagonist.

♦ **Other:** Hypocalcemia, fever, chills, dyspnea, skin rashes, urticaria, sneezing, sleepiness, flushing, hiccups, and chills

Special Considerations

♦ Ensure that the patient is sufficiently hydrated before treatment. Do not administer to patients who are dehydrated or are taking antihypertensive therapy that cannot be interrupted for 24 hours.

♦ Maintain the patient in a supine position during the infusion.

◆ Obtain a baseline blood pressure, and monitor blood pressure every 5 minutes during and 5 minutes after the infusion is completed. If the blood pressure drops below the threshold level, it may be necessary to interrupt the infusion. Restart the infusion if the blood pressure returns to threshold within 5 minutes and the patient is asymptomatic. Refer to the following manufacturer's guidelines for interruption of infusion in relation to blood pressure thresholds.

Baseline systolic BP (mm Hg)	100	100–119	120–139	140–179	>180
Amount of decrease in BP	20	25	30	40	50

◆ Infuse the drug within 15 minutes; a longer infusion period increases the incidence of side effects.
◆ Administer antiemetics before and in conjunction with amifostine. Monitor fluid balance, especially when severe emesis occurs.

◆ Aminoglutethimide

(a-meen-oh-glow-**teth**'-i-mide)   Cytadren   Pregnancy Category D

Mechanism of Action

Inhibits adrenocortical steroid synthesis by blocking the production of adrenal glucocorticoids, mineralocorticoids, estrogens, and androgens.

Indications

Suppression of adrenal function in patients with Cushing's syndrome. Unlabeled use: To cause "chemical adrenalectomy" in patients with advanced breast cancer and patients with metastatic prostate cancer.

Metabolism/Excretion

Well absorbed orally and excreted in the urine. Half-life: 11 to 16 hours.

Dosage Range

◆ **Adult:** Initial dose is 250 mg/day PO at 6-hour intervals. If cortisol suppression is not adequate, the dosage may be increased in increments of 250 mg/day at 1- to 2-week intervals to a total daily dose of 2 g. If adverse side effects occur, including extreme drowsiness or a skin rash that persists for 5 days or longer or becomes severe, or if the patient develops excessively low cortisol levels, reduce the dose or discontinue the drug.

◆ **Pediatric:** Safety and efficacy not established.

Drug Preparation/Stability

Available in 250-mg scored tablets. Protect tablets from light and dispense from a light-resistant container. Do not store above 30°C.

Drug Administration

PO

Drug Interaction

◆ Decreased effectiveness of warfarin, so dose may need to be increased.

◆ Enhanced metabolism of dexamethasone, so hydrocortisone should be used for replacement.

Side Effects and Toxicities

◆ **Cardiac:** Orthostatic hypotension, tachycardia (rare)

◆ **CNS:** Drowsiness, headache

◆ **Cutaneous:** Morbiliform rash, pruritus (may be due to allergic or hypersensitivity reactions)

◆ **Endocrine:** Adrenal insufficiency was noted in Cushing's syndrome patients who were treated for at least 4 weeks. Occasional masculinization and hirsutism in women; precocious sexual development in men.

◆ **GI:** Nausea and anorexia

◆ **Other:** Fever, myalgia

Special Considerations

◆ Avoid in patients who have hypersensitivity to the drug.

◆ Monitor adrenocortical function. If hypofunction occurs, give supplements such as hydrocortisone. Avoid dexamethasone.

◆ Monitor blood pressure at regular intervals because of the potential for hypotension. Advise patients to watch for signs of hypotension (e.g., weakness and dizziness) and teach the appropriate measures to be taken should they occur.

♦ Warn patients that drowsiness may occur and that they should not engage in activities that may be hazardous because of decreased alertness.

♦ Inform patients that effects may be potentiated by alcohol.

♦ Anastrozole

(an-**as**'-troo-zol)   Arimidex   Pregnancy Category C

Mechanism of Action

Anastrozole is a selective nonsteroidal aromatase inhibitor. Many breast cancers have estrogen receptors; the growth of these tumors is stimulated by estrogen. In postmenopausal women, the main source of estrogen is the conversion of adrenal androgen to estrogen (primarily estradiol) by aromatase in the peripheral tissues, such as the adipose tissue.

Indications

Treatment of advanced breast cancer in postmenopausal women whose disease has progressed after tamoxifen therapy.

Metabolism/Excretion

Metabolized by the hepatic system and excreted in the urine. Half-life: 7 days.

Dosage Range

♦ **Adult:** For breast cancer, 1 mg/day.
♦ **Pediatric:** Safety and efficacy not established.

Drug Preparation/Stability

Available in 1-mg tablets.

Drug Administration

PO

Drug Interaction

None known

Side Effects and Toxicities

♦ **Cardiac:** Chest pain, peripheral edema

- ◆ **CNS:** Dizziness, depression, headache
- ◆ **Cutaneous:** Rash
- ◆ **GI:** Vomiting, diarrhea, constipation, abdominal pain, anorexia, dry mouth
- ◆ **Other:** Bone pain, pharyngitis, increased cough, pelvic pain

Special Considerations

Replacement therapy with glucocorticoids or mineralocorticoids is not necessary with anastrozole because it does not affect cortisol or aldosterone secretion.

◆ Bicalutamide

(bye-ka-**loo**′-ta-myde)   Casodex   Pregnancy Category X

Mechanism of Action

Bicalutamide is a nonsteroidal antiandrogen that inhibits the uptake and binding of androgens to the androgen receptors in the prostate gland and the cancer cells. In prostatic carcinoma, the cells are androgen sensitive and respond to treatment that counteracts the effect of androgen or removes the source of androgen.

Indications

Used concomitantly with a luteinizing hormone–releasing hormone (LHRH) for the treatment of advanced prostatic cancer. Unlabeled use: Combined with orchiectomy, if orchiectomy is preferred over the LHRH analogue.

Metabolism/Excretion

Extensively metabolized in the liver and excreted in the urine and feces. Half-life: 5.8 days.

Dosage Range

With an LHRH analogue, 5 mg/day. Should be given at the same time each day.

Drug Preparation/Stability

Available as white, film-coated tablets. Store tablets at room temperature (20° to 25°C).

Drug Administration

PO

Drug Interaction

Bicalutamide is 96% bound to serum proteins and has been found to displace coumarin analogues in vitro. The prothrombin time should be monitored, and dose adjustment of the anticoagulant may be necessary.

Side Effects and Toxicities

◆ **CNS:** Anxiety, depression, hypertonia, confusion, neuropathy, somnolence, nervousness
◆ **Cutaneous:** Dry skin, pruritus, alopecia
◆ **Endocrine:** Gynecomastia, breast pain, diabetes mellitus
◆ **GI:** Constipation, diarrhea, nausea, vomiting, abnormal liver function test results
◆ **GU:** Decreased libido, urinary frequency, dysuria, urgency, retention
◆ **Hematologic:** Anemia, leukopenia
◆ **Other:** Myasthenia, arthritis, myalgia, leg cramps, dyspnea

Special Considerations

◆ Contraindicated in patients with hypersensitivity to the drug or any of its components.
◆ Monitor liver function regularly, especially in patients receiving long-term therapy. Use with caution in patients with moderate to severe hepatic impairment.
◆ Teach the patient to take the drug in combination with an LHRH analogue at the same time each day. Therapy should not be interrupted unless the physician has been consulted.

◆ Bleomycin

(blee-oh-**mye'**-sin)   Blenoxane   Pregnancy Category D

Mechanism of Action

A cell cycle–specific antitumor antibiotic that inhibits DNA, RNA, and protein synthesis.

Indications

Palliative treatment of lymphomas; squamous cell carcinoma of the cervix, skin, head and neck, and vulva; and testicular carcinoma.

Metabolism/Excretion

Rapidly inactivated in the liver and excreted by the renal system. About 70% of the dose is excreted unchanged in the urine. Half-life: 2 hours.

Dosage Range

Dose may be written in units or mg; 1 unit = 1 mg.
The first two doses for lymphoma patients should be 2 units or less because of the possibility of an anaphylactoid reaction. If none is observed, follow the regular dosage schedule as follows:

Adult

◆ **Lymphosarcoma, reticulum cell sarcoma, squamous cell carcinoma, testicular carcinoma:** 0.25 to 0.50 units/kg (10 to 20 units/m^2) given IV, IM, of SQ weekly or twice weekly.

◆ **Hodgkin's disease:** As above. After a 50% response is achieved, give a maintenance dose of 1 unit/day or 5 units/week IV or IM.

◆ Response if any will be seen within 2 weeks in patients with Hodgkin's disease or testicular carcinoma, or within 3 weeks in patients with squamous cell cancer. If no improvement is seen within these periods, it is unlikely to occur.

Pediatric

Safety and efficacy not established.

Drug Preparation/Stability

For IM or SQ administration, reconstitute contents of vial in 1 to 5 mL of sterile water for injection, sodium chloride for injection, 5% dextrose injection, or bacteriostatic water for injection. For IV use, dissolve contents of vial in 5 mL physiologic saline or glucose. The preparation is stable for 24 hours at room temperature in sodium chloride, 5% dextrose solution, and 5% dextrose with heparin (100 or 1000 units). Keep powder refrigerated.

Drug Administration

SQ, IM, IV push over 10 minutes or as a continuous 24-hour infusion.

Drug Interaction
♦ Decreases the oral bioavailability of digoxin.
♦ Decreases the pharmacologic effects of phenytoin.

Side Effects and Toxicities
♦ **Cutaneous:** Hyperpigmentation, erythema, pruritus, rash, hyperkeratosis, alopecia, nail changes
♦ **GI:** Anorexia, vomiting, weight loss, stomatitis, hepatic toxicity
♦ **GU:** Decreased renal function
♦ **Hypersensitivity:** Idiosyncratic reaction similar to anaphylaxis: hypotension, fever, chills, hypotension, and wheezing (1% noted in lymphoma patients)
♦ **Pulmonary:** Dyspnea and rales, pneumonitis; pulmonary fibrosis
♦ **Other:** Fever, chills

Special Considerations
♦ Use with caution in patients older than 70 years, those with active pulmonary disease, or those receiving oxygen.
♦ Maximum cumulative lifetime dose: 400 units.
♦ May cause irritation at the site of injection (irritant not a vesicant).
♦ Monitor closely for anaphylactoid reactions. A test dose may be needed during initial treatment.
♦ Obtain baseline and ongoing chest x-rays and pulmonary function tests to assess for pulmonary toxicity.
♦ If the patient is undergoing surgery, the anesthesiologist should be informed about bleomycin use because the pulmonary toxicity from bleomycin may be enhanced by the high intraoperative fractional-inspired oxygen (FIO_2).
♦ Advise the patient to avoid sunlight.
♦ Mix 24-hour infusions in glass, not in plastic.

♦ Busulfan

(byoo-**sul**′-fan)   Myleran   Pregnancy Category D

Mechanism of Action
Busulfan is a cell cycle–nonspecific alkylating agent that interferes with DNA replication and the transcription of RNA, resulting in the disruption of nucleic acid functioning.

Indications

◆ Chronic myelogenous leukemia: less effective in patients who lack the Philadelphia chromosome. Has been found to induce remission in 80% to 90% of patients treated. Not effective in patients in the blastic phase.

◆ Other uses: severe thrombocytopenia and polycythemia vera. Also used in the marrow-ablating regimen before bone marrow transplantation for the treatment of malignant and nonmalignant conditions.

Metabolism/Excretion

Extensively metabolized and slowly excreted in the urine. Crosses the placental barrier. Half-life: unknown.

Dosage Range

◆ **For induction of remission:** Usual adult dose is 4 to 8 mg/day, but doses of 1 to 12 mg/day have been used. Dosing is on a weight basis according to the manufacturer; dosing is the same for adults and children, with recommended daily doses of about 0.06 mg/kg or 1.8 mg/m². Continue until the leukocyte count drops to about 15,000/mm³. Patients in remission should be seen monthly. Treatment should be resumed when the leukocyte count reaches 50,000/mm³.

◆ **Maintenance therapy:** If remission is <3 months, maintenance therapy of 1 to 3 mg/day is advised. Pediatric dosage is 0.06 to 0.12 mg/kg daily. Dosage should be titrated to maintain a leukocyte count of about 20,000/mm³.

Drug Preparation/Stability

Store in a well-sealed container at 15° to 30°C.

Drug Administration

PO; available in 2-mg scored tablets.

Drug Interaction

Hepatotoxicity, esophageal varices, and portal hypertension have been reported in patients taking thioguanine concomitantly.

Side Effects and Toxicities

◆ **GI:** Dryness of the oral mucosa and cheilosis
◆ **GU:** Hyperuricemia may occur because of extensive

purine catabolism. Other reported renal effects are uric acid nephropathy, renal stones, and acute renal failure. These may be prevented by adequate hydration, alkalinization of urine, and administration of allopurinol. A wasting or Addison-like syndrome characterized by melanoderma, asthenia, hypotension, nausea, vomiting, diarrhea, fatigue, apathy, and confusion occasionally occurs and is resolved by stopping busulfan therapy.

◆ **Hematologic:** Usually dose-related and reversible after therapy is discontinued. Adverse effects include severe leukopenia, anemia, and severe thrombocytopenia. Agranulocytosis, which may occur from overdosage, may progress to pancytopenia, which can be fatal. The course can be prolonged, with recovery occurring after 1 month to 2 years. Pancytopenia is potentially reversible.

◆ **Pulmonary:** "Busulfan lung" can occur after long-term therapy (average of 4 years). This syndrome is manifested by bronchopulmonary dysplasia progressing to pulmonary fibrosis. Discontinuation of the drug and the use of corticosteroids may be helpful, but patients may die 6 months after the diagnosis of this syndrome despite these measures.

◆ **Reproductive:** Can cause fetal harm. Causes ovarian suppression and amenorrhea with menopausal symptoms in premenopausal women. Ovarian fibrosis and and atrophy have also occurred. In men, impotence, sterility, azoospermia, and testicular atrophy have been reported.

Special Considerations

◆ Give medication at the same time each day.

◆ Ensure adequate hydration before and during treatment because of the risk of hyperuricemia. Alkalinization of the urine and the administration of allopurinol may be necessary to deal with this adverse effect.

◆ Obtain periodic blood tests and respiratory tests before, during, and after therapy.

◆ Capecitabine

(kap-ah-**ceet**'-a-bean)   Xeloda   Pregnancy Category D

Mechanism of Action

Capecitabine is a prodrug to be activated preferentially at tumor sites, thus improving the therapeutic efficacy of 5-

fluorouracil (5-FU). This drug is converted to 5-FU in a three-step process. First, it is metabolized to 5'-deoxy-5-fluorocytidine (5'DFCR) by a liver enzyme. Second, 5'DFCR is converted into 5'-deoxy-5-fluoridine by the enzyme cytidine deaminase. This conversion occurs in hepatic and tumor tissues.

Indications

Patients with metastatic breast cancer refractory to paclitaxel and an anthracycline-containing regimen, or cancer resistant to paclitaxel and for whom further anthracycline therapy is not indicated.

Metabolism/Excretion

Capecitabine is metabolized in the liver and at the cellular level, and is excreted from the lungs and in the urine. Half-life: 45 minutes.

Dosage Range

◆ **Adult:** 2500 mg/m2 daily PO in two divided doses about 12 hours apart given at the end of a meal for 2 weeks followed by a one-week rest period. Given in a three-week cycle.

◆ **Pediatric:** Safety and efficacy not established.

Drug Preparation/Stability

Capecitabine is available in 150 and 500 mg tablets. No preparation is required; store at room temperature.

Drug Administration

Capecitabine is administered orally, always within 30 minutes of a meal. Have the patient swallow the tablet whole with water.

Drug Interaction

◆ Increased serum levels of capecitabine noted when administered immediately after aluminum hydroxide and magnesium hydroxide antacids.

◆ Increased toxicity and even death may occur when capecitabine is combined with leucovorin; avoid this combination.

Side Effects and Toxicities

◆ **CNS:** paresthesias, fatigue, headache, dizziness, insomnia

♦ **Cardiac:** angina, MI, arrythmias
♦ **GI:** diarrhea, sometimes severe and requiring discontinuation of the drug; nausea, vomiting, stomatitis, abdominal pain
♦ **Hematologic:** neutropenia, thrombocytopenia, anemia, lymphopenia, hyperbilirubinemia
♦ **Integumentary:** hand and foot syndrome, dermatitis, nail disorder

Special Considerations

♦ Contraindicated in the presence of known drug allergy to fluorouracil, with pregnancy or lactation.
♦ Use caution with renal or hepatic impairment and with severe diarrhea or intestinal disease; in these cases, patients are more likely to develop toxic effects. Cardiac adverse effects are more likely to occur with known coronary artery disease.
♦ Arrange to discontinue the drug if any signs of severe toxicity occur—severe nausea, diarrhea, hand and foot syndrome (characterized by numbness, paresthesias, tingling, painless or painful swelling, erythema, desquamation, blistering, and severe pain in hands and/or feet). Arrange for a rest period and consider reinitiating therapy.
♦ Monitor the patient's nutritional status and fluid and electrolyte balance. Provide supportive care and fluids as needed.
♦ To alleviate possible side effects: always administer capecitabine within 30 minutes of a meal; provide regular mouth care; encourage small and frequent meals to alleviate some of the GI effects; loperamide may be helpful for limiting the diarrhea.
♦ Laboratory tests (CBC, electrolytes) should be monitored during therapy.

♦ Carboplatin

(**kar**′-bo-pla-tin)	Paraplatin, CBDCA	Pregnancy Category D

Mechanism of Action

Carboplatin is a cell cycle–nonspecific alkylating agent that prevents cell replication by producing intra- and inter-DNA cross-links.

Indications

Ovarian cancer (advanced) previously treated with other cyto-toxic agents, including cisplatin. Endometrial cancer, relapsed and refractory acute leukemia, metastatic seminoma, small cell lung cancer, squamous cell carcinoma of the head and neck.

Metabolism/Excretion

About 70% is excreted in the urine 24 hours after administration. Plasma half-life: 1.1 to 2.0 hours. Postdistribution half-life: 2.6 to 5.9 hours.

Dosage Range

Adult

◆ **Single agent:** 360 mg/m^2 on day 1 given every 4 weeks. In general, the carboplatin dose should not be repeated until the neutrophil count is 2000/mm^3 and the platelet count is ≥100,000/mm^3.

◆ **Combination with cyclophosphamide:** 300 mg/m^2 on day 1 IV every 4 weeks.

◆ **Formula dosing:** Another method for calculating the initial carboplatin dose is the use of a mathematical formula based on the pre-existing renal function and desired platelet nadir. This approach takes into account the pretreatment renal function, which might be overlooked using the formula based on body surface. The formula, proposed by Calvert, is as follows:

$$\text{Total dose (mg)} = (\text{target AUC}) \times (\text{glomerular filtration rate} + 25)$$

AUC (area under the curve) is obtained by plotting the plasma level of a drug over time and measuring the area beneath the plotted curve. Glomerular filtration rate has a good correlation to creatinine clearance. Therefore, this value is used in the calculation for carboplatin. The target area under the curve of 4 to 6 mg/mL/ min using carboplatin as a single agent is often used.

Dose may be modified for patients with myelosuppression after prior therapy according to the following schedule:

Platelets	Neutrophils	Adjusted Dose (from Previous Course)
100,000	2000	125%
50,000–100,000	500–2000	No adjustment
<50,000	<500	75%

Baseline Creatinine Clearance	Recommended Dose (Day 1)
41–59 mL/min	250 mg/m^2
16–40 mL/min	200 mg/m^2

Pediatric
Safety and efficacy not established.

Drug Preparation/Stability

Reconstitute contents of vial with sterile water for injection, 5% dextrose in water, or sodium chloride injection. Store unopened vials at room temperature and protect from sunlight. Reconstituted preparation is stable for 24 hours; discard after 8 hours because of the lack of bacteriostatic preservative.

Drug Administration

Administer by IV infusion in 500 mL of 5% dextrose in water or normal saline over 30 minutes to 1 hour. May be infused continuously over 24, 96, and 120 hours and continuously over 21 days using an ambulatory infusion pump.

Drug Interaction

◆ Increased ototoxicity and nephrotoxicity when given with aminoglycosides.
◆ The renal effects of nephrotoxic compounds may be potentiated by carboplatin.

Side Effects and Toxicities

◆ **CNS:** Peripheral neuropathies, mild paresthesia, visual disturbances, change in taste perception
◆ **GI:** Nausea and vomiting, which usually cease within 24 hours with antiemetic therapy, abdominal pain, diarrhea, constipation, abnormal liver function (mild and reversible)
◆ **GU:** Less renal toxicity than cisplatin; abnormal renal function is usually mild and reversible.
◆ **Hematologic:** Bone marrow suppression is dose-limiting. The hematologic effects are manifested by thrombocytopenia, neutropenia, and leukopenia. The nadir occurs about day 21, with recovery by day 28.
◆ **Hypersensitivity:** Rash, urticaria, erythema, pruritus, brochospasm (rare)
◆ **Other:** Pain, asthenia, alopecia

Special Considerations

◆ Contraindicated in patients with a history of severe allergic reaction to cisplatin or other compounds containing platinum.

◆ Carboplatin is less nephrotoxic than cisplatin. It is not cross-resistant to it.

◆ Do not use aluminum needles; carboplatin can precipitate and lose its effectiveness when in contact with aluminum.

◆ Cover long infusions with a brown bag; drug is light-sensitive.

◆ Advise patient to have blood tests before and during therapy.

◆ Monitor creatinine clearance closely; dose modification may be necessary if creatinine clearance is less than 60 mL/min.

◆ Have epinephrine, corticosteroids, and antihistamines handy in case of anaphylactic reactions to the drug.

◆ Carmustine

(car-**mus**'-teen)   BCNU, BICNU   Pregnancy Category D

Mechanism of Action

A cell cycle–nonspecific alkylating agent, carmustine is a nitrosourea derivative that alkylates DNA by causing cross-links and strand breaks.

Indications

◆ Palliative treatment of primary and metastatic brain tumors
◆ Multiple myeloma
◆ Disseminated Hodgkin's disease and non-Hodgkin's lymphoma
◆ Malignant melanoma
◆ Carcinomas of the GI tract, breast, and lungs (response rate 21%)
◆ Ewing's sarcoma and Burkitt's tumor (limited studies)

Metabolism/Excretion

Rapidly metabolized and slowly excreted in the urine and in the lungs (10%). Half-life: 15 to 30 minutes.

Dosage Range

Adult
◆ **Single agent:** In untreated patients, 150 to 200 mg/m^2 every 6 weeks. May be given as a single dose or divided into daily doses of 75 to 100 mg/m^2 on 2 consecutive days.

◆ **Combined with other agents or in patients with compromised bone marrow function:** Adjust dosage according to the manufacturer's guidelines. Repeat courses should not be given until leukocyte and platelet counts reach acceptable levels (4000/mm^3 and 100,000/mm^3, respectively). An adequate number of neutrophils should also be present. Subsequent doses are usually given at 6-week intervals because of the delayed and cumulative bone marrow suppression effects.

Pediatric
Safety and effectiveness not established.

Drug Preparation/Stability

Package contains 100 mg carmustine and a vial containing 3 mL of diluent. Reconstitute the drug with the diluent plus 27 mL sterile water for injection. This solution can be further diluted with 0.9% sodium chloride or 5% dextrose. After reconstitution, the solution is stable in a glass container for 24 hours at 4°C or for 8 hours at 25°C when protected from light.

Drug Administration

IV infusion over 1 to 2 hours. Patients may experience intense pain and burning at the needle site or along the vein if the infusion is given more quickly. Can be given intra-arterially, but this method can cause ocular toxicity.

Drug Interaction

◆ Concomitant cimetidine therapy can potentiate the neutropenic and thrombocytopenic effects of carmustine.
◆ Amphotericin may enhance the cellular uptake of carmustine.

Side Effects and Toxicities

◆ **Cutaneous:** Local burning at the infusion site or along the course of the vein; vasospasm may occur. Facial flushing is observed during rapid infusion of the drug. Accidental contact with the reconstituted solution has produced transient hyperpigmentation of the exposed area.

◆ **CNS:** Dizziness, ataxia

◆ **GI:** Nausea and vomiting (2 to 4 hours after administration, lasting 24 hours), stomatitis, hepatotoxicity

◆ **GU:** Progressive renal failure has occurred in patients who received large, cumulative, and prolonged treatment.

◆ **Hematologic:** Delayed hematologic toxicity usually occurs 4 to 6 weeks after administration. Thrombocytopenia, the most severe side effect, appears and subsides earlier than any of the other hematologic toxicities.

◆ **Pulmonary:** Pulmonary infiltrate, fibrosis, or both

Special Considerations

◆ Monitor hematologic parameters before therapy and weekly during therapy.

◆ Dispense drug in a glass container; do not use plastic.

◆ Use a large vein when administering the IV infusion; do not infuse rapidly because this might cause severe pain and burning at the site.

◆ Wear gloves when handling carmustine. Accidental contact causes a brown discoloration of the skin.

◆ Chlorambucil

(klor-**am**'-byoo-sil)   Leukeran   Pregnancy Category D

Mechanism of Action

Chlorambucil is a nitrogen mustard derivative that works as an alkylating agent by interfering with DNA replication and the transcription of RNA and by disrupting the functioning of nucleic acid.

Indications

◆ Palliative treatment of chronic lymphocytic leukemia

◆ Advanced malignant (non-Hodgkin's) lymphoma

◆ Hodgkin's disease

◆ Unlabeled uses: Macroglobulinemia, polycythemia vera, trophoblastic neoplasms, ovarian neoplasms, nephrotic syndrome, advanced breast cancer

Metabolism/Excretion

Metabolized in the liver and excreted in the urine. Half-life: 1 hour.

Dosage Range

◆ **Adult:** For initiation of therapy or short courses of therapy, the usual dosage is 0.1 to 0.2 mg/kg given as a single dose for 3 to 6 weeks. The usual dosage comes out to 4 to 10 mg/day. Alternatively, adults may receive 3 to 6 mg/day. Dose modifications should be made if chlorambucil is given within 4 weeks after a full course of radiation treatment or if myelosuppression occurs. The recommended dose should not exceed 0.1 mg/kg/day or 6 mg/day. It is also believed that short courses of chlorambucil are safer than continuous maintenance therapy, although both are effective. The manufacturer states that continuous therapy may appear to maintain patients in remission and suggests that the drug should be withdrawn in those patients to determine whether maintenance therapy is necessary. The maintenance dose should not exceed 0.1 mg/kg per day and may be as low as 0.03 mg/kg or 2 to 4 mg daily.

◆ **Pediatric:** 0.1 to 0.2 mg/kg or 4.5 mg/m^2 given as a single dose daily.

Drug Preparation/Stability

Available as 2-mg tablets. Store tablets in a closed, light-resistant container at 15° to 30°C. Expiration date is 1 year after the date of manufacture. An oral suspension containing 2 mg/mL is also available and is stable for 7 days when stored in an amber glass bottle at 5°C.

Drug Administration

PO

Drug Interaction

None known

Side Effects and Toxicities

◆ **Cutaneous:** Rash or dermatitis, urticaria, alopecia
◆ **CNS:** Focal or generalized seizures, tremors, muscle

twitching, confusion, agitation, ataxia, flaccid paralysis, hallucinations

◆ **GI:** If doses of ≥20 mg are given, nausea, vomiting, diarrhea, gastric discomfort, abdominal pain, and anorexia have been seen. Hepatotoxicity with jaundice and elevated serum alkaline phosphatase and aspartate transferase may also occur.

◆ **Hematologic:** Leukopenia, thrombocytopenia; myelosuppression is dose-limiting.

◆ **Pulmonary:** May cause a syndrome of bronchopulmonary dysplasia and interstitial pneumonitis or pulmonary fibrosis manifested by cough, fever, rales, dyspnea, respiratory distress, or hypoxia.

◆ **Other:** Hyperuricemia

Special Considerations

◆ Contraindicated in patients who are hypersensitive or resistant to chlorambucil.

◆ Use with caution in patients with a seizure history or head trauma or those receiving epileptogenic drugs.

◆ Obtain CBC at least once a week while patient is receiving drug therapy. Monitor leukocyte counts every 3 to 4 days after each of the weekly CBCs for the first 3 to 6 weeks. Adjust dose or discontinue the drug temporarily if leukocyte or platelet counts decrease significantly.

◆ Advise patient to report fever, sore throat, unusual bleeding, or bruising.

◆ Cisplatin

(**sis**′-pla-teen)   CDDP, Platinol   Pregnancy Category D

Mechanism of Action

Cisplatin is a widely used heavy metal, cell cycle–nonspecific agent that interferes with cell division by binding to DNA and functioning as an alkylating agent.

Indications

◆ Metastatic testicular tumors
◆ Metastatic ovarian tumors
◆ Advanced carcinoma of the bladder

Metabolism/Excretion

Metabolized in the liver and mostly excreted in the urine; insignificant amounts of fecal excretion.

Dosage Range

Adult

♦ **Metastatic testicular tumor:** 20 mg/m^2 IV daily for 5 days.

♦ **Metastatic ovarian tumor:** As a single agent, 100 mg/m^2 IV once every 4 weeks. In combination with cyclophosphamide, 75 to 100 mg/m^2 on day 1 every 4 weeks. The cyclophosphamide dosage is given at 600 mg/m^2 on day 1 once every 4 weeks. In combination therapy, the cisplatin and cyclophosphamide doses are given sequentially.

♦ **Advanced bladder carcinoma:** Cisplatin should be given as a single agent. The dosage range is 50 to 70 mg/m^2 IV once every 3 to 4 weeks, depending on prior treatment with radiation, chemotherapy, or both. The patient must be prehydrated with 1 to 2 L of fluid given over 6 to 8 hours. Adequate urine output should be maintained for 24 hours. A repeat course should not be given until the following parameters are at acceptable levels: serum creatinine <1.5 mg/100 mL; BUN <25 mg/mL; platelets ≥100,000/mm^3; WBC count ≥4000 mm/m^3; and an audiogram within normal limits.

Pediatric

Safety and efficacy not established.

Drug Preparation/Stability

Reconstitute 10- or 50-mg vial with 10 or 50 mL of sterile water, respectively, to yield 1 mg/mL. Store unopened vials at room temperature (27°C). Reconstituted solution is stable for 24 hours at ambient temperature. Protect solution from light if it will not be used within 6 hours.

Drug Administration

IV infusion, slow or continuous, at no more than 1 mg/min. Given intraperitoneally or intra-arterially for investigational applications. The reconstituted drug is mixed in 1 to 2 L 5% dextrose in 0.45% or 0.33% normal saline with 37.5 g mannitol, and the solution is infused over 6 to 8 hours.

Drug Interaction

◆ Plasma levels of anticonvulsant drugs may become subtherapeutic with cisplatin administration.

◆ The response duration of cisplatin was adversely affected when pyridoxine was given with cisplatin and altretamine.

◆ Cisplatin produces cumulative nephrotoxicity, which is potentiated by aminoglycosides and iodine contrast.

◆ Cisplatin is incompatible in solutions that do not contain chloride ions, such as 5% dextrose in water. It is stable in dextrose 5% in 0.45 normal saline.

Side Effects and Toxicities

◆ **CNS:** Ototoxicity, manifested initially by high-frequency hearing loss; **peripheral neuropathy (dose-limiting when the cumulative dose exceeds 400 mg/m^2)** occurs 3 to 8 weeks after the last dose of cisplatin; loss of taste and muscle cramps occur.

◆ **GI:** Severe nausea and vomiting occur within 1 to 4 hours after treatment and usually last for 24 hours. Delayed nausea and vomiting have also been noted 24 hours after treatment and may persist for up to 5 days; hepatic toxicity, anorexia, and alterations in taste can also occur.

◆ **GU: Nephrotoxicity is dose-limiting and can be severe.** Electrolyte intolerances, particularly hypomagnesemia, hypocalcemia, and hypokalemia, can occur.

◆ **Hematologic:** Leukopenia, thrombocytopenia, and anemia. WBC count and platelet nadir occur in 10 to 15 days.

◆ **Hypersensitivity:** Anaphylactoid reaction

Special Considerations

◆ Contraindicated in patients with pre-existing renal and hearing impairment and myelosuppression.

◆ Monitor peripheral blood counts weekly.

◆ Perform liver function tests periodically.

◆ Assess neurologic status regularly. Ask patients about difficulty in picking up small objects or buttoning buttons, and peripheral numbness or tingling.

◆ Ensure adequate hydration and diuresis before and after treatment. Depending on the clinician's protocol, diuresis may be enhanced by the use of furosemide or mannitol. IV therapy for hydration may consist of dextrose in

0.45% normal saline with potassium or magnesium additives.

◆ Administer appropriate antiemetic regimen when giving doses of >75 mg/m² because of the highly emetogenic potential of cisplatin at this dose level.

◆ Make sure a baseline audiogram is obtained and subsequent testing is done after the initial dose. Assess patient for signs of hearing loss, manifested initially by complaints of tinnitus or buzzing in the ears.

◆ Do not use aluminum needles; a black precipitate will form and the potency of the drug is reduced.

◆ Cladribine

(kla′-drih-been)   Leustatin   Pregnancy Category D

Mechanism of Action

Unclear. A high intracellular concentration of cladribine is believed to inhibit ribonucleotide reductase, causing subsequent DNA strand breaks and inhibition of DNA synthesis and repair.

Indications

Hairy cell leukemia.

Metabolism/Excretion

Metabolized in the liver and excreted in the urine. Half-life: 5.4 hours.

Dosage Range

◆ **Adult:** 0.09 mg/kg per day for 7 consecutive days for a total dose of 0.63 mg/kg, or as a continuous 7-day infusion of the total 0.63-mg/kg dose.

◆ **Pediatric:** Safety and efficacy not established.

Drug Preparation/Stability

As a 24-hour infusion: Dilute the appropriate dose in 500 mL 0.9% sodium chloride. It is stable for 24 hours in a polyvinyl chloride bag at room temperature and ambient lighting. As a single continuous 7-day infusion: Withdraw the appropriate dose (7 × 0.09 mg/kg) from the individual vials using a 0.22-micron filter, and add to the infusion reservoir. Dilute with bacteriostatic 0.9% sodium chloride containing benzyl alcohol preservative, drawn through a 0.22-micron syringe filter to a total volume of 100 mL. Do not use dextrose in water as a diluent because it accelerates the degradation of the drug. Stable for 7 days in the Pharmacia Deltec medication cassette.

Drug Administration

As a 24-hour infusion daily for 7 consecutive days or as a single infusion for the total 7-day dose.

Drug Interaction

None known

Side Effects and Toxicities

◆ **Cardiac:** Edema and tachycardia were reported in 6% of patients during the first 2 weeks after initiation of treatment.

◆ **CNS:** Fatigue, headache

◆ **Cutaneous:** Rash was reported in 27% of treated patients after 2 weeks of initial therapy. The rash was mild and occurred in patients who were previously treated with drugs known to cause rash. Pain, erythema, and phlebitis were felt at the site of injection.

◆ **GI:** Mild nausea (28%), decreased appetite (17%), vomiting (13%), diarrhea (10%), and constipation (9%); all effects occurred 2 weeks after initiation of treatment. Patients with advanced malignancy also had transient increases in aspartate transferase.

◆ **GU:** Acute renal insufficiency is dose-related.

◆ **Hematologic: Severe bone marrow depression as evidenced by neutropenia, anemia, and thrombocytopenia is dose-limiting.**

◆ **Metabolic:** Tumor lysis syndrome and hyperuricemia were found in patients with a large tumor burden. These were alleviated by the administration of allopurinol.

◆ **Musculoskeletal:** Myalgia (7%), arthralgia (5%)

◆ **Pulmonary:** Abnormal breath sounds (11%), cough (10%), abnormal chest sounds (9%), shortness of breath (7%)

Special Considerations

◆ Contraindicated in patients with known hypersensitivity to the drug or any drug.

◆ Administer with caution to patients with renal or hepatic dysfunction.

◆ Monitor hematologic profile carefully and frequently during and after therapy.

◆ Neutropenic fevers frequently occur during the first month of treatment, so watch patients carefully.

◆ Tumor lysis and hyperuricemia can occur. Consider the empiric use of allopurinol.

◆ Cyclophosphamide

(cy-klo-**foss**'-fa-mide)   Cytoxan,   Pregnancy Category D
                             Neosar

Mechanism of Action

Cyclophosphamide is a cell cycle–nonspecific nitrogen mustard derivative that acts as an alkylating agent by interfering with DNA replication and transcription of RNA, ultimately resulting in the disruption of nucleic acid function.

Indications

Acute or chronic lymphocytic leukemia, acute myeloblastic leukemia, breast cancer, Hodgkin's disease, lymphoma, multiple myeloma, mycosis fungoides, neuroblastoma, ovarian cancer, retinoblastoma.

Metabolism/Excretion

Metabolized in the liver and excreted in the urine. Half-life: 4 to 6 hours.

Dosage Range

Adult

◆ **Induction** (for patients with no hematologic deficiencies): 40 to 50 mg/kg is usually administered IV in divided doses over a course of 2 to 5 days. If the patient has bone marrow deficiency, reduce the initial loading dose by 33% to 50%. PO, give 1 to 5 mg/kg daily.

◆ **Maintenance:** Various IV dosing schedules include 10 to 15 mg/kg (350 to 550 mg/m^2) every 7 to 10 days and 3 to 5 mg/kg (110 to 185 mg/m^2) twice weekly.

Pediatric

- ◆ **Induction:** PO or IV, 2 to 8 mg/kg or 60 to 250 mg/m² daily.
- ◆ **Maintenance:** PO, 2 to 5 mg/kg or 50 to 150 mg/m², administered twice weekly.

Drug Preparation/Stability

Use sterile water for injection or bacteriostatic water for injection containing parabens to yield a final concentration of 20 mg/mL. The reconstituted solution may be given by slow IV push through a running IV. Higher doses (>600 mg) are infused in 50 mL 5% dextrose in water over 30 minutes to 3 hours. Use the reconstituted solution within 24 hours if stored at room temperature or within 6 days if refrigerated. For oral use, dissolve the powder for injection in aromatic elixir; solutions containing 1 to 5 mg/mL are generally used. The solution should be refrigerated in a glass container and used within 14 days.

Drug Administration

PO or IV; in some cases, given intraperitoneally in doses of 200 to 500 mg.

Drug Interaction

- ◆ Potentiates cardiotoxic effects of other drugs such as doxorubicin.
- ◆ Prolongs the neuromuscular blocking activity of succinylcholine.
- ◆ Decreases serum digoxin level and therapeutic effect, necessitating an increased digoxin dose.

Side Effects and Toxicities

- ◆ **Cardiac:** In high-dose therapy (120 to 270 mg/kg), as a single agent or as part of a combination regimen, deaths have been reported from diffuse hemorrhagic myocardial necrosis and from acute myopericarditis syndrome. Other cardiotoxic effects observed with high doses include severe and sometimes fatal congestive heart failure that occurs within a few days of initial therapy and hemipericardium secondary to hemorrhagic myocarditis and myocardial necrosis.
- ◆ **Cutaneous:** Alopecia begins 3 weeks after initiation of therapy. There is transverse ridging, retarded growth, or

hyperpigmentation of fingernails, and skin pigmentation and nonspecific dermatitis.

◆ **GI:** Anorexia, nausea, and vomiting (dose-related; these occur 2 to 4 hours after administration and peak in 12 hours; they are relieved by antiemetics). Occasionally, diarrhea, hemorrhagic colitis, mucosal irritation, hepatotoxicity, and oral ulceration have been reported.

◆ **GU:** Sterile hemorrhagic cystitis can occur, especially in children receiving long-term therapy. Hematuria usually resolves after the drug is discontinued but may last for several months. Bladder fibrosis with or without hemorrhagic cystitis has also been reported.

◆ **Hematologic: The hematologic adverse effects are leukopenia, thrombocytopenia, hypoprothrombinemia, and anemia, which are dose-limiting** and reversible when the drug is discontinued. Leukopenia nadir occurs within 2 weeks, recovery after 3 to 4 weeks.

◆ **Metabolic:** Hyperuricemia, especially in patients with non-Hodgkin's lymphoma and leukemia, syndrome of inappropriate diuretic hormone (SIADH) excretion, hyponatremia, and hypokalemia

◆ **Pulmonary:** Interstitial pulmonary fibrosis

◆ **Reproductive:** Interferes with oogenesis and spermatogenesis. Amenorrhea, gonadal suppression, sterility, and ovarian fibrosis can occur.

◆ **Other:** Headache, dizziness, and myxedema. Faintness, facial flushing, and diaphoresis have occurred with IV use. Anaphylactic reaction (rare) has also been reported.

Special Considerations

◆ Contraindicated in patients with severely compromised bone marrow function and with known hypersensitivity to the drug.

◆ Consider dose modification in patients with impaired renal, hematopoietic, and hepatic function.

◆ Monitor hematologic status carefully at least weekly during the few months of therapy and until maintenance therapy is set, and then at intervals of 2 to 3 weeks. For high-dose therapy, ECG should be checked and documented before administration.

◆ To prevent hemorrhagic cystitis, ensure adequate hydration. Have the patient drink 10 to 12 glasses a day before, during, and for at least 24 hours after treatment; encourage the patient to void frequently, especially at bedtime, to avoid contact of metabolites with bladder wall.

◆ Advise the patient to take oral doses on an empty stomach in the morning.

◆ Cytarabine

(cye-**tar**'-a-been)   ARA-C, cytosine   Pregnancy Category D
                 arabinoside,
                 Cytosar-UR

Mechanism of Action

Cytarabine is a cell cycle–specific (S phase) antimetabolite that inhibits cell development from the G1 to the S phase.

Indications

◆ Induction of remission in acute myelogenous (non-lymphocytic) leukemia
◆ Induction of remission in acute lymphocytic leukemia
◆ Meningeal leukemia and other meningeal neoplasms
◆ Chronic myelogenous leukemia

Metabolism/Excretion

Rapidly and extensively metabolized, mainly in the liver, and excreted in the urine. Half-life: 1 to 3 hours.

Dosage Range

◆ **Induction of remission in acute leukemia:** As a single agent, 200 mg/m² by continuous IV infusion for 5 days at 2-week intervals. In combination therapy, the usual dosage is 2 to 6 mg/kg daily or 100 to 200 mg/m² daily by continuous IV infusion or in 2 or 3 divided doses by rapid injection or IV infusion for 5 to 10 days until remission is attained.

◆ **Maintenance therapy:** Usually given as a single dose of 1.0 or 1.5 mg/kg IM or SQ at intervals of 1 to 4 weeks or at 70 to 200 mg/m² daily by rapid injection or continuous IV infusion for 2 to 5 days at monthly intervals.

◆ **Refractory acute leukemia or non-Hodgkin's lymphoma:** IV infusion of 3 g/m² every 12 hours for up to 12 doses. IV infusion can be given over 1 to 3 hours.

◆ **Meningeal leukemia/neoplasms:** Intrathecal injection of 5 to 75 mg/m^2 or 30 to 100 mg/m^2 once every 4 days until cerebrospinal fluid findings return to normal; give one additional dose. Modify dose in the presence of systemic toxicity.

◆ Doses for adult and pediatric patients are usually the same. Safety and efficacy in infants not established.

Drug Preparation/Stability

Reconstitute 100-mg vial with 5 mL bacteriostatic water for injection, yielding 20 mg/mL. Add 10 mL of bacteriostatic water to a 500-mg vial to yield 50 mg/mL. Admixture can be further diluted with 5% dextrose in water or 0.9% sodium chloride. Mixed solutions are stable for 8 days; however, if a slight haze is noticed in the solution, the solution should be properly discarded.

Drug Administration

IV infusion, SQ injection, or intrathecally. There is no clinical advantage of one route over the other.

Drug Interaction

◆ GI absorption of oral digoxin may be substantially reduced with concomitant use with cytarabine.

◆ May interfere with concomitant therapy with aminoglycosides given to treat *Klebsiella pneumoniae*.

Side Effects and Toxicities

◆ **Cardiac:** Chest pain, cardiopathy

◆ **CNS:** Dizziness, somnolence, neuritis

◆ **Cutaneous:** Rash, freckling, skin ulceration, alopecia, reactions at the injection site (pain, inflammation, phlebitis, or cellulitis)

◆ **GI:** Nausea and vomiting are more severe with rapid infusion of the drug than with continuous infusion. Diarrhea, anorexia, and oral and anal inflammation and ulceration occur; less frequently, abdominal pain, sore throat, esophagitis, esophageal ulceration, GI hemorrhage, and hepatic dysfunction occur.

◆ **GU:** Urinary retention, renal dysfunction

◆ **Hematologic:** Myelosuppression, as evidenced by megaloblastosis, reticulocytopenia, leukopenia, and thrombocytopenia. Severity depends on the dose and the schedule of administration. After a 5-day course, the WBC count initially decreases after 24 hours, with a nadir at 7 to 9 days. This nadir is biphasic; a rise in the WBC count is noted, and it peaks at about 12 days. A second nadir then occurs in 15 to 24 days, followed by a rise to above the baseline count in 10 days.

◆ **Intrathecal administration:** Nausea, vomiting, fever, and transient headaches are usually mild and self-limiting. In rare cases, meningism, paresthesia, paraplegia, spastic paraparesis, and seizures have occurred. There have been reports of blindness, necrotizing leukoencephalopathy (children), and progressive ascending paralysis (children) when intrathecal cytarabine was used in conjunction with CNS irradiation and other drugs.

◆ **High-dose regimens:** Cerebral and cerebellar dysfunction manifested by somnolence, coma, and personality changes, which are reversible; hemorrhagic conjunctivitis and corneal toxicity occur. Peripheral motor and sensory neuropathies have occasionally occurred, manifested by gait disturbances, writing difficulties, paresthesia, numbness, and myalgia.

◆ **Other:** "Cytarabine syndrome" is manifested by fever, myalgia, bone pain, maculopapular rash, conjunctivitis, malaise, and occasional chest pain. Usually occurs 6 to 12 hours after administration and is relieved by corticosteroids. Hyperuricemia has also been reported.

Special Considerations

◆ Contraindicated in patients with known hypersensitivity to the drug.

◆ Assess renal and hepatic function periodically.

◆ Monitor hematologic status closely.

◆ Because of increased potential for infections and hematologic complications, instruct the patient to report fever, sore throat, or unusual bruising or bleeding.

◆ Administer a prophylactic corticosteroid ophthalmic solution before the high-dose regimen (6 hours before initial therapy and every 6 hours for the next 24 hours).

◆ Obtain a baseline neurologic assessment, including upper and lower extremity function, ocular movements, speech, gait, and fine hand coordination. Assess neurologic status before each dose.

◆ Do not administer cytarabine reconstituted with bacteriostatic water for an injection containing benzyl alcohol to neonates.

◆ Dacarbazine

(de-**kar**'-ba-zeen)   DTIC-Dome   Pregnancy Category C

Mechanism of Action

The activity may be the result of three mechanisms: alkylation, antimetabolite activity as a purine precursor, and interaction with sulfhydryl groups in proteins. DTIC appears to be more active in the G2 phase but is not particularly phase-specific.

Indications

◆ Metastatic melanoma
◆ Advanced Hodgkin's disease (combination therapy)
◆ Unlabeled use: In combination with cyclophospha- mide and vincristine, for malignant pheochromocytoma. More effective when coadministered with tamoxifen for metastatic malignant melanoma.

Metabolism/Excretion

Extensively metabolized in the liver; biphasic half-life: 9 minutes, then 5 hours. Excreted in the urine; 30% to 46% of the dose is excreted after 6 hours.

Dosage Range

Adult

◆ **Malignant melanoma:** 2.0 to 4.5 mg/kg daily for 10 days at 4-week intervals, or 250 mg/m^2 daily for 5 days at 3-week intervals.
◆ **Hodgkin's disease:** 150 mg/m^2 daily for 5 days in combination with other drugs at 4-week intervals, or 375 mg/m^2 on the first day in combination with other drugs and repeated every 15 days.

Pediatric

Safety and efficacy not established.

Drug Preparation/Stability

Reconstitute a 100-mg vial with 9.9 mL sterile water for in- jection or add 19.7 mL of the same to a 200-mg vial. The re- sultant solution yields 10 mg/mL and can be further diluted with 250 mL of D$_5$W or 0.9% normal saline and given as a

15 to 30-minute infusion. Drug vials should be protected from light and refrigerated at 2° to 8°C. Reconstituted solutions are stable for 96 hours when refrigerated and protected from light, 24 hours if not refrigerated but protected from light, and approximately 4 hours when not refrigerated or protected from light.

Drug Administration

IV push with a running line of dextrose in water or 0.9% sodium chloride, or IV infusion given over 15 to 30 minutes. Assess venous patency before, during, and after the infusion because this drug has vesicant properties. Given experimentally by intra-arterial infusion.

Drug Interaction

◆ Incompatible with heparin, lidocaine, and hydrocortisone.
◆ Decreased effectiveness with phenytoin and phenobarbital.
◆ Toxicity may be enhanced when given concomitantly with allopurinol, azathiopine, or mercaptopurine.

Side Effects and Toxicities

◆ **CNS:** Confusion, lethargy, blurred vision, seizures, headache
◆ **Cutaneous:** Facial flushing; alopecia; erythematous, macular, papular, or urticarial rashes; photosensitivity reactions
◆ **GI:** Severe nausea, vomiting, and anorexia, which occur within 1 hour after the initial dose and persist for 12 hours; these symptoms lessen with each subsequent dose. Diarrhea, stomatitis, intractable nausea and vomiting, and hepatic toxicity rarely occur.
◆ **Hematologic:** Leukopenia and thrombocytopenia occur 2 to 4 weeks after the last dose.
◆ **Local:** Pain, burning, and irritation along the site of injection if the drug extravasates; may cause tissue damage.
◆ **Other:** Flulike syndrome is manifested by fever, myalgia, and malaise occurring about 7 days after treatment and lasting 1 to 3 weeks.

Special Considerations

◆ Has vesicant properties. Check for venous patency before, during, and after treatment. Diluting the drug in 100 to 250 mL dextrose in water and slowly infusing it will minimize venous discomfort. Apply hot compresses if extravasation occurs.

◆ Monitor hematologic and hepatic function regularly.

◆ Protect the drug from sunlight; drug deactivates by 50% if left in room light for >4 hours.

◆ Teach the patient to stay away from the sun and to use skin protection with an SPF of 15 or greater.

◆ Advise the patient not to eat for 4 to 6 hours before treatment because of the high incidence of emesis. Premedicate with antiemetics.

◆ Ensure adequate hydration at least 1 hour before treatment.

◆ Dactinomycin

(dak-tee-no-**my**'-seen) Actinomycin, Pregnancy Category C
Cosmegen

Mechanism of Action

Dactinomycin is a cell cycle–nonspecific, antitumor antibiotic that interferes with RNA synthesis.

Indications

◆ Wilms' tumor

◆ Rhabdomyosarcoma

◆ Ewing's sarcoma

◆ Trophoblastic neoplasms (choriocarcinoma and chorioadenoma destruens)

◆ Testicular carcinoma

◆ As an adjunct (given by regional isolation perfusion) to surgery or as palliative treatment of various carcinomas and sarcomas that have not responded to systemic chemotherapy

Metabolism/Excretion

Slightly metabolized; excreted in urine and bile. Half-life: 36 hours.

Dosage Range

◆ Depends on the patient's tolerance, the clinical response, and whether other cytotoxic drugs or treatments are being given concomitantly. The drug must be given in short courses. When calculating the dose for obese or edematous patients, use the body surface area to relate dosage to lean body mass. Dosage for adults and children should not exceed 15 mcg/kg or 400 to 600 mcg/m² daily IV for 5 days. For adults and children, repeat courses have been given every 2 to 4 weeks, depending on the resolution of drug toxicities.

◆ **Adult:** 500 mcg/day for a maximum of 5 days.

◆ **Pediatric:** 15 mcg/day (to a maximum of 500 mcg) IV for 5 days; alternatively, a total of 2.5 mg/m² in divided doses over 1 week.

◆ **Regional isolation perfusion:** 50 mcg/kg for the pelvis or lower extremity and 35 mcg/kg for an upper extremity.

Drug Preparation/Stability

Reconstitute the powder by adding 1.1 mL sterile water for injection without preservatives for a yield of 500 mcg/mL. For pediatric use, mix the vial with 5 mL sterile water for injection without preservatives for a yield of 100 mcg/mL. Reconstituted solution may be further added to IV solutions of 5% dextrose or 0.9% sodium chloride. Protect powder from sunlight and store at 30°C. The drug should be reconstituted immediately before use, and any unused portion should be discarded. Do not use a filter, because it will remove the drug.

Drug Administration

Can be given by direct IV injection using two sterile needles, one for withdrawing the drug from the vial and the other for direct administration. However, it is preferable to administer the drug through a running IV line over 2 to 3 minutes. Do not administer by IM or SC injection.

Drug Interaction

None reported

Side Effects and Toxicities

◆ **Cutaneous:** Alopecia (7 to 10 days after administration); pruritic, maculopapular rash; acne and acneiform eruptions

◆ **GI:** Nausea and vomiting (within a few hours after administration; can last up to 24 hours), anorexia, abdominal pain, diarrhea, oral and GI ulcerations, hepatic toxicity

◆ **Hematologic:** Dose-limiting hematologic toxicity is manifested by leukopenia and thrombocytopenia. Myelosuppression occurs 1 to 7 days after course is completed. Leukocyte and platelet nadirs occur 14 to 21 days after end of course; counts return to normal in 21 to 25 days.

◆ **Local:** Drug has vesicant properties; pain and erythema can occur at injection site. Inadvertent infiltration causes severe tissue damage, and an appropriate antidote should be administered. Alopecia, radiation recall reaction, acne, hyperpigmentation, and increased sensitivity to sunlight also occur.

Special Considerations

◆ Contraindicated in patients with chicken pox or herpes zoster.

◆ Avoid extravasation.

◆ Advise patient to stay out of the sun and to wear sunscreen with SPF 15 or greater.

◆ The drug has a narrow therapeutic index; do not exceed the recommended dose.

◆ Monitor hepatic and renal function.

◆ Teach the patient to report fever, sore throat, unusual bleeding, or bruising.

◆ Monitor hematologic function frequently to determine myelosuppression. If severe myelosuppression occurs, the drug may have to be discontinued to allow bone marrow recovery.

◆ Daunorubicin Hydrochloride

(daw-no-**roo**′bi-sin)   Cerubidine,   Pregnancy Category D
                          Rubidomycin
                          Hydrochloride

Mechanism of Action

Daunorubicin is a cytotoxic, anthracycline antibiotic that inhibits the synthesis of DNA. It has antimitotic and immunosuppressive properties.

Indications

♦ Induction of remission in acute myelogenous leukemia (AML) in adults
♦ Induction of remission of acute lymphocytic leukemia (ALL) in adults and children

Metabolism/Excretion

Extensively metabolized in the liver and excreted in the urine and bile. Half-life: 18.5 hours.

Dosage Range

Total dose should not exceed 500 to 600 mg/m^2 in adults because of the incidence of cumulative cardiotoxicity. In both adults and children, the actual dose planned should take into account past and concurrent therapies, including radiation and other cytotoxic agents that are cardiotoxic. If the patient has had cardiac irradiation, the total dose should be reduced to 400 to 450 mg/m^2. If the patient has hepatic or renal impairment, as evidenced by abnormal serum bilirubin and creatinine values, the dose modification is as follows: for a serum bilirubin value of 1.2 to 3.0 mg%, 75% of the normal dose; for a serum bilirubin value of >3 mg% and a serum creatinine value of >3 mg%, half the normal dose.

Adult

♦ AML: As a single agent, 60 mg/m^2 IV daily for 3 days and repeated every 3 to 4 weeks. In combination therapy, the dosage for adults younger than 60 years is 45 mg/m^2 IV for the first 3 days of a course of induction therapy. For patients older than 60 years, the dosage is usually 30 mg/m^2 given daily for 3 days during the first course of induction and for 2 days during subsequent therapy.
♦ ALL: In combination therapy, three daily doses of 45 mg/m^2 IV for the first course of induction for remission.

Pediatric

For remission induction in ALL, 25 mg/m^2 IV as combination therapy. Frequency depends on the specific protocol. For children 2 years or younger or whose body surface area is <0.5 mg/m^2, the dose should be based on body weight.

Drug Preparation/Stability

Reconstitute by adding 4 mL sterile water for injection to a 20-mg vial; this will yield 5 mg/mL. The reconstituted solution is stable for 24 hours at room temperature and for 48 hours refrigerated. Protect the solution from light.

Drug Administration

The reconstituted dose can be further diluted by drawing the desired dose into a syringe containing 10 to 15 mL normal saline. The drug is then injected into the side arm of a free-flowing IV line. Do not give the drug IM or IV because of its vesicant properties.

Drug Interaction

Incompatible with heparin.

Side Effects and Toxicities

◆ **Cardiac:** Congestive heart failure occurs in adults at a cumulative dose >550 mg/m^2; the limit is lower for patients who have received prior radiation therapy to the heart. At doses <550 mg/m^2, rare instances of pericarditis/myocarditis have been reported. Children and infants are more susceptible than adults to the cardiotoxic effects of anthracycline therapy, including daunorubicin. The manifestations of cardiotoxicity in children are impaired left ventricular systolic performance, reduced contractility, congestive heart failure, and death. These conditions may occur months to years after treatment.
◆ **Cutaneous:** Reversible alopecia
◆ **GI:** Mild nausea and vomiting, mucositis 3 to 7 days after administration, diarrhea
◆ **Hematologic:** Bone marrow suppression; WBC and platelet nadir occurs in 10 to 14 days
◆ **Local:** Tissue necrosis if extravasation occurs
◆ **Other:** Hyperuricemia caused by rapid lysis of leukemic cells

Special Considerations

◆ Assess hematologic, hepatic, cardiac, and renal function before, during, and after treatment. Consider dose modification if problems occur.
◆ Advise the patient to expect a transient reddish coloration in the urine.
◆ Avoid extravasation; ensure good venous access and patency.

◆ Monitor uric acid levels and give allopurinol if necessary.

◆ Dexrazoxane

(dex-**ra**'-zoo-zayne)   Zinecard   Pregnancy Category C

Mechanism of Action

Dexrazoxane is a chelating agent that interferes with iron-mediated radicals thought to be responsible for anthracycline-induced cardiotoxicity.

Indications

Reduction of the incidence and severity of cardiomyopathy associated with doxorubicin therapy in women with metastatic breast cancer who have received a cumulative dose of 300 mg/m^2 and who could benefit from continued doxorubicin therapy.

Metabolism/Excretion

Not bound to plasma proteins; 42% of the dose is excreted in the urine.

Dosage Range

◆ **Adult:** Ratio of dexrazoxane to doxorubicin of 10:1.
◆ **Pediatric:** Safety and efficacy not investigated.

Drug Preparation/Stability

Available in 230- and 500-mg single-use vials. Should not be mixed with other medications. Reconstitute with 0.167 molar sodium lactate injection to yield a concentration of 10 mg/mL. The reconstituted formulation is transferred to a bag and remains stable for 6 hours at room temperature (15° to 30°C) or if refrigerated at 2° to 8°C. Discard unused solution.

Drug Administration

Slow IV push or IV drip over 15 minutes. After dexrazoxane is completed, the doxorubicin should be given so that both drugs are infused over a 30-minute period.

Drug Interaction

None known; does not interfere with the pharmacokinetics of doxorubicin.

Side Effects and Toxicities

◆ **Hematologic:** May add to the myelosuppressive effects of doxorubicin, causing more severe leukopenia, thrombocytopenia, and granulocytopenia than when given without dexrazoxane.

◆ **Other:** Pain at the injection site, which may be ameliorated by giving the drug as a rapid infusion rather than by slow IV push and by using a central venous access device.

Special Considerations

◆ Do not give with nonanthracycline-based chemotherapy.

◆ Monitor hematologic profile. Dexrazoxane's myelosuppressive effect is mild, but because it is administered with cytotoxic agents that are myelosuppressive, it can have an additive effect on the patient's reserves.

◆ There is clinical evidence that dexrazoxane can interfere with the clinical efficacy of the FAC (fluorouracil, Adriamycin, and cyclophosphamide) regimen during the first cycle. This use is therefore not recommended.

◆ Monitor cardiac function with multigated radionuclide angiography (MUGA) periodically.

◆ Diethylstilbestrol Diphosphate

(diey-e-thil-stil-**bes**'-trol)   Stilphostrol   Pregnancy
Category D

Mechanism of Action

Unknown. Diethylstilbestrol is an estrogen that affects the hormonal milieu of the body.

Indications

◆ Inoperable prostate cancer
◆ Postmenopausal metastatic carcinoma of the breast (oral therapy)

Metabolism/Excretion

Metabolized mainly in the liver and undergoes enterohepatic circulation.

Dosage Range

Adult

◆ **PO:** Initially, 50 mg three times a day; increase the dose to 200 mg, depending on the patient's tolerance. Maximum daily dose is 1 g/day. Give IV if oral dosing is not effective.

◆ **IV:** 0.5 g for 5 days; after the first cycle, 0.25 to 0.50 g once or twice weekly.

Pediatric
Not recommended

Drug Preparation/Stability

Dissolve the drug in 250 mL normal saline or dextrose in water. Keep at room temperature and away from light. A solution kept under these conditions will be stable for 5 days. Discard if cloudiness and precipitation occur.

Drug Administration

For the first 10 to 15 minutes, infuse the IV solution slowly at 1 to 2 mL/min; then adjust the rate so that the entire amount is infused over 1 hour.

Drug Interaction

Incompatible with calcium gluconate.

Side Effects and Toxicities

◆ **Cardiovascular:** Thromboembolic complications with long-term and high doses; increased risk of cardiovascular-related deaths in men receiving high-dose estrogens; hypertension, edema, weight gain

◆ **Cutaneous:** Hepatic cutaneous porphyria, erythema nodosum, erythema multiforme

◆ **GI:** Nausea and vomiting, cholestatic jaundice, weight loss

◆ **GU:** *Male:* Gynecomastia, loss of libido, impotence, voice change. *Female:* Breast engorgement, uterine prolapse, exacerbation of pre-existing uterine fibroids, urinary incontinence.

◆ **Other:** Headache, hyperglycemia, hypercalcemia

Special Considerations

◆ Obtain baseline cardiovascular status and monitor during therapy.

◆ Instruct the patient about possibility of fluid retention and bloating; instruct the patient to monitor weight.

◆ Emphasize the importance of maintaining a low-sodium diet.

◆ Review with the patient the possible changes in sexual function. Explore the patient's feelings about the impact of these changes on his or her sexual patterns. Provide support and counseling as needed.

◆ Teach the patient to report signs and symptoms of dyspnea, edema, pain and tenderness in calf muscles, and weight gain.

◆ Instruct the breast cancer patient to report signs and symptoms of hypercalcemia—drowsiness, increased urine output, increased thirst, and constipation.

◆ Ensure that the patient has antiemetic medications.

◆ Docetaxel

(doh-see-**tax**′-el)   Taxotere   Pregnancy Category D

Mechanism of Action

Docetaxel belongs to the taxoid family and acts by disrupting the microtubular network in the cells, which is essential for their mitotic and interphase functions.

Indications

Locally advanced or metastatic breast carcinoma after progression of the disease with anthracycline-based therapy or relapse during anthracycline-based adjuvant treatment.

Metabolism/Excretion

The oxidative metabolites, which are metabolized in the liver, are excreted in the urine and feces, mainly in the feces. Half-life: 11 hours.

Dosage Range

◆ **Adult:** 60 to 100 mg/m^2 IV every 3 weeks. Patients who are initially given 100 mg/mL and experience neutropenic fevers, a neutrophil count of <500 cells/mm^3 for more than 1 week, severe or cumulative cutaneous reactions, or severe peripheral neuropathy should have the dose reduced to 75 mg/m^2. If symptoms persist at the new level, the dose may be further reduced to 50 mg/m^2 or discontinued. Patients who are started at a lower dose of 60 mg/m^2 and who do not experience the above symptoms may be given higher doses.

◆ **Pediatric:** Safety and efficacy not established.

Drug Preparation/Stability

Available in 20- and 80-mg vials with diluents, which when reconstituted will ensure a premix concentration of 10 mg/mL. The premixed solution can be further diluted with 250 mL 0.9% sodium chloride solution or 5% dextrose solution to produce a final concentration of 0.3 to 0.9 mg/mL of docetaxel. If a dose >240 mg is needed, use a larger volume of the infusion so that a concentration of 0.9 mg/mL is not exceeded. Diluted docetaxel should be mixed in a glass bottle or plastic bag (polypropylene, polyolefin) and administered through polyethylene-lined administration sets. Premixed or fully prepared solutions should be used as soon as possible after reconstitution. However, the premixed solution is stable for 8 hours at room temperature (15° to 25°C) or refrigerated at 2° to 8°C.

Drug Administration

IV infusion over 1 hour at room temperature with ambient lighting. The patient should be premedicated with an oral corticosteroid such as dexamethasone 8 mg twice a day for 5 days starting 1 day before docetaxel administration. This reduces the incidence and severity of fluid overload and possible hypersensitivity reactions.

Drug Interaction

No clinical studies conducted.

Side Effects and Toxicities

◆ **Cardiac:** Hypotension, fluid retention as evidenced by edema and weight gain and less frequently pleural effusion, pericardial effusion, or ascites

◆ **Cutaneous:** Reversible rash and localized eruptions on the feet or hands, arms, face, or thorax associated with pruritus within 1 week of infusion; alopecia

◆ **GI:** Nausea and vomiting, diarrhea, stomatitis

◆ **Hematologic:** Neutropenia is the dose-limiting toxicity; nadir occurs on day 8, with recovery in 7 days.

Special Considerations

◆ Monitor weight and observe for signs and symptoms of fluid retention.

◆ Advise the patient that possible weight gain or fluid retention subsides when the drug is discontinued. Administer antidiuretic therapy (spironolactone, furosemide) if ordered by the physician.

◆ Observe the blood count, particularly the neutrophil count, before each dose. If a growth factors test is ordered, ascertain that the patient knows how to self-administer an SQ injection.

◆ Administer premedications as ordered to avoid hypersensitivity reactions.

◆ Doxorubicin Hydrochloride

(dox-oh-**roo**′-bih-sin)   Adriamycin   Pregnancy Category D

Mechanism of Action

Doxorubicin is an anthracycline antibiotic that binds to nucleic acids by intercalating with the DNA double helix.

Indications

◆ Acute lymphoblastic leukemia
◆ Acute myeloblastic leukemia
◆ Wilms tumor, neuroblastoma
◆ Soft tissue and bone sarcoma
◆ Carcinoma of the breast and ovaries, and transitional cell bladder, thyroid, and gastric cancer
◆ Hodgkin's disease, malignant lymphoma, bronchogenic cancer (small cell)

Metabolism/Excretion

Metabolized in the liver; excreted in the urine, bile, and feces. May discolor urine from 1 to 48 hours.

Dosage Range

◆ **Adult:** *As a single agent,* 60 to 75 mg/m^2 IV as a single dose every 21 days, or 30 mg/m^2 IV for 3 days every 4 weeks. When used in *combination therapy,* 40 to 50 mg/m^2 as a single IV injection every 21 to 28 days. The dose should

be adjusted if the patient has inadequate bone marrow reserve caused by old age, prior therapy, or neoplastic marrow infiltration. Dose modifications are recommended for the following serum bilirubin levels: for 1.0 to 2.3 mg, reduce dose by 50%; for 3.1 to 5.0 mg, reduce dose by 75%.
◆ **Pediatric:** Safety and efficacy not established.

Drug Preparation/Stability

Reconstitute the 50- or 100-mg vials with 25 or 50 mL, respectively, of 0.9% sodium chloride or sterile water for injection. The diluted solution yields 2 mg/mL of the drug. The reconstituted drug is stable for 24 hours at room temperature or for 48 hours if refrigerated at 36° to 46°F. It should be protected from sunlight.

Drug Administration

Slow IV push through a free-flowing IV solution over 3 to 5 minutes or as a continuous 24-hour infusion using a central venous access device. Doxorubicin is a parenteral vesicant; avoid extravasation.

Drug Interaction

Do not mix with heparin because of the danger of precipitate formation. It is also incompatible with aminophylline, cyclosporine, dexamethasone, diazepam, furosemide, and streptozocin.

Side Effects and Toxicities

◆ **Cardiac:** Cardiomyopathy with high cumulative doses ($>$550 mg/m^2 or 450 mg/m^2 with concurrent cardiotoxic or radiation therapy)
◆ **Cutaneous:** Alopecia (complete but reversible), radiation recall, photosensitivity, hyperpigmentation of nail beds and dermal creases, facial flushing, local tissue necrosis if extravasation occurs
◆ **GI:** Nausea, vomiting, mucositis, diarrhea, anorexia
◆ **GU:** Reddish discoloration of urine, hyperuricemia, dysuria, urgency
◆ **Hematologic:** Bone marrow depression; leukocyte nadir occurs in 10 to 14 days with recovery by day 21.
◆ **Hypersensitivity:** Fever, chills, urticaria, flulike syndrome

Special Considerations

◆ Avoid extravasation because of the drug's vesicant potential. Use large veins with a new peripheral line.

◆ Teach the patient to report pain or burning. Extravasation can occur with a good venous return and without initial complaints of stinging at the injection site. Discontinue infusion immediately and start a new line if suspected extravasation occurs.

◆ Advise the patient to expect a red discoloration of the urine, which is harmless.

◆ Monitor hepatic function; assess renal and hematologic function.

◆ The maximum cumulative lifetime dose is 550 mg/m²; however, if the patient has had myocardial irradiation or prior cytotoxic medications, the cumulative lifetime dose is 400 mg/m².

◆ Assess cardiac function before, during, and after treatment. Any significant changes in the ECG and echocardiogram should be evaluated because of the potential for irreversible cardiac damage.

◆ Doxorubicin Hydrochloride Liposome

(dox-oh-**roo**′-bih-sin)   Doxil   Pregnancy Category D

Mechanism of Action

The active ingredient is doxorubicin hydrochloride, which exerts its cytotoxic effect by binding DNA and inhibiting nucleic acid synthesis. Doxorubicin hydrochloride is encapsulated in liposomal vesicles consisting of one or more concentric lipid bilayers surrounding aqueous compartments. This form allows slow release of the drug, decreases rapid exposure to sensitive organ systems, and provides specific target delivery. It is hypothesized that because of their small size and persistence in the circulation, the pegylated liposomes can penetrate tumor vasculature.

Indications

◆ AIDS-related Kaposi's sarcoma in patients with disease that has progressed with prior combination chemotherapy or in patients who are intolerant to such therapy

◆ Metastatic carcinoma of the ovary refractory to both paclitaxel and platinum-based regimens.

Metabolism/Excretion

The major metabolite of doxorubicin, doxorubicinol, was detected at very low levels in the plasma of patients who were given a 10- or 20-mg/m^2 dose. Terminal half-life: 55 hours.

Dosage Range

◆ **Adult:** 20 mg/m^2 IV once every 3 weeks for patients with Kaposi's sarcoma; 50 mg/m^2 IV every 4 weeks for ovarian cancer. The initial rate should be 1 mg/min to minimize the risk of acute infusion-related reactions for ovarian cancer patients; if no reactions are noted, the infusion can be given in an hour.

◆ **Pediatric:** Safety and efficacy not investigated.

Drug Preparation/Stability

Available in single-dose 10-mL vials equivalent to 2 mg/mL. The solution appears translucent and is red. The appropriate dose up to 90 mg must be diluted with 5% dextrose injection only. Other diluents and bacteriostatic agents should not be used. The diluted formulation should be refrigerated at 2° to 8°C and given within 24 hours. Unopened vials should be refrigerated at similar temperatures. Short-term freezing (<1 month) does not have a deleterious effect on the drug.

Drug Administration

IV infusion. Do not use in-line filters. Do not give as a bolus or without dilution. Do not give IM or SQ. Doxil should be considered an irritant, so take proper precautions in administration.

Drug Interaction

No formal studies conducted, but may potentiate the cytotoxic effects of radiation therapy and chemotherapeutic agents such as cyclophosphamide and 6-mercaptopurine.

Side Effects and Toxicities

◆ **Cardiac:** Arrhythmia (nonspecific), cardiomyopathy, heart failure, pericardial effusion, tachycardia

◆ **Cutaneous:** Radiation recall, alopecia, palmar-plantar

erythrodysesthesia characterized by swelling, pain, erythema, and desquamation on the hands and feet
♦ **Hematopoietic:** Leukopenia, anemia, thrombocytopenia
♦ **Infusion reaction:** Acute reaction (with first infusion) manifested by flushing, shortness of breath, facial swelling, headache, chills, back pain, tightness in the throat and chest, or hypotension. Extravasation may occur at the injection site with or without a stinging or burning sensation.

Special Considerations

♦ Monitor cardiac, hematologic, and hepatic function. Use reduced dosage in patients with impaired hepatic function.
♦ Avoid extravasation.
♦ Observe warnings related to the conventional formulation of doxorubicin hydrochloride, particularly in relation to its cardiac toxicity.

♦ Epirubicin HCl

(ep-ee-**roo**'-bi-sin)　　Ellence　　Pregnancy Category D

Mechanism of Action

Epirubicin, closely related to doxorubicin and daunorubicin, is a cytotoxic anthracycline that binds to DNA and inhibits DNA and protein synthesis, leading to cell death. It also interferes with replication and transcription by inhibiting DNA helicase and generates cytotoxic free radicals.

Indications

Epirubicin is used as adjunctive therapy in patients with axillary node tumor involvement following resection of primary breast cancer.

Metabolism/Excretion

Epirubicin is metabolized in the liver and is excreted in bile, feces, and urine. Half-life: 12 minutes, then 3.3 hours, then 29.6 hours.

Dosage Range

◆ **Adult:** 50–120 mg/m2 IV; dose is individualized.
◆ **Pediatric:** Safety and efficacy not established.

Drug Preparation/Stability

Reconstitute 50-mg vial with 0.9% sodium chloride or sterile water for injection. The reconstituted solution is stable for 24 hours at toom temperature or 48 hours if refrigerated. Protect solution from sunlight. Take appropriate precautions in handling and disposing of vials.

Drug Administration

Administer epirubicin slowly into tubing of a freely running IV infusion of sodium chloride injection or 5% dextrose injection. Attach the tubing to a butterfly needle inserted in a large vein; avoid using veins over joints, or those in extremities with poor perfusion. The rate of administration depends on the vein and the dosage, but do not give in less than 3–5 minutes. Facial flushing and red streaking over the vein are often signs that administration has been too rapid.

Drug Interaction

◆ Increased toxicity if epirubicin is given in conjunction with cardiotoxic, hepatotoxic, or cytotoxic agents; avoid such combinations.
◆ Risk of severe toxicity if given with cimetidine. Discontinue cimetidine before administering epirubicin.

Side Effects and Toxicities

◆ **Cardiac:** Cardiac toxicity, congestive heart failure, phlebosclerosis, delayed cardiomyopathy
◆ **GI:** Nausea, vomiting, mucositis, anorexia, diarrhea
◆ **Hematologic:** myelosuppression, hyperuricemia due to cell lysis
◆ **Dermatologic:** Complete but reversible alopecia, hyperpigmentation of nailbeds and dermal creases, facial flushing
◆ **Local:** Severe local cellulitis, vesiccation and tissue necrosis if extravasation should occur
◆ **Hypersensitivity:** Fever, chills, urticaria, anaphylaxis
◆ **Other:** Carcinogenesis, including leukemia

Special Considerations

◆ Do baseline monitoring for cardiac status, bone marrow function, renal and hepatic function.

◆ Do not administer if neutrophil count is <1500 cell/mm³.

◆ Before beginning therapy, premedicate the patient with antiemetics, allopurinol, trimethoprim/sulfamethoxozole or a fluorquinolone.

◆ Ensure adequate hydration during therapy to prevent hyperuricemia; alkalinize urine.

◆ Monitor the injection site for extravasation. If patient reports burning or stinging, discontinue infusion immediately and restart in another vein. For local subcutaneous extravasation: infiltration with corticosteroid may be ordered; flood area with normal saline and apply cold compress. If ulceration begins, arrange consultation with plastic surgeon.

◆ Monitor patient's response to therapy: serum uric acid level, cardiac output (listen for S³). CBC changes may require a decrease in the dose; consult with a physician.

◆ Monitor nutritional status and weight loss.

◆ Epoetin-alfa

(e-poe-e′-tin)   Epogen, Procrit,   Pregnancy Category C
                  EPO, erythropoietin

Mechanism of Action

Stimulates red blood cell production.

Indications

Anemia associated with chronic renal failure, anemia in HIV patients receiving zidovudine, and anemia associated with cancer chemotherapy.

Metabolism/Excretion

Metabolized in the serum and excreted in the urine. After IV administration, the circulating half-life is 4 to 13 hours. Serum concentrations peak within 5 to 24 hours after SQ administration.

Dosage Range

Adult

♦ **Chronic renal failure:** Initially, 50 to 100 units/kg three times a week. Reduce dose as the hematocrit approaches 36% or increases by more than 4 points in any 2-week period. Dosage is individualized to maintain the hematocrit in target range. Administer IV in dialysis patients; inject SQ or administer IV in patients not receiving dialysis. Unless clinically indicated, dosage adjustments should not be made more frequently than once a month. Maintenance dose is titrated to maintain hematocrit target range.

♦ **HIV patients receiving zidovudine:** Determine serum erythropoietin level before administration. Starting dose for patients with serum erythropoietin levels <500 mUnits/mL who are receiving <4,200 mg zidovudine per week: 100 units/kg as an IV infusion or SQ injection administered three times a week for 8 weeks. If desired response is not achieved after 8 weeks of therapy, increase by 50 to 100 units/kg three times a week. Maintenance dose is titrated to maintain hematocrit target range.

♦ **Anemia associated with cancer chemotherapy:** Starting dose is 150 units/kg SQ three times a week. If desired response is not achieved after 8 weeks, increase to 300 units/kg three times a week.

♦ If the hematocrit exceeds 40%, withhold the dose until it falls to 36%; then reduce dose by 25% and titrate to maintain desired hematocrit.

Pediatric

Safety and efficacy not established.

Drug Preparation/Stability

Supplied in solution for injection: single-dose preservative-free 1-mL vial containing 2000, 3000, 4000, or 10,000 units epoetin-alfa. Do not re-enter the vial, and discard unused portions. Also supplied in multidose, preserved 2-mL vial containing 20,000 units epoetin-alfa. Discard 21 days after initial entry. Store in the refrigerator at 2° to 8°C (36° to 46°F). Do not shake or freeze.

Drug Administration

SQ injection or IV infusion.

Drug Interaction

None observed during clinical trials.

Side Effects and Toxicities

- ◆ **Constitutional:** Headache, arthralgia, fatigue, fever
- ◆ **CNS:** Seizures, dizziness
- ◆ **GI:** Nausea, diarrhea, vomiting
- ◆ **Integumentary:** Redness, swelling, or itching at site of injection, clotted access, rash
- ◆ **Pulmonary and cardiovascular:** Hypertension, chest pain, cough, shortness of breath, congestion, upper respiratory infection
- ◆ **Other:** Asthenia, edema, paresthesia.

Special Considerations

- ◆ Contraindicated in patients with uncontrolled hypertension and known allergy to mammalian cell-derived products and human albumin.
- ◆ Decrease dose if the hematocrit increases 4 points in any 2-week period.
- ◆ Monitor and control blood pressure.
- ◆ Assess neurologic symptoms closely during the first 90 days of treatment because of a higher incidence of seizures during this time.
- ◆ During hemodialysis, increased anticoagulation with heparin may be needed to prevent clotting.
- ◆ Monitor hematologic parameters regularly. In chronic renal failure patients, the hematocrit should be measured twice a week; in others, it should be measured once a week until the hematocrit has been stabilized, then periodically.
- ◆ Evaluate iron status, including transferrin saturation and serum ferritin, before and during therapy. Practically all patients require iron supplements.
- ◆ For home use, instruct patient regarding SQ administration. Provide a puncture-resistant container with guidelines on disposal of used syringes and needles.

◆ Estramustine Phosphate Sodium

(ess-tra-**muss**'-teen)   Emcyt   Pregnancy Category D

Mechanism of Action

The estrogen portion facilitates the selective uptake of the drug into the cells, enhancing the alkylating effect in tissue with estrogen-positive receptor cells. This drug is cell cycle–nonspecific.

Indications

Palliative treatment of metastatic or progressive prostate carcinoma.

Metabolism/Excretion

Metabolized in the liver and excreted in the feces. Half-life: 20 hours.

Dosage Range

14 mg/kg per day in three or four divided doses. Patients should be treated for 30 to 90 days before the physician determines the possible benefits of continued treatment. Patients have been maintained on therapy for more than 3 years at dosages of 10 to 16 mg/kg per day.

Drug Preparation/Stability

Store at 36° to 46°F (2° to 8°C).

Drug Administration

Available as white opaque capsules for oral administration. Drug should be taken with water at least 1 hour before or 2 hours after meals. Do not take milk or any calcium-rich products simultaneously.

Drug Interaction

Calcium-rich products may impair absorption.

Side Effects and Toxicities

◆ **Cardiac:** Edema, dyspnea, leg cramps, thrombophlebitis, congestive heart failure, myocardial infarction, hypertension
◆ **Cutaneous:** Pruritus, easy bruising, dry skin
◆ **GI:** Nausea, vomiting, minor GI upset, anorexia, elevated hepatic enzymes
◆ **Hematologic:** Leukopenia
◆ **Other:** Breast changes, including tenderness and mild to moderate enlargement

Special Considerations

◆ Contraindicated in patients with known hypersensitivity to estradiol or nitrogen mustard. Do not use in patients with thromboembolic disorders, except where the cause of these disorders is from the tumor mass and the benefits of therapy outweigh the risks.

◆ Use caution in patients with cerebral or coronary artery disease.

◆ Closely monitor diabetic patients because the drug may cause decreased glucose tolerance.

◆ Etoposide

(e-toe-**poe**'-side)   VePesid, VP-16   Pregnancy Category D

Mechanism of Action

Etoposide is a cell cycle–specific plant alkaloid that inhibits DNA synthesis in the S and G2 phases so that cells do not enter mitosis and prophase.

Indications

Refractory testicular tumors, small cell lung cancer.

Metabolism/Excretion

Metabolized in the liver and rapidly excreted mostly by the kidneys and to a smaller extent in the bile. Half-life: 4 to 11 hours.

Dosage Range

◆ **Adult:** *In combination therapy for testicular cancer,* 50 to 100 mg/m² IV on days 1 to 5 or 100 mg/m² IV on days 1, 3, and 5. *In combination therapy for small cell lung cancer,* 35 mg/m² day for 4 days or 50 mg/m² per day for 5 days. Repeat courses are given at 3- to 4-week intervals. PO, twice the IV dose, rounded to the nearest 50 mg.

◆ **Pediatric:** Safety and efficacy not established.

Drug Preparation/Stability

Dilute the injection form with 5% dextrose or 0.9% normal saline to yield a concentration of 0.2 to 0.4 mg/mL. If the drug is diluted to yield a concentration of more than 0.4 mg/mL, precipitation might occur. Plastic devices made of ABS (acrylonitrile, butadiene, and styrene) have been reported to crack or leak when in contact with the undiluted formulation of etoposide. The diluted solution at a concentration of 0.2 and 0.4 mg/mL is stable for 96 and 24 hours, respectively, at room temperature and normal fluorescent light. Refrigerate the oral form; it is stable for 24 months at 2° to 8°C.

Drug Administration

Do not administer as a rapid infusion because of the danger of hypotension. Give over 30 to 60 minutes; may be administered over a longer period depending on the volume of the infusion. The oral form is available in 50-mg pink capsules.

Drug Interaction

◆ Concurrent use of warfarin increases the prothrombin time.
◆ Synergistic effect with cisplatin.

Side Effects and Toxicities

◆ **Cardiac:** Hypotension has been noted. This is not related to cardiac pathology; it is attributed to rapid infusion of the drug and can be ameliorated by stopping the infusion and giving the patient IV fluids and other appropriate supportive therapy.
◆ **Cutaneous:** Reversible alopecia
◆ **GI:** Mild to moderate nausea and vomiting controlled by appropriate antiemetics. GI toxicities are more common with oral administration. Hepatic toxicity is associated with doses higher than recommended.
◆ **Hematologic:** Myelosuppression is dose-related and dose-limiting and is manifested by granulocytopenia, which reaches a nadir in 7 to 14 days; platelet nadir occurs in 9 to 16 days. Recovery is noted in 20 days.
◆ **Hypersensitivity:** Anaphylactic reaction characterized by chills, fever, tachycardia, bronchospasm, dyspnea, and hypotension. These respond well to drug discontinuation and corticosteroids, antihistamines, and volume expanders. Other hypersensitivity reactions are facial and tongue swelling.

Special Considerations

◆ Contraindicated in patients with known hypersensitivity to etoposide.

◆ Administer the infusion over 30 to 60 minutes to avoid hypotension.

◆ Obtain CBC before and during therapy.

◆ Monitor prothrombin time when given with warfarin.

◆ Etoposide Phosphate

(e-to-**poe**'-side)   Etopophos   Pregnancy Category D

Mechanism of Action

Induces DNA strand breaks by an interaction with DNA-topoisomerase II or the formation of free radicals.

Indications

◆ Refractory testicular tumors (as combination therapy with other approved agents in patients who have already received appropriate surgery, chemotherapy, and radiation therapy)

◆ Small cell lung cancer (in combination with other approved agents as first-line treatment)

Metabolism/Excretion

Similar to that of etoposide.

Dosage Range

Equivalent to the etoposide doses previously mentioned. Modify dosage in patients with renal impairment and when myelosuppression occurs as a result of prior radiation and chemotherapy treatment.

Drug Preparation/Stability

Reconstitute the contents of the vial with 5 or 10 mL sterile water for injection, 5% dextrose injection, 0.9% sodium chloride injection, bacteriostatic water for injection with benzyl alcohol, or bacteriostatic sodium chloride with alcohol to a concentration equivalent to 20 or 10 mg/mL etoposide (22.7 or 11.4 mg/mL etoposide phosphate), respectively. The reconstituted formulation can be infused without further dilution or can be diluted to concentrations as low as 0.1

mg/mL with 5% dextrose injection or 0.9% sodium chloride injection. When reconstituted, store the solution in a glass or plastic container at 20° to 25°C or under refrigeration at 2° to 8°C. Use the refrigerated solution immediately on return to room temperature.

Drug Administration

IV infusion over 5 to 210 minutes. The short infusion time is an advantage over etoposide, which requires 30 to 60 minutes.

Drug Interaction

Use with caution with agents known to inhibit phosphatase activity (e.g., levamisole hydrochloride). High-dose cyclosporine (>2 g/mL) administered with oral etoposide has led to an 80% increase in the exposure to etoposide, with a 38% decrease in total body clearance of etoposide compared with etoposide alone.

Side Effects and Toxicities

◆ **Cutaneous:** Reversible alopecia, rash, urticaria, pruritus
◆ **GI:** Nausea and vomiting, mild to moderate; constipation
◆ **Hematologic:** Myelosuppression is dose-related and dose-limiting, with the leukocyte nadir occurring at day 15 to 22, the granulocyte nadir at day 12 to 19, and the platelet nadir at day 10 to 15. Marrow recovery usually occurs by day 21 but may be delayed. Cumulative myelotoxicity has not been reported.
◆ **Other:** Anaphylactic-like reactions at the initiation of treatment, manifested by facial and tongue swelling, fever, chills, back pain, loss of consciousness, cyanosis, coughing, diaphoresis, and laryngospasm

Special Considerations

◆ Monitor CBC at initiation of therapy and periodically throughout.
◆ Instruct the patient about the possibility of anaphylactic reactions. Review the signs and symptoms with the patient. At initiation of treatment, stay with the patient. Have available emergency equipment and drugs to treat anaphylaxis.
◆ Patients with low albumin levels may be at increased risk for etoposide-associated toxicities.

◆ Exemestane

(ex-e-**mes**'-tayne)   Aromasin   Pregnancy Category D

Mechanism of Action

Exemestane is an irreversible steroidal agent that inactivates aromatase, which converts androgens to estrogens, the primary source of estrogen in postmenopausal women. Estrogen depletion is the main objective when treating estrogen-dependent breast cancer.

Indications

◆ Treatment of advanced breast cancer in postmenopausal women whose disease has progressed following tamoxifen therapy.

Metabolism/Excretion

Exemestane is metabolized in the liver and excreted in the bile and feces. Half-life: 22–24 hours.

Dosage Range

The recommended dose is 25 mg once daily after a meal.

Drug Preparation/Stability

Exemestane is available in 25 mg tablets. No preparation is needed.

Drug Administration

This drug is given orally once a day after a meal.

Drug Interaction

Decreased effectiveness is noted if exemestane is combined with any estrogen-containing agents.

Side Effects and Toxicities

◆ **GI:** Nausea, vomiting, increased appetite
◆ Other side effects: Fatigue, hot flashes, pain, depression, insomnia, and increased sweating

Special Considerations

◆ Do not administer to premenopausal women or coadminister with estrogen-containing agents.

◆ Filgrastim

(fill-**grass**'-tim) Neupogen, G-CSF Pregnancy Category C
(granulocyte colony-
stimulating factor)

Mechanism of Action
Increases the number of neutrophils in the bone marrow.

Indications
◆ To reduce the incidence of infection in patients with nonmyeloid malignancies who are receiving myelosuppressive anticancer drugs that have a significant incidence of severe neutropenia with fever
◆ To reduce the duration of neutropenia in patients with nonmyeloid malignancies who are undergoing bone marrow transplant
◆ For patients undergoing peripheral blood progenitor cell collection (for mobilization of hematopoietic progenitor cells in the peripheral blood for collection by leukopheresis)
◆ For treatment of severe chronic neutropenia (congenital, cyclic, or idiopathic neutropenia)

Metabolism/Excretion
Metabolism unknown. Elimination half-life: 210 minutes for IV administration and 210 minutes for SQ injection.

Dosage Range

Adult
◆ **Cancer patients receiving myelosuppressive chemotherapy:** Starting dose, 5 mcg/kg per day SQ or slow IV infusion (over 15 to 30 minutes). Administer ≥24 hours after the administration of cytotoxic chemotherapy. Obtain CBC with differential before initiating filgrastim and twice weekly during therapy. May increase in increments of 5 mcg/kg for each chemotherapy cycle. Administer for up to 2 weeks until the neutrophil count has reached $10,000/mm^3$ after the expected chemotherapy-induced neutrophil nadir.
◆ **Cancer patients undergoing bone marrow transplant:** 10 mcg/kg per day as an IV infusion over 4 or 24

hours, or as a continuous 24-hour SQ infusion. Administer ≥24 hours after cytotoxic chemotherapy and ≥24 hours after bone marrow infusion. Obtain CBC with differential at least three times a week.

◆ **Patients undergoing peripheral blood progenitor cell collection:** 10 mcg/kg per day SQ. Give for ≥4 days before first leukopheresis procedure and continue until the last leukopheresis.

◆ **Severe chronic neutropenia:** For congenital neutropenia, 6 mcg/kg SQ twice a day; for idiopathic or cyclic neutropenia, 5 mcg/kg SQ once a day. Chronic daily administration may be required. Base dose adjustments on the clinical course and the neutrophil count. Obtain CBC with differential twice a week for the first 4 weeks and during the 2 weeks after any dose adjustments. After patient is clinically stable, may monitor every month.

Pediatric
Safety and efficacy not established.

Drug Preparation/Stability

Supplied in solution for injection: preservative-free, single-use vial containing 300 mcg/mL filgrastim or 480 mcg/1.6 mL filgrastim. Do not re-enter the vial. Discard unused portions. Store in the refrigerator at 2° to 8°C (36° to 46°F). Do not shake or freeze.

Drug Administration
SQ or IV.

Drug Interaction

Not fully evaluated. Use cautiously with drugs that potentiate the release of neutrophils (e.g., lithium).

Side Effects and Toxicities

◆ **Constitutional:** Fever, fatigue, headache
◆ **GI:** Nausea, vomiting, diarrhea, constipation, mucositis, anorexia, stomatitis
◆ **Hematologic:** Elevations in uric acid, lactate dehydrogenase, and alkaline phosphatase; anemia; thrombocytopenia
◆ **Musculoskeletal:** Medullary bone pain
◆ **Other:** Alopecia, dyspnea, cough, skin rash, chest pain

Special Considerations

◆ Contraindicated in patients with known allergy to *Escherichia coli*–derived proteins, filgrastim, or any component of the product.

◆ If dilution is required, dilute only in 5% dextrose. Do not dilute with saline because product may precipitate.

◆ In cancer patients, discontinue filgrastim if neutrophil count exceeds $10,000/mm^3$ after the chemotherapy-induced neutrophil nadir has occurred.

◆ Do not use within 24 hours before or after cytotoxic chemotherapy.

◆ Avoid simultaneous use of filgrastim with chemotherapy and radiation therapy.

◆ Avoid use in myeloid malignancies.

◆ Monitor CBC with differential regularly.

◆ For home use, instruct patient regarding SQ administration. Provide a puncture-resistant container with guidelines on disposal of used syringes and needles.

◆ Floxuridine

(flox-**yur**'-i-deen)   FUDR   Pregnancy Category D

Mechanism of Action

Floxuridine is a cytotoxic antimetabolite that acts primarily by interfering with the synthesis of DNA; to a lesser extent, it inhibits the formation of RNA.

Indications

Palliative management of GI adenocarcinoma metastatic to the liver (when given by regional intra-arterial infusion) for patients considered incurable by surgery or other means.

Metabolism/Excretion

Metabolized in the liver; excreted in the urine; also expired as respiratory carbon dioxide. It has a biphasic half-life: initial = 10 to 20 minutes; terminal = 20 hours.

Dosage Range

◆ **Adult:** 0.1 to 0.6 mg/kg per day. If is given by hepatic artery infusion, the dosage is 0.4 to 0.6 mg/kg per day because the liver metabolizes the drug, reducing systemic toxicities. Therapy can continue when side effects have resolved and should be maintained as long as a therapeutic response is observed.

◆ **Pediatric:** Safety and effectiveness not studied.

Drug Preparation/Stability

Reconstitute each vial with 5 mL sterile water for injection to yield a concentration of about 100 mg/mL. The solution can be further diluted with 5% dextrose in water or 0.9% sodium chloride to a volume appropriate to the infusion device. Store the sterile powder at 59° to 86°C. Store the reconstituted solution at 2° to 8°C for ≤ 2 weeks.

Drug Administration

By a surgically implanted catheter directed to the major artery supplying the tumor. A pump is used to ensure appropriate delivery of the drug to the intended site at a uniform rate.

Drug Interaction

None significant

Side Effects and Toxicities

◆ **Cardiac:** Myocardial ischemia
◆ **CNS:** Lethargy, malaise, vertigo, nystagmus, cerebellar ataxia, blurred vision, photophobia
◆ **Cutaneous:** Alopecia, dermatitis, hyperpigmentation, nail changes, rash
◆ **Hematologic:** Leukopenia, thrombocytopenia, anemia
◆ **GI:** Mild and infrequent nausea and vomiting, diarrhea, cramps, duodenal ulcer, gastritis, stomatitis, bleeding, glossitis, pharyngitis, abdominal pain, chemically induced hepatitis manifested by elevated alkaline phosphatase
◆ **Intra-arterial infusion:** Infection, bleeding, leakage at insertion site, dislodgement of catheter, arterial aneurysm, arterial ischemia, necrosis, abscesses

Special Considerations

◆ Use with caution in patients who are poor risks, such as those with impaired renal or hepatic function, a history of pelvic irradiation, or previous use of antineoplastic agents.

- ◆ Discontinue the drug when one of the following conditions appears:
  - ◆ Myocardial ischemia
  - ◆ Leukopenia <3500/mm³ or rapidly falling levels, thrombocytopenia <100,000 mm³
  - ◆ Intractable vomiting, diarrhea
  - ◆ Stomatitis or esophagopharyngitis (first visible sign)
  - ◆ GI bleeding, ulcer
  - ◆ Hemorrhage from any site
- ◆ Inform the patient of the possibility of reversible alopecia.

◆ Fludarabine Phosphate

(floo-**dar**'-a-been)   Fludara   Pregnancy Category D

Mechanism of Action

Fludarabine is an antimetabolite that inhibits DNA synthesis by inhibiting ribonucleic reductase, DNA polymerase, and DNA primase.

Indications

Used in patients with B-cell chronic lymphocytic leukemia (CLL) whose disease is refractory to treatment or whose disease has not progressed during treatment with at least one standard alkylating agent. Low grade lymphoma; mycosis fungoides.

Metabolism/Excretion

Converted to its active metabolite, 2-fluoro-ara-A, in the liver; primarily eliminated by the kidneys. Half-life: 10 hours.

Dosage Range

- ◆ **Adult:** 25 mg/m² as a 30-minute IV infusion for 5 consecutive days. Each course is given every 28 days. Adjust dosage because of toxicities or other conditions that may increase toxicities, such as old age, renal impairment, and bone marrow suppression.
- ◆ **Pediatric:** Safety and efficacy not established.

Drug Preparation/Stability

Add 2 mL of sterile water for injection to the lyophilized powder to get a concentration of 25 mg/mL. The powder is refrigerated. Once the drug is reconstituted, it is stable for only 8 hours.

Drug Administration

Desired dose may be further dissolved in 100 mL 5% dextrose in water or normal saline and infused IV over 30 minutes.

Drug Interaction

Do not give with pentostatin because of the severe risk of pulmonary toxicity.

Side Effects and Toxicities

- ◆ **Cardiac:** Peripheral edema, pericardial effusion, angina
- ◆ **CNS:** Weakness, agitation, confusion, peripheral neuropathy, visual disturbances, coma
- ◆ **Cutaneous:** Skin rashes, pruritus
- ◆ **GI:** Nausea, vomiting, diarrhea, stomatitis, bleeding, anorexia
- ◆ **GU:** Hemorrhagic cystitis (rare)
- ◆ **Hematologic:** Anemia, bone marrow depression
- ◆ **Metabolic:** Tumor lysis syndrome
- ◆ **Pulmonary:** Pneumonia, pulmonary hypersensitivity manifested by dyspnea, cough, and interstitial infiltrate

Special Considerations

- ◆ Contraindicated in patients with known sensitivity to the drug.
- ◆ Pay careful attention to administering the correct dose; in 36% of patients who received a dose four times greater than the recommended dose, blindness, coma, and death were reported.
- ◆ Monitor hematologic and neurologic status closely.

◆ Fluorouracil

(flure-oh-**yoor'**-a-seel) 5-FU, Adrucil Pregnancy Category D

Mechanism of Action

Interferes with DNA synthesis and formation of RNA, which are essential for cell division and growth. Causes a thymine deficiency, which leads to unbalanced growth and death of the cell.

Indications

◆ Carcinoma of the colon, rectum, breast, stomach, and pancreas

◆ Orphan drug uses: In combination with interleukin-2a recombinant for esophageal and advanced colorectal carcinoma; with leucovorin for colorectal metastatic adenocarcinoma.

Metabolism/Excretion

Primarily metabolized by the liver; excreted by the kidneys and lungs. Half-life: 8 to 20 minutes.

Dosage Range

Adult

Give 12 mg/kg for 4 consecutive days with a daily dose limit of 800 mg. If no toxicity occurs, give a 6-mg/kg dose on days 6, 8, 10, and 12. The drug is then discontinued even if there are no signs of toxicity. *For high-risk patients or those who do not have adequate nutritional status,* give 6 mg/kg for 3 consecutive days. If no toxicity is observed, give 3 mg/kg on days 5, 7, and 9 unless toxicity occurs. The daily dose should not exceed 400 mg.

For maintenance therapy, when toxicity is not a problem, follow the following dosing schedule:

1. Repeat the dosage given for the first course of treatment every 30 days after the last day of the previous course.

2. When toxic signs from the initial course have subsided, give a maintenance dose of 10 to 15 mg/kg/week as a single dose. Do not exceed 1 g/week.

Monitor the patient's response to previous treatment and make dose modifications accordingly. Patients have had 9 to 45 courses within a period of 12 to 60 months.

Pediatric

Safety and efficacy not established.

Drug Preparation/Stability

No dilution needed. Store the solution at controlled room temperature and protect it from light. A slight discoloration may occur during storage; the potency and safety of the drug are not affected. If a precipitate is noted caused by low-temperature storage, the solution should be resolubilized by heating it to 140°F, shaking it vigorously, and allowing it to cool to body temperature before administration.

Drug Administration

Infused slowly into a running IV line. Discontinue the infusion if the patient reports pain, and restart it using a new site.

Drug Interaction

Leucovorin calcium may enhance the toxicity of fluorouracil.

Side Effects and Toxicities

- ◆ **Cardiovascular:** Myocardial ischemia, angina
- ◆ **Cutaneous:** Alopecia; pruritic and maculopapular rash noted on the extremities, dry skin; fissuring photosensitivity manifested by erythema; increased pigmentation of the skin, including the veins; nail changes, including loss of nails
- ◆ **GI:** GI ulceration and bleeding
- ◆ **Hematopoietic:** Leukopenia nadir occurs between days 9 and 14 after the initial course of treatment; it is uncommonly delayed up to 20 days, with rebound happening by the 30th day. Pancytopenia, anemia, thrombocytopenia, and agranulocytosis are also noted.
- ◆ **Hypersensitivity:** Anaphylaxis, generalized allergic reactions
- ◆ **Neurologic:** Acute cerebellar syndrome (which may persist even after the drug is stopped), disorientation, confusion, headache, nystagmus
- ◆ **Ophthalmic:** Photophobia, lacrimal duct stenosis, lacrimation, visual changes
- ◆ **Other:** Thrombophlebitis, epistaxis

Special Considerations

- ◆ Contraindicated in patients with a poor nutritional status, decreased bone marrow reserve, potentially serious infection, or a known hypersensitivity to the drug.
- ◆ Do not give >800 mg/day.
- ◆ Discontinue therapy if any of the following toxicities occur:
    - ◆ Stomatitis and esophagopharyngitis (first visible signs)

◆ Leukopenia (WBC count <3,500) or a rapidly drop-
ping WBC count
◆ Thrombocytopenia (platelet count <100,000)
◆ Intractable vomiting
◆ Diarrhea
◆ GI ulceration and bleeding
◆ Bleeding from any site
◆ Advise patients of the possibility of transient alopecia
and the major manifestations of the side effects.
◆ Monitor hematologic status, especially the WBC count
with differential, before each dose.

◆ Flutamide

(**floo**′-ta-mide)   Eulexin   Pregnancy Category D

Mechanism of Action

This drug is a potent nonsteroidal agent that acts by inhibiting the uptake of androgen or the nuclear binding of androgen to target tissues.

Indications

Metastatic prostate cancer in combination with luteinizing
hormone–releasing hormone agonists such as leuprolide acetate.

Metabolism/Excretion

Metabolized in the hepatic system; excreted in the urine.
Half-life: 6 hours.

Dosage Range

◆ **Adult:** Two capsules three times a day at 8-hour intervals. The total daily dose is equivalent to 750 mg.
◆ **Pediatric:** Safety and efficacy not tested.

Drug Preparation/Stability

Store the opaque, two-toned capsules at 2° to 30°C and protect them from moisture.

Drug Administration

PO

Drug Interaction

Increases in prothrombin time have been noted when flutamide is given concomitantly with warfarin.

Side Effects and Toxicities

◆ **Cutaneous:** Rash, photosensitivity
◆ **GI:** Nausea, vomiting, diarrhea; hepatic injury, including hepatic encephalopathy, hepatic necrosis; abnormal liver function tests; cholestatic jaundice
◆ **GU:** Impotence, elevated BUN and serum creatinine levels, loss of libido
◆ **Hematologic:** Hemolytic anemia, macrocytic anemia, methemoglobinemia
◆ **Other:** Gynecomastia

Special Considerations

◆ Advise patients to take flutamide and the drug used for medical castration concomitantly. They cannot interrupt or stop taking these drugs without consulting their physician.
◆ Monitor liver function carefully. Obtain appropriate tests when initial signs and symptoms of possible hepatic injury are noted. Consider dosage reduction or discontinuation if hepatic dysfunction becomes severe.

◆ Gemcitabine

(gem-**see**'-ta-bean)   Gemzar   Pregnancy Category D

Mechanism of Action

Gemcitabine is a cell cycle–specific (S phase) cytotoxic agent that kills cells in the S phase undergoing DNA synthesis. It also blocks cells through the G1/S phase boundary.

Indications

First-line therapy for locally advanced, nonresectable stage II, III, or IV adenocarcinoma of the pancreas; also for patients previously treated with 5-fluorouracil.

Metabolism/Excretion

Active metabolite is excreted in the urine. Half-life: 1.7 to 19.4 hours.

Dosage Range

◆ **Adult:** 1000 mg/m² once a week for 7 weeks or until a dose modification is needed because of toxicities. Give subsequent cycles once a week for 3 weeks out of every 4 weeks. Modify the dosage depending on the degree of hematologic toxicity:

Absolute Granulocyte Count	Platelet Count	% of Full Dose
>1000	and >100,000	100
500–999	or 50,000–99,000	75
<500	or <50,000	HOLD

Patients who complete the first 7 weeks of treatment or the subsequent 3-week cycle can receive an escalated dose of 25% of the full dose equivalent to 1250 mg/m², provided that the absolute granulocyte count is >1500, the platelet count is >150,000, and the nonhematologic toxicity is not greater than World Health Organization grade 1. A subsequent dose escalation at 1500 mg/m² for the next cycle can be given if the same parameters are maintained.

◆ **Pediatric:** Not studied.

Drug Preparation/Stability

Add 5 mL 0.9% sodium chloride injection to the 200-mg vial or 25 mL of the same diluent to the 1-g vial. The dilutions will yield a gemcitabine concentration of 40 mg/mL. Concentrations of >40 mg/mL should not be attempted because of the danger of incomplete dissolution. The desired dose may be further diluted with 0.9% normal saline to concentrations as low as 0.1 mg/mL. Unopened vials are stable until the expiration date specified by the manufacturer when maintained at 20° to 25°C. The reconstituted solution is stable for 24 hours at 20° to 25°C. Do not refrigerate because of the possibility of crystallization.

Drug Administration

IV infusion over 30 minutes; may be given in an outpatient setting.

Drug Interaction

None known

Side Effects and Toxicities

◆ **Cardiac:** Myocardial infarction, arrhythmia, hypertension, cerebrovascular accident, peripheral edema

◆ **CNS:** Mild paresthesia

◆ **Cutaneous:** Mild alopecia, rash, pruritus

◆ **GI:** Mild to moderate nausea and vomiting, diarrhea, stomatitis, elevated serum transaminases

◆ **GU:** Mild proteinuria, mild hematuria, hemolytic uremic syndrome

◆ **Hematologic:** Bone marrow suppression, which is dose-limiting, manifested by anemia, leukopenia, and thrombocytopenia

◆ **Pulmonary:** Dyspnea, believed to be due to pulmonary problems from underlying cancer

◆ **Other:** Flulike syndrome consisting of fever, asthenia, anorexia, headache, cough, chills, and myalgia

Special Considerations

◆ Contraindicated in patients with a known hypersensitivity to the drug.

◆ Use with caution in patients with renal or hepatic impairment.

◆ Do not prolong drug infusion longer than 60 minutes and do not give more frequently than once a week because of the danger of increased toxicities.

◆ Monitor hematologic status before commencing treatment and on subsequent cycles.

◆ Check renal and hepatic function, including serum transaminase and serum creatinine levels, before administration and periodically afterward.

◆ Goserelin Acetate

(**goe**'-se-rel-in)   Zoladex   Pregnancy Category X

Mechanism of Action

This drug is an analogue for luteinizing hormone–releasing hormone and acts on the pituitary hormone to inhibit the secretion of gonadotropin, causing chemical orchiectomy within 2 to 4 weeks.

Indications

◆ Advanced prostatic cancer when orchiectomy or estrogen administration is not indicated

   ◆ Endometriosis
   ◆ Advanced breast cancer

Metabolism/Excretion

Metabolized in the liver; excreted in the urine. Half-life: 4.2 hours.

Dosage Range

Adult

   ◆ **Men:** A 3.6-mg implant every 28 days or a 10.8-mg implant every 12 weeks; intended for long-term administration.
   ◆ **Women:** A 3.6-mg implant every 28 days; recommended duration is 6 months.

Pediatric

Safety and efficacy not established.

Drug Preparation/Stability

Available as a preloaded, sterile, disposable syringe with a 14-gauge needle. The unit is contained in a sealed, light- and moisture-proof, aluminum foil laminate pouch containing a desiccant capsule. The pouch should be stored at room temperature.

Drug Administration

Administered SQ into the upper abdominal wall using an aseptic technique, as follows:

   1. Inspect the syringe for any damage. Make sure the drug is visible through the translucent chamber.
   2. Select an area on the upper abdominal wall and cleanse with an alcohol swab. Use a local anesthetic if needed.
   3. Stretch the skin with one hand, and with the dominant hand insert the needle at a 45° angle into the subcutaneous tissue.
   4. Change the direction of the needle so it parallels the abdominal wall. Push the needle until the hub touches the skin.
   5. Withdraw the needle 1 cm to create a space to discharge the drug; fully depress the plunger to discharge the drug into the site.
   6. Withdraw the needle and confirm discharge by ensuring that the tip of the plunger is visible within the tip of the needle.

7. Bandage the site.
8. Document administration.

Drug Interaction

None known

Side Effects and Toxicities

◆ **Cardiovascular:** Arrhythmia, cerebrovascular accident, hypertension, pulmonary embolus, cerebral ischemia, angina pectoris, edema
◆ **CNS:** Dizziness, headache, insomnia, emotional lability, paresthesia, asthenia
◆ **Cutaneous:** Rash, acne, seborrhea, pruritus, herpes simplex
◆ **GI:** Nausea, anorexia, constipation, diarrhea, ulcer, hematemesis
◆ **GU:** Sexual dysfunction, decreased libido, vaginal bleeding, gynecomastia, urinary tract impairment, breast tenderness and swelling
◆ **Other:** Hot flashes, bone pain, pelvic pain, flulike syndrome, osteoporosis, voice alterations

Special Considerations

◆ Use in pregnancy is contraindicated in women being treated for endometriosis.
◆ Obtain baseline vital signs, heart rate, and kidney function tests.
◆ Teach the patient to report shortness of breathing, dyspnea, palpitations, and problems with urination and defecation.
◆ Assess normal sexual patterns. Explore the patient's feelings about possible sexual dysfunction. Offer support and sexual counseling if needed.
◆ Instruct the female patient that menstruation should stop with effective doses of the drug. If regular menstruation occurs, the patient should notify her physician. Breakthrough menstrual bleeding may occur with one or more successive missed doses.
◆ Advise the patient to use nonhormonal contraception. If the patient becomes pregnant during therapy, discontinue the drug and advise the patient about the risks to the fetus.

◆ Monitor the patient during the first month of treatment because transient worsening of symptoms or occurrence of additional signs and symptoms of prostate and breast cancer (spinal cord compression, ureteral obstruction, bone pain, hypercalcemia) may occur.

◆ Initiate standard treatment for the preceding; in the case of spinal cord compression or renal impairment, consider an immediate orchiectomy.

◆ Emphasize the importance of adhering to the dosage schedule.

◆ Hydroxyurea

(hye-drox-ee-yoor-**ee**′-ya)   Hydrea   Pregnancy Category D

Mechanism of Action

Unknown. It is thought to cause an immediate inhibition of DNA synthesis without interfering with the synthesis of RNA or protein.

Indications

◆ Melanoma
◆ Resistant chronic myelocytic leukemia
◆ Recurrent, inoperable, metastatic carcinoma of the ovary
◆ Local control (concomitant with irradiation) of primary squamous cell (epidermoid) carcinoma of the head and neck, excluding the lip

Metabolism/Excretion

Metabolized in the liver; excreted through the kidneys. Half-life: 3 to 4 hours.

Dosage Range

Adult

Dosage determination should be based on the patient's actual or ideal weight, whichever is less.

◆ **Solid tumors:** Intermittent therapy: 80 mg/kg PO as a single dose every 3 days. Continuous therapy: 20 to 30 mg/kg PO as a single dose daily. Concomitant therapy with irradiation: Carcinoma of the head and neck: 80

mg/kg PO as a single dose every third day. Give the hydroxyurea dose ≥7 days before initiating radiation therapy; therapy is continued indefinitely provided that the patient can be monitored closely for adverse effects. The dose of radiation therapy does not need to be adjusted when given concurrently with hydroxyurea.

◆ **Resistant chronic myelocytic leukemia:** The dose given for continuous therapy in solid tumors should be followed until dosing studies for intermittent therapy for chronic myelocytic leukemia are completed. The trial period for determining hydroxyurea's efficacy is 6 weeks. If therapeutic response as evidenced by tumor regression is noted, the treatment should be continued indefinitely. If the WBC count falls to $<2,500/mm^3$ or the platelet count drops to $<100,000/mm^3$, hydroxyurea should be interrupted for a few doses. Because hematopoietic rebound is prompt, counts should be checked in 3 days. If rebound does not occur with concurrent irradiation, irradiation may also be interrupted, although this is rarely necessary.

Pediatric

Not established because of the rarity of these indications in children.

Drug Preparation/Stability

Available in capsules; keep in a tightly closed container at room temperature.

Drug Administration

PO. If the patient cannot swallow the capsules, empty the contents of the capsule into a glass of water and give immediately. Advise the patient that the contents of the capsule may not be fully dissolved because of the drug's formulation.

Drug Interaction

None known

Side Effects and Toxicities

◆ **CNS:** Headache, dizziness, disorientation, hallucinations, convulsions
◆ **Cutaneous:** Maculopapular rash, facial erythema, alopecia, radiation recall
◆ **GI:** Stomatitis, diarrhea, vomiting, elevated liver enzymes, constipation

◆ **GU:** Dysuria; temporary impairment of the renal tubules; elevated BUN, creatinine, and uric acid levels
◆ **Hematologic:** Bone marrow depression, including leukopenia, anemia, and thrombocytopenia
◆ **Other:** Fever, chills, malaise

Special Considerations

◆ Contraindicated in patients with markedly depressed bone marrow reserve.
◆ Monitor renal, hepatic, and hematopoietic function before and periodically during treatment. The decision to interrupt treatment should be based on recommended parameters.
◆ If the patient is anemic, whole blood replacement can be given without interrupting therapy.
◆ If the patient prefers to empty the contents of the capsules in water, advise him or her to be careful when handling a cytotoxic agent. The patient should avoid letting the drug touch the skin or mucous membranes.

◆ Idarubicin Hydrochloride

(eye-da-**roo**'-bee-sin)   Idamycin   Pregnancy Category D

Mechanism of Action

Idarubicin is an intercalating analogue of daunorubicin, which inhibits nucleic acid synthesis and interacts with the enzyme topoisomerase.

Indications

Acute myeloid leukemia in combination with other antileukemic drugs.

Metabolism/Excretion

Excreted mainly in the bile and urine. Half-life: 6.0 to 9.4 hours.

Dosage Range

◆ **Adult:** For induction therapy in acute myeloid leukemia, 12 mg/m^2 daily for 3 days IV with cytarabine 100 mg/m^2 daily by continuous infusion for 7 days, or with cytarabine 25 mg/m² by IV bolus followed by cytarabine 200 mg/m² daily for 5 days as continuous infusion. A repeat course may be given to patients with unequivocal evidence of leukemia. Reduce the dose to 25% lower than the normal dose if severe mucositis occurs. Dosage should be modified in patients with renal or hepatic impairment.

◆ **Pediatric:** Safety and efficacy not established.

Drug Preparation/Stability

Reconstitute the 5- or 10-mg vials with 5 or 10 mL 0.9% sodium chloride injection, respectively, to yield a final concentration of 1 mg/mL. The reconstituted solution is stable for 7 days under refrigeration (2° to 8°C) or for 3 days at room temperature of 15° to 30°C. Discard unused reconstituted solution.

Drug Administration

Slow IV push through the side arm of a free-flowing IV infusion of sodium chloride 0.9% or 5% dextrose injection.

Drug Interaction

Do not give with any other drugs. Precipitate may form if given with heparin. Prolonged contact with any solution having an alkaline pH will result in degradation of the product.

Side Effects and Toxicities

◆ **Cardiac:** Congestive failure, serious dysrhythmias, including atrial fibrillation, chest pain, myocardial infarction, and asymptomatic declines in left ventricular ejection fraction. These symptoms are reported in patients older than 60 years and in patients who have a pre-existing heart condition.

◆ **Cutaneous:** Alopecia

◆ **GI:** Nausea and vomiting, mucositis, abdominal pain, diarrhea

◆ **Hematologic:** Severe myelosuppression

Special Considerations

◆ Hyperuricemia may occur because of lysis of the leukemic cells. Implement appropriate preventive measures before therapy.

◆ Assess CBC and hepatic and renal function periodically.

◆ Idarubicin has vesicant properties. Extravasation and tissue damage can occur with or without stinging or burning pain at the infusion site.

◆ Ifosfamide

(eye-**fos**'-fa-myde)   Ifex   Pregnancy Category D

Mechanism of Action

Ifosfamide is an alkylating agent that is cell cycle–nonspecific. It is an analogue of cyclophosphamide that acts by alkylating DNA and interfering with replication of susceptible cells.

Indications

Third-line therapy for germ cell testicular carcinoma, in combination with other cytotoxic agents. Unlabeled uses: lung, breast, ovarian, pancreatic, and gastric cancer, bone and tissue sarcoma.

Metabolism/Excretion

Extensively metabolized in the liver. Most of the drug is excreted in the urine almost completely unchanged. Half-life: 15 hours.

Dosage Range

◆ **Adult:** 1.2 g/m^2 day for 5 consecutive days. Give repeat cycles every 3 weeks after hematopoietic recovery (platelets >100,000, WBC count >4000). Larger single doses of 5.0 g/m^2 can be given over 24 hours. Patients should be vigorously hydrated, PO or IV, with ≥2 L fluid per day.

◆ **Pediatric:** Safety and efficacy not established.

Drug Preparation/Stability

Mixed with sterile water for injection or bacteriostatic water for injection. The amount of diluent is as follows:

Dosage Strength	Diluent	Final Concentration
1 g	20 mL	50 mg/mL
3 g	60 mL	50 mg/mL

The diluted solution can be further mixed to yield concentrations of 0.6 to 20 mg/mL with 5% dextrose injection, 0.9% sodium chloride injection, lactated Ringer's injection, or sterile water for injection. Keep reconstituted solutions refrigerated and use within 24 hours.

Drug Administration

Slow IV infusion over ≥30 minutes; may also be given as a continuous infusion. Because of the danger of hemorrhagic cystitis, the patient should be well hydrated. *A uroprotective agent such as mesna is mandatory. When ifosfamide is given as a continuous infusion, a dose of mesna equal to the ifosfamide dose (mg/kg) is given admixed with ifosfamide. If ifosfamide is given as an IV bolus, a loading dose of mesna, which is equivalent to 20% of the ifosfamide dose, is given. The same dose of mesna is repeated 4 and 8 hours after the ifosfamide.*

Drug Interaction

None significant.

Side Effects and Toxicities

- ◆ **CNS:** Somnolence, confusion, depression, psychosis, hallucinations
- ◆ **Cutaneous:** Alopecia, hyperpigmentation, ridging of the nails
- ◆ **GI:** Nausea and vomiting, anorexia, diarrhea, constipation, elevated liver enzyme and bilirubin levels
- ◆ **GU:** Urotoxicity manifested by hemorrhagic cystitis, dysuria, urinary frequency, and hematuria. Abnormalities in serum and urine chemistries such as elevated BUN or serum creatinine levels or a decrease in creatinine clearance, as well as proteinuria and acidosis, are rare occurrences.
- ◆ **Hematologic:** Myelosuppression is dose-related and dose-limiting, manifested mostly by leukopenia. To a lesser degree, thrombocytopenia may occur. Dose adjustments should be made when ifosfamide is given concomitantly with myelosuppressive drugs. Patients with severe myelosuppression are also prone to infections.

Special Considerations

- ◆ Give cautiously in patients with depressed bone marrow reserves and impaired renal or hepatic function. Optimal dose schedules for patients with these conditions are not established.

◆ Ensure adequate hydration by making sure the patient receives at least 2 L/day of IV or oral fluids.

◆ Administer a uroprotective agent such as mesna or ethyol.

◆ Consider fractionating the daily dose to reduce the incidence of renal toxicity.

◆ Administer antiemetics as needed.

◆ Before and during treatment, assess the hematologic profile.

◆ Ifosfamide may interfere with normal would healing.

◆ Interferon-alfa-2a

(in-ter-**feer**'-on) Roferon-A, rIFN-A   Pregnancy Category C

Mechanism of Action

Not clearly understood; exerts antitumor activity through antiviral, antiproliferative, and immunomodulatory biologic effects.

Indications

◆ Hairy cell leukemia and AIDS-related Kaposi's sarcoma in patients 18 years and older

◆ pH-positive chronic myelogenous leukemia in chronic phase with minimal pretreatment (1 year of diagnosis)

Metabolism/Excretion

Metabolized in the kidney and liver; excreted in the urine. Elimination half-life: 3.7 to 8.5 hours for IV infusion. Peak serum concentrations: 3.8 hours and 7.3 hours for IM and SQ administration, respectively.

Dosage Range

Adult

◆ **Hairy cell leukemia:** Induction dose is 3 million IU daily for 16 to 24 weeks injected SQ or IM. Maintenance dose is 3 million IU three times a week. Monitor patients periodically to determine response to treatment; discontinue treatment if patient has not responded within 6 months. Dosage may need to be halved or withheld with severe reactions.

♦ **AIDS-related Kaposi's sarcoma:** Induction dose is 36 million IU daily for 10 to 12 weeks injected SQ or IM. Maintenance dose is 36 million IU three times a week. Dosage may need to be halved or temporarily withheld with severe reactions. Continue treatment until there is no further evidence of tumor or discontinuation is required.

♦ **Chronic myelogenous leukemia:** Initial dose is 9 million units daily injected SQ or IM. Continue treatment until disease progression. Optimal dose and duration not determined. Dosage may need to be reduced or withheld with severe reactions.

Pediatric

Safety and efficacy not established.

Drug Preparation/Stability

Supplied in injectable solution: 3, 9, 18, or 36 million IU per vial. Supplied in sterile powder for injection: 18 million IU per vial. Reconstitute powder with 3 mL diluent and gently swirl to dissolve. One milliliter of reconstituted powder will contain 6 million IU of interferon-alfa. Reconstituted powder must be used within 30 days. Store sterile powder, diluent, reconstituted powder, and injectable solution in the refrigerator at 2° to 8°C (36° to 46°F). Do not shake or freeze.

Drug Administration

SQ or IM injection.

Drug Interaction

♦ Reduces the clearance of theophylline.
♦ Synergistic myelosuppressive effects noted when used in combination with zidovudine.

Side Effects and Toxicities

♦ **Constitutional:** Flulike syndrome, fever, fatigue, myalgia, headache, chills, weight loss
♦ **CNS:** Dizziness, depression, sleep disturbance, decreased mental status, anxiety, visual disturbance, confusion, involuntary movements

◆ **GI:** Anorexia, nausea, vomiting, diarrhea, abdominal pain, change in taste
◆ **Hematologic:** Leukopenia, neutropenia, thrombocytopenia, anemia; elevated serum phosphorus, liver transaminase, alkaline phosphatase, and uric acid levels; decreased serum calcium level
◆ **Integumentary:** Skin rash, diaphoresis, partial alopecia, dry skin, pruritus
◆ **Musculoskeletal:** Myalgia, joint or bone pain, paresthesia, numbness
◆ **Pulmonary and cardiovascular:** Coughing, dyspnea, chest pain, edema, hypertension, hypotension, dysrhythmia
◆ **Other:** Throat irritation or dryness, rhinorrhea, sinusitis

Special Considerations

◆ Contraindicated in patients with known allergy to interferon-alfa, mouse immunoglobulin, or any component of the product. Should not be used during pregnancy or lactation.
◆ Give with caution in patients with cardiac, renal, or hepatic disease, seizure disorders, myelosuppression, or CNS dysfunction.
◆ Monitor for depressive symptoms. Dose reduction or withholding may lead to resolution of depressive symptoms.
◆ Obtain laboratory tests (CBC with differential, hairy cells and bone marrow hairy cells, and liver function tests) before and periodically during therapy. Patients with heart disease should have an ECG before and during treatment.
◆ For home use, instruct patient regarding SQ or IM administration. Provide a puncture-resistant container and guidelines on the proper disposal of used syringes and needles.
◆ To alleviate possible side effects, have patient take acetaminophen before injection.
◆ Some of the flulike symptoms may be minimized by administering the drug at bedtime.
◆ Ensure that the patient is well hydrated, especially during initiation of therapy.

◆ Interferon-alfa-2b

(in-ter-**feer**'-on)   Intron-A,   Pregnancy Category C
                              IFN-alpha 2

Mechanism of Action

Interferon exerts antitumor activities through antiviral replication, immunomodulatory, and antiproliferative biologic effects. Its direct antiproliferative properties may explain its activity in certain malignancies.

Indications

Hairy cell leukemia, condylomata acuminata, AIDS-related Kaposi's sarcoma, chronic hepatitis non-A, non-B/C, and chronic hepatitis B, and as adjuvant treatment for malignant melanoma with no evidence of disease but at high risk for recurrence. All patients must be 18 years or older.

Metabolism/Excretion

Metabolized in the kidneys; excretion unknown. Elimination half-life after SQ or IM injection: about 2 to 3 hours; serum concentrations peak from 3 to 12 hours after injection and are undetectable by 16 hours after injection. Elimination half-life after IV infusion: about 2 hours; serum concentrations peak at the end of a 30-minute infusion and are undetectable by 4 hours.

Dosage Range

Adult

◆ **Hairy cell leukemia:** Two million IU/m^2 three times a week injected IM or SQ. Continue treatment unless rapid progression of disease or severe intolerance occurs. May need to reduce dose by half or temporarily withhold until adverse reactions resolve.

◆ **Condylomata acuminata:** Reconstitute vial containing 10 million IU powder for injection with 1 mL diluent (bacteriostatic water); then inject 1.0 million IU (0.1 mL of reconstituted solution) into each lesion (intralesionally) three times a week for 3 weeks using a tuberculin syringe with a 25- to 20-gauge needle. Maximum response may take up to 4 to 8 weeks after initiation of treatment.

A second course of treatment may be needed if a satisfactory response is not achieved after 12 to 16 weeks.

◆ **AIDS-related Kaposi's sarcoma:** Thirty million IU/m^2 three times a week injected SQ or IM. Continue treatment until complete response is achieved. Discontinue treatment with severe opportunistic infection or adverse reactions. May need to reduce dose by half or temporarily withhold until adverse reactions resolve.

◆ **Chronic hepatitis non-A, non-B/C:** Three million IU/m^2 three times a week injected SQ or IM. Those responding to treatment should complete 6 months of treatment. May consider discontinuing treatment if no response is noted after 16 weeks of treatment. May need to reduce dose by half or temporarily withhold until adverse reactions resolve.

◆ **Chronic hepatitis B:** Thirty to 35 million IU/m^2 per week injected SQ or IM, either as 5 million IU/m^2 daily or as 10 million IU/m^2 three times a week for 16 weeks. May need to reduce dose by half or temporarily withhold until adverse reactions resolve.

◆ **Malignant melanoma:** Induction treatment is 20 million IU/m^2 for 5 consecutive days per week for 4 weeks as an IV infusion. Maintenance dose is 10 million IU/m^2 three times a week injected SQ for 48 weeks. If granulocytes are <500/mm^3 or aspartate transferase/alanine transferase is >5 times the upper normal limit, withhold treatment until laboratory values return to normal.

Pediatric

Safety and efficacy not established.

Drug Preparation/Stability

Store powder and solution for injection in the refrigerator at 2° to 8°C (36° to 46°F). After reconstitution of powder, solution is stable for 1 month if refrigerated. Do not shake or freeze.

When reconstituting powder for injection, use diluent (bacteriostatic water). Use the strengths listed for the appropriate indications:

Vial Strength	mL Diluent	Final Concentration
3 million IU	1.0	3 million IU/mL
5 million IU	1.0	5 million IU/mL
10 million IU	2.0	5 million IU/mL
18 million IU multidose	3.8	6 million IU/mL
25 million IU	5.0	5 million IU/mL

Vial Strength	mL Diluent	Final Concentration
10 million IU	1.0	10 million IU/mL

Vial Strength	mL Diluent	Final Concentration
50 million IU	1	50 million IU/mL

Vial Strength	mL Diluent	Final Concentration
3 million IU	1.0	3 million IU/mL
18 million IU multidose	3.8	6 million IU/mL

Vial Strength	mL Diluent	Final Concentration
5 million IU	1.0	5 million IU/mL
10 million IU	1.0	10 million IU/mL

Vial Strength	mL Diluent	Final Concentration
3 million IU	1.0	3 million IU/mL
5 million IU	1.0	5 million IU/mL
10 million IU	1.0	10 million IU/mL
18 million IU	1.0	18 million IU/mL
25 million IU	5.0	5 million IU/mL
50 million IU	1.0	50 million IU/mL

If the drug is supplied in solution for injection, it does not need to be reconstituted. Use only in hairy cell leukemia, chronic hepatitis non-A, non-B/C, and chronic hepatitis B:

Vial Strength	Solution	Final Concentration
10 million IU	2.0 mL	5 million IU/mL
18 million IU multidose	5.0 mL	5 million IU/mL
25 million IU	5.0 mL	5 million IU/mL

Drug Administration

SQ or IM injection; IV infusion.

Drug Interaction

◆ Use caution when giving with other myelosuppressive agents, such as zidovudine.
◆ Incompatible with 5% dextrose solution.

Side Effects and Toxicities

 ◆ **Constitutional:** Flulike syndrome, fever, fatigue, myalgia, headache, chills, weight loss, rigors, malaise
 ◆ **CNS:** Depression, paresthesia, confusion, irritability, somnolence, insomnia, dizziness, impaired concentration
 ◆ **GI:** Anorexia, diarrhea, nausea, vomiting, taste alteration, dry mouth, abdominal pain
 ◆ **Hematologic:** Leukopenia, neutropenia, thrombocytopenia, anemia; elevated serum phosphorus, liver transaminase, alkaline phosphatase, and uric acid levels; decreased serum calcium level
 ◆ **Integumentary:** Skin rash, diaphoresis, alopecia, dry skin, pruritus, increased sweating
 ◆ **Musculoskeletal:** Arthralgia, asthenia, back pain
 ◆ **Pulmonary and cardiovascular:** Coughing, dyspnea, chest pain, edema, hypertension, hypotension, dysrhythmia

Special Considerations

 ◆ Contraindicated in patients with known allergy to interferon-alfa or any component of the product. Should not be used during pregnancy or lactation.
 ◆ Do not give to patients with pre-existing psychiatric conditions, especially depression. Discontinue use in patients developing severe depression or other psychiatric disorders.
 ◆ Use with caution in patients with pulmonary disease, diabetes mellitus, coagulation disorders, cardiovascular disease, or severe myelosuppression.
 ◆ Monitor the WBC count in patients who are myelosuppressed or receiving other myelosuppressive medications.
 ◆ For home use, instruct patient regarding SQ or IM administration. Provide a puncture-resistant container and guidelines on disposal of used syringes and needles.
 ◆ To alleviate possible side effects, have patient take acetaminophen before injection and every 4 hours after the initial injection.
 ◆ Flulike symptoms may be minimized by administering the drug at bedtime.
 ◆ Ensure that the patient is well hydrated, especially during initiation of therapy.
 ◆ Obtain laboratory tests (CBC with differential, elec-

trolytes, liver function tests, thyroid-stimulating hormone) before and during therapy. Patients with malignant melanoma should have CBCs with differential and liver function tests every week during the induction phase and then monthly during the maintenance phase.
◆ Patients with heart disease or advanced cancer should have an ECG before and during treatment.
◆ All patients should have a baseline chest x-ray.
◆ Assess fatigue level and performance status regularly. Dose adjustments may be made depending on the severity of fatigue. Teach patient about strategies to combat fatigue, such as moderation of activities, proper diet, maintaining sleep hygiene, and conserving energy.

◆ Interferon-beta-1a

(in-ter-**feer**′-on)   Avonex   Pregnancy Category C

Mechanism of Action

Not clearly understood; exerts biologic activities by binding to cell surface receptors.

Indications

To decrease physical disability and reduce the frequency of clinical exacerbations in relapsing forms of multiple sclerosis.

Metabolism/Excretion

After IM injection, serum levels peak between 3 and 15 hours with an elimination half-life of 10 hours. After SQ injection, serum levels peak between 3 to 18 hours with an elimination half-life of 8.6 hours.

Dosage Range

◆ **Adult:** 30 mcg injected IM once a week.
◆ **Pediatric:** Safety and efficacy not established.

Drug Preparation/Stability

Supplied in powder for injection: A single-use vial containing 33 mcg (6.6 million IU) of interferon-beta-1a to be reconstituted with 1.1 mL of provided diluent (sterile water). Use 1.0 mL for administration. Store vials in the refrigerator at 2° to 8°C (36° to 46°F); if a refrigerator is not available, can be stored at 25°C (77°F) for up to 30 days. After reconstitution, use as soon as possible or within 6 hours if stored at 2° to 8°C (36° to 46°F). Do not shake or freeze.

Drug Administration

IM injection.

Drug Interaction

Synergistic myelosuppressive effects noted when used in combination with zidovudine.

Side Effects and Toxicities

- ◆ **Constitutional:** Flulike syndrome, fever, fatigue, myalgia, headache, chills, weight loss, rigors, malaise
- ◆ **CNS:** Sleep difficulties, dizziness
- ◆ **GI:** Abdominal pain, nausea, diarrhea, dyspepsia, anorexia
- ◆ **Hematologic:** Anemia
- ◆ **Integumentary:** Urticaria
- ◆ **Musculoskeletal:** Muscle aches, arthralgia, muscle spasm, asthenia
- ◆ **Pulmonary and cardiovascular:** Chest pain, upper respiratory tract infection, sinusitis, dyspnea
- ◆ **Other:** Infection, pain, otitis media

Special Considerations

- ◆ Contraindicated in patients with known allergy to interferon-beta, human albumin, or any component of the drug.
- ◆ Use caution in patients with pre-existing seizure disorders and cardiac disease.
- ◆ Monitor for depressive symptoms. Advise patient to report symptoms of depression immediately. Consider stopping interferon if depression develops.
- ◆ For home use, instruct patient in IM administration and provide a puncture-resistant container with guidelines on the proper disposal of used syringes and needles.
- ◆ To alleviate possible side effects, have patient take acetaminophen before injection.
- ◆ Some of the flulike symptoms may be minimized by administering at bedtime.
- ◆ Monitor laboratory tests (CBC with differential, blood chemistries, including liver function tests) during therapy.

◆ Interferon-beta-1b

(in-ter-**feer**′-on) Betaseron, rIFN-B Pregnancy Category C

Mechanism of Action

Not clearly understood; exerts antiviral and immunoregulatory biologic activities by binding to cell surface receptors.

Indications

To reduce the frequency of clinical exacerbations in ambulatory patients with relapsing/remitting multiple sclerosis.

Metabolism/Excretion

Metabolized in the kidney and liver and excreted in the urine. Serum concentrations peak between 1 to 8 hours after SQ injection and IV infusion. Elimination half-life: 8 minutes to 4.3 hours.

Dosage Range

◆ **Adult:** 0.25 mg (8 million IU) injected SQ every other day. Discontinue with unremitting disease progression of ≥6 months.

◆ **Pediatric:** Safety and efficacy not established.

Drug Preparation/Stability

Supplied as powder for injection: Single-use vial containing 0.3 mg (9.6 million IU) of interferon-beta-1b. Reconstitute with 1.2 mL of provided diluent (sodium chloride). Inject 1 mL of reconstituted solution. Use solution within 3 hours of reconstitution. Store powder and reconstituted solution in the refrigerator at 2° to 8°C (36° to 46°F). Do not shake or freeze.

Drug Administration

SQ injection.

Drug Interaction

Not fully evaluated.

Side Effects and Toxicities

◆ **Constitutional:** Flulike syndrome, fever, fatigue, headache, chills, malaise

◆ **CNS:** Dizziness, hypertonia, anxiety, nervousness, somnolence, abnormal vision

- ◆ **GI:** Abdominal pain, diarrhea, constipation, GI disorder
- ◆ **GU:** Dysmenorrhea, menstrual disorder, metrorrhagia, cystitis, menorrhagia
- ◆ **Hematologic:** Increase in alanine transferase, total bilirubin, urine protein; decrease in glucose, lymphocytes, neutrophils, WBCs
- ◆ **Integumentary:** Injection site reaction, necrosis
- ◆ **Musculoskeletal:** Pain, asthenia, pelvic pain, myalgia, myasthenia
- ◆ **Pulmonary and cardiovascular:** Sinusitis, dyspnea, laryngitis; migraine, palpitation, hypertension, tachycardia, peripheral vascular disorder
- ◆ **Other:** Generalized edema, lymphadenopathy, conjunctivitis, breast pain

Special Considerations

- ◆ Contraindicated in patients with known allergy to interferon-beta, human albumin, or any other component of the product.
- ◆ Monitor for depressive symptoms. Advise patient to report symptoms of depression immediately. Consider stopping interferon if depression develops.
- ◆ For home use, instruct patient in SQ administration and provide a puncture-resistant container with guidelines on the proper disposal of used syringes and needles.
- ◆ To alleviate possible side effects, have patient take acetaminophen before injection.
- ◆ Some of the flulike symptoms may be minimized by administering at bedtime.
- ◆ Obtain laboratory tests (CBC with differential, blood chemistries, including liver function tests) before and during therapy.

◆ Interferon-gamma

(in-ter-**feer**′-on)   Actimmune   Pregnancy Category C

Mechanism of Action

Exerts immunomodulatory properties by phagocyte-activating effects; acts as a lymphokine of the interleukin type; enhances oxidative metabolism of tissue macrophages, antibody-dependent cellular cytotoxicity, and natural killer cell activity.

Indications

To reduce the frequency and severity of serious infections associated with chronic granulomatous disease.

Metabolism/Excretion

Metabolized in the liver and kidneys and excreted in the urine. Mean elimination half-life after IV infusion is 38 minutes; after SQ injection, 5.0 hours; and after IM injection, 2.9 hours. Serum concentrations peak in 7 hours after SQ injection and in 4 hours after IM injection.

Dosage Range

◆ **Adult:** 50 mcg/m^2 (1.5 million units/m^2) for patients whose body surface area is >0.5 m^2; 1.5 mcg/kg per dose for patients whose body surface area is ≤ 0.5 m^2; inject SQ three times a week.

◆ **Pediatric:** Safety and efficacy not established in patients younger than 1 year.

Drug Preparation/Stability

Supplied in solution for injection: Single-dose vial. Each 0.5-mL vial contains 100 mcg (3 million units) of interferon-gamma-1b. Store in the refrigerator at 2° to 8°C (36° to 46°F). Do not shake or freeze.

Drug Administration

SQ injection.

Drug Interaction

Not fully evaluated. Use with caution with other drugs that cause myelosuppression.

Side Effects and Toxicities

Fever, headache, rash, chills, injection site erythema or tenderness, fatigue, diarrhea, vomiting, nausea, weight loss, myalgia, anorexia.

Special Considerations

◆ Contraindicated in patients with known allergy to interferon-gamma, *Escherichia coli*–derived products, or any component of the product.

◆ Use cautiously in patients with cardiac disease, seizure disorders, or CNS dysfunction.

◆ For home use, instruct patient in SQ administration and provide a puncture-resistant container with guidelines on the proper disposal of used syringes and needles.
◆ To alleviate possible side effects, have the patient take acetaminophen before injection.
◆ Some of the flulike symptoms may be minimized by administering at bedtime.
◆ Obtain laboratory tests (CBC with differential, blood chemistries, including renal and liver function tests, urinalysis) before and every 3 months during therapy.

◆ Irinotecan

(eye-ree-**no**′-tee-kan)   Camptosar,   Pregnancy Category D
                            CPT-11

Mechanism of Action

A plant alkaloid that inhibits the topoisomerase I enzyme. This enzyme plays a critical role in DNA replication and transcription. Irinotecan is the second most recently approved topoisomerase inhibitor that has become available; the first one is topotecan.

Indications

Metastatic carcinoma of the colon or rectum that has progressed or recurred after treatment with 5-fluorouracil. Phase II trials are underway using this drug in ovarian cancer.

Metabolism/Excretion

Converted to its active metabolites in the liver; excreted through the biliary and renal system. Half-life: 6 hours.

Dosage Range

◆ **Adult:** 125 mg/m^2 given weekly by IV infusion for 4 weeks, followed by 2 weeks of rest before repeat cycles are given.
◆ **Pediatric:** Safety and efficacy not studied.

Drug Preparation/Stability

Dilute, preferably with 5% dextrose injection or 0.9% sodium chloride injection, to yield a final concentration of 0.12 to 1.1 mg/mL. The solution is usually infused in 500 mL

5% dextrose in water. The reconstituted solution is stable for up to 24 hours at room temperature (25°C) and in ambient fluorescent lighting. If refrigerated at approximately 2° to 8°C, the drug when diluted with 5% dextrose injection is stable for 48 hours, protected from sunlight. Admixtures with 0.9% sodium chloride should not be refrigerated because of the possibility of particulates. Do not freeze irinotecan or its admixtures because of precipitation.

Drug Administration

IV infusion over 90 minutes. The infusion is given once a week for 4 consecutive weeks followed by a 2-week rest period. Repeat cycles are given every 6 weeks—that is, 4 weeks on therapy and 2 weeks off therapy. The doses may be escalated to as much as 150 mg/m^2 or reduced to as low as 50 mg/m^2, depending on the patient's tolerance to treatment.

Drug Interaction

Not formally studied, but dexamethasone, when given as part of an antiemetic regimen before irinotecan administration, may enhance lymphocytopenia or hyperglycemia.

Side Effects and Toxicities

  ◆ **Cardiovascular:** Vasodilation (flushing) has been observed during drug infusion.
  ◆ **CNS:** Insomnia, dizziness
  ◆ **Cutaneous:** Alopecia, rashes
  ◆ **GI:** Diarrhea, nausea, and vomiting can be severe. These events have happened during or after administration. Liver enzyme abnormalities have been noted in patients with hepatic metastases.
  ◆ **Hematologic:** Neutropenia, leukopenia including lymphocytopenia, anemia
  ◆ **Other:** Asthenia or fatigue, fever, abdominal pain

Special Considerations

  ◆ Do not use with irradiation.
  ◆ Manage diarrhea, a common side effect, according to its onset. For patients who experience it early (during or within 24 hours of administration), give 0.25 mg to 1 mg atropine to ameliorate the cholinergic nature of the diarrhea. For late-onset diarrhea, give 4 mg loperamide every 2 hours until patient is diarrhea free for 12 hours.

◆ Monitor fluid and electrolyte balance, especially when diarrhea and vomiting are severe.

◆ Advise patients to refrain from using laxatives or diuretics because they may exacerbate diarrhea or dehydration.

◆ Discontinue treatment if the patient has a neutropenic fever or if the absolute neutrophil count falls to <500/mm³. Modify the dose if the hemoglobin count is <8 g/dL or the platelet count is <100,000. GSF is efficacious in significant cases of neutropenia. Monitor CBC before treatment.

◆ Avoid extravasation. Irinotecan is not a vesicant, but mild to moderate erythema has been observed after infiltration. Monitor the infusion site for these signs. Occasionally, patients have reported pain or soreness at the site.

◆ Teach patient fatigue-management strategies, such as sleep hygiene, energy conservation, proper nutrition, moderate exercise, and symptomatic management of pain, nausea, and vomiting if relevant.

◆ Leucovorin Calcium

(loo-koh-**vor'**-in)   Citrovorum   Pregnancy Category C
                        factor, folinic acid

Mechanism of Action

Essential for purine and DNA synthesis; bypasses the inhibitor action of folic acid antagonists.

Indications

◆ Folinic acid rescue after high-dose methotrexate for osteosarcoma, epidermoid tumors, and various refractory tumors

◆ Megaloblastic anemias due to nutritional deficiency, pregnancy, infancy, and sprue

◆ Palliative treatment with 5-fluorouracil for metastatic colorectal cancer

Metabolism/Excretion

Metabolized in the liver; primarily excreted in urine, small amounts in feces.

Dosage Range

◆ **After high-dose methotrexate:** 12 to 15 g/m2 IV or PO, followed by 10 mg/m2 PO every 6 hours for 72 hours; 24 hours after methotrexate, if serum creatinine is 50% greater than premethotrexate level or if serum methotrexate level exceeds 5×10^{-8} M, increase dose to 100 mg/m every 3 hours until methotrexate level is $< 5 \times 10^{-8}$ M

◆ **Megaloblastic anemia:** maximum dose 1 mg/day IM.

◆ **Metastatic colon cancer (palliative treatment):** 200 mg/m² slow IV drip or slow IV push immediately before 5-fluorouracil.

Drug Preparation/Stability

Reconstitute 50-mg vial with 5 mL or the 100-mg vial with 10 mL of bacteriostatic or sterile water for injection to obtain a solution of 10 mg/mL. Because the bacteriostatic water contains benzyl alcohol, it is stable for 7 days if protected from light. If reconstituted with sterile water for injection, use immediately.

Oral solution contains a 60-mg vial and 60 mL Aromatic Elixir NF.

Also available in oral tablets, 10 and 15 mg.

Drug Administration

IV slowly over 3 to 5 minutes, continuous infusion, PO, IM.

Drug Interaction

None known

Side Effects and Toxicities

◆ **GI:** Nausea, vomiting
◆ **Dermatologic:** Rash, pruritus, erythema
◆ **Pulmonary:** Bronchospasm
◆ **Other:** Hypersensitivity, allergic reactions

Special Considerations

◆ Contraindicated in patients with previous allergy on exposure, pernicious anemias or other megaloblastic anemias with a vitamin B_{12} deficiency, lactation.

◆ Coordinate dose and timing of leucovorin with the high-dose methotrexate protocol.

◆ Leuprolide

(loo-**proe**'-lide)   Lupron, Lupron   Pregnancy Category X
                        Depot, Lupron
                        Depot-Ped

Mechanism of Action

GnRH agonist that binds to gonadotrophin-releasing hormone cell surface receptors in the pituitary.

Indications

Palliative treatment of prostate cancer; metastatic breast cancer; refractory ovarian and endometrial cancer; endometriosis; precocious puberty.

Metabolism/Excretion

Unclear

Dosage Range

Adult

 ◆ **Palliative prostate cancer:** 1 mg (0.2 mL) every day subcutaneously.
 ◆ **Metastatic breast cancer:** 1 to 10 mg every day subcutaneously
 ◆ **Ovarian and endometrial cancer:** 1 mg every day subcutaneously
 ◆ **Depot:** 7.5 mg IM every 28 to 33 days using a 21- or 22-gauge needle.

Pediatric

Not recommended.

Drug Preparation/Stability

 ◆ A 5-mg/mL solution for SQ administration given undiluted (data on stability and admixture not available).
 ◆ Depot suspension: add 1 mL of the provided diluent to the 7.5-mg leuprolide vial, shake thoroughly until it has a milky appearance; stable for 24 hours.

Drug Administration

Lupron: 5 mg/1 mL solution SQ; Lupron-Depot: suspension IM.

Drug Interaction

Not available

Side Effects and Toxicities

◆ **Cardiac:** Arrhythmias, congestive heart failure, myocardial infarction, peripheral edema, thrombophlebitis

◆ **CNS:** Dizziness, headache, pain, paresthesia, visual changes, fatigue, lethargy, memory impairment, insomnia, dysuria

◆ **Dermatologic:** Pruritus, alopecia, erythema, rash

◆ **GI:** Nausea, vomiting, anorexia, constipation, GI bleeding, sour taste

◆ **GU:** Elevated BUN and creatinine, frequency, hematuria, decrease in testes size

◆ **Pulmonary:** Difficulty breathing, pleural rub, pulmonary fibrosis

◆ **Other:** Diaphoresis, hot flashes, bone pain

Special Considerations

◆ Contraindicated in patients with previous allergy to leuprolide, pregnancy, lactation.

◆ Use with caution in patients with a history of cardiac problems, pulmonary problems, or GI hemorrhage.

◆ Assess cardiac, pulmonary, and kidney function before administration.

◆ Instruct patient on use of contraception.

◆ Levamisole

(lev-**am**′-ih-sole)   Ergamisol   Pregnancy Category C

Mechanism of Action

Mediates the potentiation of monocyte, macrophage, T-lymphocyte, and antibody production.

Indications

Combined with 5-fluorouracil for patients with Duke's C resected colon cancer.

Metabolism/Excretion

Metabolized in the liver; excreted in urine.

Dosage Range

♦ **Adult:** Initial therapy: 7 to 30 days after resection, levamisole 50 mg PO every 8 hours for 3 days; 21 to 34 days after resection, 5-fluorouracil 450 mg/m^2 per day IV for 5 days. Maintenance therapy: levamisole 50 mg PO, 5-fluorouracil 450 mg/m^2 per day once weekly with levamisole 50 mg every 2 weeks.

♦ **Pediatric:** Not recommended.

Drug Preparation/Stability

No preparation required. Tablets are stable as packaged for 5 years.

Drug Administration

PO

Drug Interaction

Increased phenytoin levels with possible toxicity; possible disulfiram-like reaction with alcohol.

Side Effects and Toxicities

♦ **CNS:** Dizziness, headache, paresthesia, depression, somnolence, altered taste perception

♦ **Dermatologic:** Dermatitis, alopecia

♦ **GI:** Nausea, diarrhea, stomatitis, abdominal pain, constipation, anorexia

♦ **Hematologic:** Bone marrow depression

♦ **Other:** Fever, rigors, fatigue, infections, arthralgia

Special Considerations

♦ Monitor CBC before, during, and after therapy.

♦ Hold administration of 5-fluorouracil for WBC count <3,500/mm^3.

♦ Instruct patient on use of contraception.

♦ Lomustine

(loe-**mus**'-teen)   CCNU, CeeNu   Pregnancy Category D

Mechanism of Action

Nitrosourea alkylating agent that prevents alkylation of DNA and RNA, which inhibits DNA, RNA, and protein synthesis.

Indications

Brain tumors, Hodgkin's disease, non–small cell lung carcinoma, GI carcinoma, multiple myeloma.

Metabolism/Excretion

Metabolized in the liver; excreted in urine.

Dosage Range

Single dose of 130 mg/m² PO every 6 weeks. Defer dose for platelet count $<100,000/mm^3$ and leukocytes $<4000/mm^3$.

Drug Preparation/Stability

No preparation needed. Available in 100-, 40-, and 10-mg capsules. Store in closed containers at room temperature. Avoid exposure to heat and moisture. Check package lot labels for expiration date.

Drug Administration

PO on an empty stomach to avoid GI upset.

Drug Interaction

To maximize lomustine absorption, avoid concurrent administration with other potentially nauseating medications and alcohol.

Side Effects and Toxicities

◆ **CNS:** Lethargy, confusion, ataxia, dysarthria
◆ **Dermatologic:** Alopecia
◆ **GI:** Delayed nausea and vomiting 2 to 6 hours after administration, stomatitis, anorexia, diarrhea
◆ **GU:** Nephrotoxicity
◆ **Hematologic:** Delayed myelosuppression (4 to 6 weeks)
◆ **Pulmonary:** Pulmonary fibrosis
◆ **Reproductive:** Possible infertility

Special Considerations

◆ Contraindicated in patients with previous hypersensitivity to lomustine, bone marrow depression, pregnancy, lactation, radiation therapy.
◆ Instruct patient on use of contraception.

◆ Mechlorethamine Hydrochloride

(me-klor-**eth**'-a-meen) Mustargen,   Pregnancy Category D
                        nitrogen
                        mustard

Mechanism of Action

Cell cycle–nonspecific alkylating agent that causes abnormal base pairing of guanine and thymine, DNA cross-linking, and impaired RNA and protein synthesis, causing cell lysis.

Indications

Lung carcinoma, chronic lymphocytic leukemia, chronic myelocytic leukemia, Hodgkin's disease, lymphosarcoma, malignant effusions, mycosis fungoides.

Metabolism/Excretion

Metabolized immediately on administration to active drug that is taken up by cells; excreted in urine.

Dosage Range

Adults

 ◆ IV 0.4 mg/kg per course as single dose or in divided doses of 0.1 to 0.2 mg/kg per day; dose based on ideal body weight.
 ◆ **Intracavitary injections:** 0.2 to 0.4 mg/kg.
 ◆ **Topical:** 0.01% to 0.02% solution or ointment.

Pediatric

Limited use in children; safety and effectiveness not proved.

Drug Preparation/Stability

Reconstitute 10-mg vial with 10 mL sterile water or normal saline injection to yield a concentration of 1 mg/mL. Use within 15 minutes after reconstitution; drug rapidly decomposes on standing. Prepare drug immediately before use.

Drug Administration

Slow IV push over 20 to 30 minutes or IV push over 1 to 3 minutes into tubing of rapidly running IV solution; intracavitary; topical (for mycosis fungoides).

Drug Interaction

Tendency to raise uric acid levels may decrease the effectiveness of antigout medication.

Side Effects and Toxicities

- ◆ **CNS:** Vertigo, tinnitus, diminished hearing
- ◆ **Dermatologic:** Alopecia, tissue damage secondary to drug extravasation, phlebitis
- ◆ **GI:** Severe nausea and vomiting, metallic taste in mouth, diarrhea, jaundice
- ◆ **Hematologic:** Bone marrow depression
- ◆ **Reproductive:** Infertility, azoospermia
- ◆ **Other:** Hyperuricemia leading to acute renal failure, secondary malignancy

Special Considerations

- ◆ Contraindicated in patients with previous sensitivity to mechlorethamine, pregnancy, lactation.
- ◆ This drug is a potent vesicant; avoid extravasation. Treat extravasation by infiltrating the area with sodium thiosulfate.
- ◆ Instruct patient on use of contraception.

◆ Medroxyprogesterone Acetate

(me-drox-ee-proe-**jess**'-te-rone)	Amen, Curretab, Provera, Depo-Provera	Pregnancy Category X

Mechanism of Action

A progestin that promotes differentiation and maintenance of the endometrium, inhibits growth of sensitive malignancies, prevents ovulation through inhibition of pituitary gonadotropin secretion, and prevents spontaneous uterine contraction.

Indications

Contraceptive treatment of breast cancer; secondary amenorrhea; palliation and adjunctive therapy of inoperable recurrent and metastatic renal and endometrial carcinomas; abnormal uterine bleeding without an organic etiology.

Metabolism/Excretion

Metabolized in the liver; excretion unclear.

Dosage Range

Adult

◆ **Secondary amenorrhea:** 5 to 10 mg/day PO for 5 to 10 days; may begin therapy at any time.

◆ **Renal or endometrial carcinoma:** 400 to 1000 mg/wk IM.

◆ **Abnormal uterine bleeding:** start on the 16th or 21st day of the menstrual cycle, 5 to 10 mg/day PO for 5 to 10 days.

Pediatric

Safety and effectiveness not established.

Drug Preparation/Stability

Tablets: 2, 5, and 10 mg. Injection: 100-mg/mL and 400-mg aqueous suspension. May crystallize on storage at low temperature.

Drug Administration

PO tablets. Rotate IM injection sites.

Drug Interaction

May alter hepatic metabolism of other drugs.

Side Effects and Toxicities

◆ **Cardiac:** Cerebrovascular disorders, retinal thrombosis, pulmonary embolism, thromboembolic and thrombotic disease, thrombophlebitis, elevated blood pressure

◆ **CNS:** Loss of vision, diplopia, proptosis, migraine, depression, insomnia, somnolence, pyrexia

◆ **Dermatologic:** Acne, alopecia, hirsutism, photosensitivity, melasma, chloasma, rash, pruritus

◆ **GI:** Nausea, jaundice

◆ **GU:** Amenorrhea, breakthrough bleeding, spotting, changes in menstrual flow and cervical secretions, breast tenderness

◆ **Other:** Weight loss or gain, fluid retention, edema, decreased glucose tolerance

Special Considerations

◆ Contraindicated in patients with previous allergy to progestins, pregnancy, lactation, asthma, history of migraine, epilepsy, cardiac or renal dysfunction, hepatic disease, carcinoma of the breast or genital organs, thrombophlebitis, thromboembolic disorders, cerebral hemorrhage.

◆ Perform history and physical before and twice yearly during treatment.

◆ Obtain pregnancy test before treatment.

◆ Discontinue medication and consult physician if any of the following occurs: loss of vision, retinal lesions, papilledema, leg pain or swelling, shortness of breath, peripheral perfusion changes, severe headache.

◆ Instruct patient to avoid sun exposure and to wear protective clothing and sunscreen.

◆ Drug may alter accuracy of hepatic and endocrine function tests.

◆ Megestrol Acetate

(me-**jess**′-trole)　　　Megace　　　Pregnancy Category X

Mechanism of Action

Synthetic derivative of the naturally occurring steroid hormone progesterone with an unknown mechanism of antineoplastic activity.

Indications

Breast carcinoma, endometrial carcinoma, AIDS-associated cachexia, appetite stimulator.

Metabolism/Excretion

Metabolized in the liver; excreted in urine and feces.

Dosage Range

Adult

◆ **Breast cancer:** tablets, 160 mg/day in divided doses of 40 mg four times a day.

◆ **Endometrial carcinoma:** tablets, 40 to 320 mg/day in four divided doses.

◆ **AIDS cachexia:** 400 to 800 mg/day suspension divided in four doses (40 mg/mL).

Pediatric

Not recommended.

Drug Preparation/Stability

Scored tablets: 20, 40 mg; suspension: 40 mg/mL. A plastic dosage cup with 10- and 20-mL markings is provided with suspension. Store suspension at 25°C or less and dispense in a tight container. Protect tablets and suspension from heat.

Drug Administration

PO only. Available in tablets or in a lemon/lime-flavored suspension.

Drug Interaction

Not investigated

Side Effects and Toxicities

◆ **Cardiac:** Cardiomyopathy, palpitation, peripheral edema
◆ **CNS:** Paresthesia, confusion, convulsion, depression, neuropathy, hyperesthesia, abnormal thinking
◆ **Dermatologic:** Alopecia, herpes, pruritus, vesiculo-bullous rash, diaphoresis, skin disorder
◆ **GI:** Constipation, dry mouth, hepatomegaly, increased salivation, oral moniliasis
◆ **GU:** Albuminuria, urinary incontinence, urinary tract infection, gynecomastia
◆ **Hematologic:** Leukopenia
◆ **Pulmonary:** Dyspnea, cough, pharyngitis, lung disorder
◆ **Other:** Abdominal pain, edema, elevated level of lactate dehydrogenase (LDH), chest pain, infection, moniliasis, sarcoma, amblyopia, teratogenic changes

Special Considerations

◆ Contraindicated in patients with pregnancy, lactation, lung disorders.
◆ Use with caution in patients with a history of thromboembolic disease.
◆ Obtain pregnancy test before using.
◆ Use in cachexia only after treatable causes of weight loss are sought and addressed.
◆ Monitor serum levels of LDH.
◆ Instruct patient on use of contraception.

◆ Melphalan

(**mel**'-fa-lan)   Alkeran   Pregnancy Category D

Mechanism of Action

Cell cycle–nonspecific alkylating agent that alkylates and impairs DNA replication, causing cell lysis.

Indications

Ovarian carcinoma; multiple myeloma; bone marrow transplant cytoreduction for neuroblastoma, melanoma, lymphoma, myeloma, and colon cancer.

Metabolism/Excretion

Metabolized by hydrolysis in plasma; excreted in urine and feces.

Dosage Range

Adult

◆ **Ovarian carcinoma:** 0.2 mg/kg per day for 5 days, repeated every 4 to 5 weeks

◆ **Multiple myeloma:** 6 mg/day for 2 weeks; subsequent doses depend on recovery from previous course. IV dose: 16 mg/m^2 every 3 weeks for four doses, then every 4 weeks.

◆ **Bone marrow transplant cytoreduction:** Tremendous variation in protocol dosage, to 200 mg/m^2.

Pediatric

Safety and effectiveness not established.

Drug Preparation/Stability

Reconstitute the 50-mg vial with the supplied 10 mL of diluent and shake until solution is clear. Reconstituted solution yields a concentration of 5 mg/mL. Dilute in 100 to 200 mL of 0.45% or 0.9% sodium chloride solution. Stability before reconstitution in sodium chloride is rapid. Once reconstituted in sodium chloride, administer within 60 minutes. Also available in 2-mg tablets; store at room temperature.

Drug Administration

PO, or as an IV infusion over 30 to 60 minutes.

Drug Interaction

◆ Corticosteroids may enhance antitumor effects.
◆ Misonidazole enhances DNA cross-linking from melphalan.
◆ Cimetidine decreases oral melphalan bioavailability.
◆ Ingestion of food reduces oral melphalan bioavailability.

Side Effects and Toxicities

◆ **Dermatologic:** Alopecia, urticaria, maculopapular skin rash
◆ **GI:** Nausea and vomiting, stomatitis
◆ **Hematologic:** Bone marrow depression (14 to 21 days after administration), hyperuricemia
◆ **Pulmonary:** Pulmonary fibrosis, bronchopulmonary dysplasia
◆ **Reproductive:** Teratogenic effects, amenorrhea
◆ **Other:** Secondary malignancy, hypersensitivity, anaphylaxis

Special Considerations

◆ Contraindicated in patients with previous hypersensitivity reaction, pregnancy, lactation, bone marrow depression.
◆ Use caution in patients with impaired renal function.
◆ This drug is a potent irritant.
◆ IV administration is highly emetogenic. Start antiemetic regimen before administration.
◆ Tablets must be taken on an empty stomach to ensure adequate bioavailability.
◆ Instruct patient on use of contraception.

◆ 6-Mercaptopurine

(mer-kap-toe-**pyoor**'-een)   Purinethol   Pregnancy Category D

Mechanism of Action

Cell cycle–specific (S phase) purine antagonist antimetabolite that inhibits RNA and DNA synthesis.

Indications

Acute lymphocytic leukemia, acute myelocytic leukemia, acute myelomonocytic leukemia.

Metabolism/Excretion

Metabolized in the liver; excreted in urine.

Dosage Range

Initial dose 2.5 mg/kg per day PO as a single dose. When in hematologic remission, start maintenance dose at 1.5 to 2.5 mg/kg per day as a single dose. If patient is to receive concurrent allopurinol, reduce 6-mercaptopurine dose to one-third or one-fourth usual dose.

Drug Preparation/Stability

Available in 50-mg oral tablets. Store tablets at room temperature and protect from light. Dilute 500-mg vial with 50 mL sterile water (10 mg/mL 6-mercaptopurine). Further dilute in 0.09% sodium chloride or 5% dextrose to a concentration of 1 to 2 mg/mL. Stable for 24 hours.

Drug Administration

50-mg tablet for oral administration. Investigational: IV, IT.

Drug Interaction

◆ Concomitant use with allopurinol requires a dose reduction to one-third or one-fourth the usual dose; allopurinol enhances the toxicity of oral administration.

◆ Warfarin's anticoagulant effects are antagonized by 6-mercaptopurine.

Side Effects and Toxicities

◆ **Dermatologic:** Skin ulceration at injection site, alopecia, vasculitis

◆ **GI:** Nausea and vomiting, mild anorexia, mouth sores

◆ **Hematologic:** Bone marrow depression

◆ **Pulmonary:** Pulmonary toxicity

◆ **Reproductive:** Infertility

◆ **Other:** Hypersensitivity

Special Considerations

◆ Contraindicated in patients with previous hypersensitivity reaction, pregnancy, lactation, bone marrow depression.

◆ Use with caution in patients with impaired renal or hepatic function or those taking allopurinol.

- ◆ Assess hematopoietic status before and during therapy.
- ◆ Teach patient to drink adequate fluids (≥8 glasses/day) to avoid hyperuricemia.
- ◆ Instruct patient on use of contraception.

◆ Mesna

(**mes′**-na)   Mesnex   Pregnancy Category B

Mechanism of Action

Converted to its metabolite, mesna disulphide, which in the kidneys then is converted to the free thiol, mesna. The free thiol reacts chemically with the urotoxic ifosfamide metabolites, resulting in their detoxification.

Indications

As a prophylactic agent in reducing the incidence of hemorrhagic cystitis associated with ifosfamide therapy. Orphan drug use: Reduction of hemorrhagic cystitis in cyclophosphamide therapy.

Metabolism/Excretion

Excreted by the kidneys. Half-life: 0.36 to 1.7 hours.

Dosage Range

For adults and children, the recommended dose of mesna is equivalent to 20% of the ifosfamide dose. The mesna dose is given at the time of the ifosfamide infusion and at 4 hours and 8 hours after. With this fractionated dosing schedule, the total daily dose is equivalent to 60% of the ifosfamide dose. The cycle is repeated on each day of ifosfamide administration. If the ifosfamide dose is adjusted, the same should be done with the mesna dose. Mesna may be given orally at twice the IV dose. For higher doses of ifosfamide, Mesna at 100% of the ifosfamide dose is admixed with ifosfamide and given as a continuous infusion.

Drug Preparation/Stability

Dilute with 5% dextrose, 5% dextrose and 0.2% sodium chloride injection, 5% dextrose and 0.33% sodium chloride injection, 5% dextrose and 0.45% sodium chloride injection, 0.92% sodium chloride injection, or lactated Ringer's injection. The final concentration yields 20 mg/mL mesna. The reconstituted solution is stable for 24 hours at 25°C. Use the solution within 8 hours.

Drug Administration

IV bolus injection.

Drug Interaction

Incompatible with cisplatin. Produces a false-positive result for urinary ketones.

Side Effects and Toxicities

Nausea, vomiting, diarrhea.

Special Considerations

♦ Contraindicated in patients with known hypersensitivity to mesna or other thiol compounds.
♦ Use with caution in older children.
♦ Do not use the multidose vial in neonates and infants because of its benzyl alcohol content.
♦ Mesna does not prevent hemorrhagic cystitis in all patients. Test for hematuria before each day's ifosfamide therapy. If hematuria occurs despite mesna, ifosfamide doses should be adjusted or discontinued.

♦ Methotrexate

(meth-oh-**trex**'-ate)   MTX,   Pregnancy Category X
                     amethopterin

Mechanism of Action

Cell cycle–specific (S phase) antimetabolite that inhibits folic acid reductase by blocking the enzyme dihydrofolate reductase. Arrests DNA, RNA, and protein synthesis.

Indications

Trophoblastic neoplasms; acute leukemia; meningeal leukemia; breast carcinoma; head, neck, and lung neoplasms; Burkitt's lymphoma; osteosarcoma; lymphosarcoma; mycosis fungoides.

Metabolism/Excretion

Hepatic and intracellular metabolism; excreted primarily through the kidneys.

Dosage Range

Methotrexate is given by numerous dosing schedules; consult literature and manufacturer's guidelines for dosing.

Adult

◆ **Trophoblastic neoplasms:** three to five cycles of 15 to 30 mg/day IM or PO for 5 days.

◆ **Leukemia induction:** 3.3 mg/m^2 per day with prednisone 60 mg/m^2 per day.

◆ **Leukemia maintenance:** 2.5 mg/kg IV every 14 days or 15 mg/m^2 PO or IM twice a week.

◆ **Lymphoma:** *Burkitt's stage I or II:* 10 to 25 mg/day PO for 4 to 8 days; *stage III,* concurrently with combination therapy.

◆ **Mycosis fungoides:** 2.5 to 10 mg/day PO for variable lengths of time (weeks to months); 50 mg IM every week or 25 mg IM twice a week.

◆ **Osteosarcoma:** 12 to 15 g/m^2 IV, IM, or PO concurrently with leucovorin.

Pediatric

Safety and effectiveness established in osteosarcoma at 8 to 12 g/m^2 IV.

Drug Preparation/Stability

Reconstitute with sterile water, 0.9% sodium chloride, or 5% dextrose injectable solution. For preservative-free powder, use preservative-free 0.9% sodium chloride. 20 mL in 20-mg vial = 1 mg/mL; 20 mL in 50-mg vial = 2.5 mg/mL; 20 mL in 100-mg vial = 5 mg/mL; 19.4 mL in 1-g vial = 50 mg/mL. Use as soon as possible after reconstitution. Stable for 7 days after reconstitution, but discard after 24 hours because of lack of preservative. Vials and 2.5-mg tablets are stable for 2 years at room temperature. Protect from light.

Drug Administration

IV push, IV infusion, IV continuous infusion, IM, intrathecal, intra-arterial. Refer to the specific protocol and manufacturer's guidelines for dose and schedule guidelines.

Drug Interaction

◆ Enhanced methotrexate toxicity is common with phenytoin, salicylates, nonsteroidal anti-inflammatory drugs, and sulfonamides.

◆ Increased hepatotoxicity with alcohol.

◆ Consult literature regarding the many potential drugs that react with methotrexate.

Side Effects and Toxicities

◆ **Dermatologic:** Alopecia, urticaria, telangiectasia, acne, photosensitivity, folliculitis
◆ **GI:** Nausea and vomiting, stomatitis, GI ulceration, diarrhea, hepatotoxicity
◆ **GU:** Renal failure, hemorrhagic cysts
◆ **Hematologic:** Bone marrow suppression (cumulative)
◆ **Pulmonary:** Interstitial pneumonitis
◆ **Other:** Fever, malaise, chills

Special Considerations

◆ Contraindicated in patients with previous hypersensitivity, renal or hepatic disorder, myelosuppression, pregnancy, lactation.
◆ Due to potential for teratogenicity, instruct patient to use birth control during treatment and for ≥2 months after.
◆ Initiate antiemetic regimen before administration.
◆ Assess CBC, creatinine studies (BUN, urine, and serum creatinine), and liver function tests before, during, and after administration.
◆ Administer leucovorin and sodium bicarbonate concomitantly with high-dose methotrexate (see leucovorin for dosage).
◆ After high-dose methotrexate, assess specific gravity, urine output volume, and urinary pH; administer PO or IV leucovorin and sodium bicarbonate every 6 hours for 72 hours; and maintain urine pH >7 for 72 hours. Methotrexate precipitates in acid urine. Monitor serum methotrexate levels for 72 hours.
◆ Administer leucovorin rescue PO or IV for methotrexate toxicity.

◆ Mitomycin

(mye-toe-**mye**′-sin)   Mutamycin,   Pregnancy Category D
MTC,
Mitomycin-C

Mechanism of Action

Cell cycle–nonspecific antitumor antibiotic that inhibits DNA, RNA, and protein synthesis, causing cell lysis.

Indications

Part of combination or palliative therapy for disseminated adenocarcinoma of the stomach or pancreas. Unlabeled uses: Ovarian, cervical, or breast carcinoma; head and neck cancer; and non–small cell lung cancer.

Metabolism/Excretion

Metabolized in the liver; primarily excreted in urine.

Dosage Range

◆ **Adult:** Initially, 20 mg/m^2 IV as a single dose through a functioning IV catheter. Re-evaluate the patient after each course; reduce the dose if any toxicity is experienced. The following dosage schedule may be used at 6- to 8-week intervals:

Leukocytes/mm^3	Platelets	Percentage of Prior Dose to Be Given
>4000	>100,000	100%
>3000–3999	>75,000–99,999	100%
>2000–2999	>25,000–74,999	70%
<2000	<25,000	50%

◆ **Pediatric:** Safety and effectiveness not established.

Drug Preparation/Stability

Unreconstituted and stored at room temperature, stable for lot life on package. Avoid excessive heat. Reconstitute with sterile water for injection to a concentration of 0.5 mg/mL. Stable for 14 days refrigerated or 7 days at room temperature. Can be diluted in various IV fluids at room temperature to a concentration of 20 to 40 µg/mL:

IV Fluid	Stability
5% dextrose injection	3 h
0.9% sodium chloride injection	12 h
Sodium lactate injection	24 h

Each vial contains mitomycin 5 mg and mannitol 10 mg, mitomycin 20 mg and mannitol 40 mg, or mitomycin 40 mg and mannitol 80 mg. To administer, add sterile water for injection, 10, 40, or 80 mL, respectively. Shake to dissolve. If it does not dissolve, allow it to stand at room temperature until solution is obtained.

Drug Administration

IV. Mitomycin is a vesicant, so give carefully.

Drug Interaction

Enhanced toxicity often results when administered in combination with other myelosuppressive drugs.

Side Effects and Toxicities

- ◆ **Cardiac:** Congestive heart failure
- ◆ **CNS:** Confusion, headache, blurry vision, drowsiness, syncope
- ◆ **Dermatologic:** Cellulitis at injection site, stomatitis, alopecia, rashes, tissue necrosis and sloughing with extravasation
- ◆ **GI:** Nausea and vomiting, anorexia, diarrhea
- ◆ **GU:** Elevated creatinine and BUN, hemolytic uremic syndrome
- ◆ **Hematologic:** Delayed myelosuppression (4 to 8 weeks), cumulative myelosuppression
- ◆ **Pulmonary:** Dyspnea with nonproductive cough, radiographic evidence of pulmonary infiltrates, respiratory distress syndrome
- ◆ **Other:** Pain, fatigue, edema, thrombophlebitis, hypersensitivity, anaphylaxis

Special Considerations

- ◆ Contraindicated in patients with previous sensitivity to mitomycin, thrombocytopenia, coagulation disorder, increased bleeding tendency from other causes, pregnancy, lactation.
- ◆ Acute shortness of breath and severe bronchospasm have been reported after administration of vinca alkaloids in patients who have simultaneously or previously received mitomycin.
- ◆ Monitor blood counts before, during, and after treatment.
- ◆ Cumulative myelosuppression may occur. Follow recommended dosage reductions. No repeat doses should be given until the leukocyte count has returned to 4000/mm^3 and the platelet count to 100,000/mm^3.

◆ Stop administration if disease progresses through two courses of mitomycin.

◆ This drug is a potent vesicant. Assess for signs of extravasation; intervene immediately if present.

◆ Instruct patient on use of contraception.

◆ Mitotane

(**mye'**-toe-tane)   Lysodren   Pregnancy Category C

Mechanism of Action

Unknown. Appears to reduce levels of urinary and plasma adrenocorticosteroids and causes lysis of adrenal cortical cells.

Indications

Adrenal cortex carcinoma.

Metabolism/Excretion

Metabolized in the liver; excreted in urine and bile.

Dosage Range

◆ **Adult:** Initial dose 2 to 6 g/day PO in three or four divided doses, increased to 8 to 10 g/day until toxicities interfere. Maximum tolerated dose varies from 2 to 16 g/day; usual range is 8 to 10 g/day.

◆ **Pediatric:** Not recommended.

Drug Preparation/Stability

500-mg tablet needs no additional preparation. Stable until expiration date. Store at room temperature.

Drug Administration

PO

Drug Interaction

Questionable in metabolism of warfarin, phenytoin, cortisol, barbiturates.

Side Effects and Toxicities

◆ **CNS:** Depression, lethargy, dizziness, somnolence

◆ **Dermatologic:** Skin toxicity, transient skin rashes

- ◆ **GI:** Nausea and vomiting, anorexia, diarrhea
- ◆ **Other:** Adrenal crisis, adrenal insufficiency

Special Considerations

- ◆ Contraindicated in patients with adrenal insufficiency, pregnancy, lactation.
- ◆ Discontinue if severe trauma, shock, or sepsis occurs.
- ◆ Supplemental corticosteroids may be necessary.
- ◆ Instruct patient on use of contraception.

◆ Mitoxantrone Hydrochloride

(mye-toe-**zan**'-trone)   Novantrone   Pregnancy Category D

Mechanism of Action

Cell cycle–nonspecific agent that interacts with DNA and inhibits the DNA enzyme topoisomerase, causing cell lysis.

Indications

Acute monocytic leukemia, acute myelocytic leukemia, acute promyelocytic leukemia.

Metabolism/Excretion

Metabolized in the liver; primarily excreted in urine and feces.

Dosage Range

- ◆ **Adult:** 12 mg/m² per day for 2 to 3 days in combination therapy with cytosine arabinoside 100 mg/m² continuous infusion for 5 to 7 days. Cumulative cardiac dose is 120 to 140 mg/m², depending on history of mediastinal radiation or anthracycline therapy.
- ◆ **Pediatric:** Safety and effectiveness not established.

Drug Preparation/Stability

Sterile solution in vials containing 20, 25, or 30 mg of a 2-mg/mL concentration. Dilute in ≥50 mL 5% dextrose or 0.9% sodium chloride injection. Concentrations of 20 to 500 μg/mL in PVC containers are stable refrigerated or at room temperature for 1 week.

Drug Administration

IV infusion over at least 3 minutes through a free-flowing IV solution of 5% dextrose or 0.9% sodium chloride.

Drug Interaction

Synergistic effect of cytosine arabinoside and mitoxantrone.

Side Effects and Toxicities

◆ **Cardiac:** Congestive heart failure, tachycardia, chest pain, ECG changes
◆ **Dermatologic:** Alopecia, rash, urticaria
◆ **GI:** Mild to moderate nausea and vomiting, stomatitis, mucositis
◆ **Hematologic:** Myelosuppression
◆ **Reproductive:** Teratogenic effects
◆ **Other:** Bluish-green urine and bluish sclera, phlebitis, hypersensitivity

Special Considerations

◆ Contraindicated in patients with previous hypersensitivity, severe cardiovascular disease, pregnancy, lactation.
◆ Monitor blood counts before, during, and after therapy.
◆ Perform cardiac monitoring before treatment and at predetermined intervals after treatment.
◆ Inform patient that urine and sclera may become bluish for 1 to 2 days after administration.
◆ Increased potential for cardiotoxicity if patient received previous mediastinal radiation or anthracycline therapy.
◆ Instruct patient on use of contraception.

◆ Muromonab-CD3

(mew-**ro'**-mon-ab)   Orthoclone,   Pregnancy Category C
OKT3

Mechanism of Action

Functions as an immunosuppressant by blocking the function of all T cells.

Indications

Acute allograft rejection in renal transplant patients; steroid-resistant acute allograft rejection in cardiac and hepatic transplant patients.

Metabolism/Excretion

Mean time of appearance of IgG antibodies is 20 ± 2 days.

Dosage Range

- ◆ **Adult:** 5 mg/day in a single bolus as an IV injection for 10 to 14 days.
- ◆ **Pediatric:** Safety and efficacy not established.

Drug Preparation/Stability

Supplied in solution for injection: 5-mL ampule contains 5 mg of muromonab-CD3. Store in the refrigerator at 2° to 8°C (36° to 46°F). Do not shake or freeze. Once the ampule is opened, use immediately and discard unused portion.

Drug Administration

IV administration as a bolus in <1 minute. Do not administer by IV infusion or in conjunction with other drug solutions.

Drug Interaction

- ◆ Indomethacin: encephalopathy and other CNS effects
- ◆ Corticosteroids: psychosis and infections
- ◆ Azathioprine: infections and malignancies
- ◆ Cyclosporine: seizures, encephalopathy, infections, malignancies, thrombotic event

Side Effects and Toxicities

- ◆ **CNS:** Seizures, encephalopathy, cerebral edema, aseptic meningitis
- ◆ **GU:** Decline in glomerular filtration rate, decreased urine output
- ◆ **Hematologic:** Pancytopenia, aplastic anemia, neutropenia, leukopenia, thrombocytopenia, lymphopenia, leukocytosis; increased transaminases, BUN, and serum creatinine
- ◆ **Hypersensitivity:** Cardiovascular collapse, cardiorespiratory arrest, loss of consciousness, hypotension, tachycardia, tingling, angioedema, airway obstruction, bronchospasm, dyspnea, urticaria, pruritus
- ◆ **Integumentary:** Rash, erythema, flushing, diaphoresis
- ◆ **Musculoskeletal:** Arthralgia, arthritis, myalgia, stiffness, aches, pains
- ◆ **Pulmonary and cardiovascular:** Pulmonary edema, apnea, wheezing, shortness of breath, hypoxemia, angina, bradycardia, hypertension, arrhythmias, chest pain or tightness
- ◆ **Other:** Cytokine release syndrome, characterized by

high fevers, chills and rigors, headache, tremor, nausea and vomiting, diarrhea, abdominal pain, malaise, muscle and joint aches and pains, and generalized weakness; infections, malignancies, lymphoproliferative disorders

Special Considerations

◆ Contraindicated in patients with known allergy to muromonab-CD3 or any other product of murine origins, antimouse antibody titer >1:1000, uncompensated heart failure or fluid overload, history of seizures, pregnancy, lactation.

◆ Treat patients in an area equipped and staffed for cardiopulmonary resuscitation.

◆ Assess fluid volume status before treatment. There should be no evidence of heart failure or fluid overload seen on chest x-ray or a weight gain >3% within the week before treatment.

◆ Monitor vital signs frequently.

◆ Monitor for serious allergic events, including anaphylactic reactions. Serious acute hypersensitivity reactions may require emergency treatment with epinephrine, oxygen treatment, IV fluids, antihistamines, and corticosteroids.

◆ Monitor laboratory test results (renal, hepatic, hematopoietic function) periodically.

◆ May need to premedicate with methylprednisolone sodium succinate 8.0 mg/kg 1 to 4 hours before first dose.

◆ Discontinue drug with an acute hypersensitivity reaction (usually occurs within 10 minutes of administration).

◆ To prepare for injections, use a low protein-binding 0.2- or 0.22-micron filter.

◆ Do not infuse simultaneously with other drugs. IV line should be flushed with saline before and after infusion.

◆ Paclitaxel

(pass-leh-**tax**'-el)   Taxol   Pregnancy Category D

Mechanism of Action

A novel antimicrotubule cytotoxic agent that promotes microtubule assembly and inhibits the microtubule reorganization that is essential for interphase and mitotic function.

Indications

Metastatic carcinoma of ovary after failure of first-line or subsequent chemotherapy; breast carcinoma after failure of combination chemotherapy for metastatic disease or relapse within 6 months of adjuvant chemotherapy.

Metabolism/Excretion

Metabolized in the liver; excreted in bile.

Dosage Range

Adult

◆ **Breast carcinoma:** 175 mg/m^2 IV over 24 hours every 3 weeks.

◆ **Ovarian carcinoma:** 135 mg/m^2 or 175 mg/m^2 IV over 3 hours every 3 weeks.

◆ Do not repeat the dose until the neutrophil count is ≥1500/mm^3 and the platelet count is ≥100,000 cells/mm^3. Patients with severe neutropenia (neutrophil count <500/mm^3 for 1 week or longer) or with severe peripheral neuropathy from paclitaxel should receive a 20% dose reduction for subsequent doses.

Pediatric

Safety and effectiveness not established.

Drug Preparation/Stability

Dilute concentrate before infusion in 0.9% sodium chloride, 5% dextrose, 5% dextrose plus 0.9% sodium chloride, or 5% dextrose in Ringer's injection to a final concentration of 0.3 to 1.2 mg/mL. Diluted solution is physically and chemically stable for up to 27 hours at room temperature. Refrigerate intact vials; they are stable until the date indicated on the package. Solutions should be prepared and stored in glass, polypropylene, or polyolefin containers only. Use non-PVC administration sets; PVC contains the extractable plasticizer di-(2-ethylhexyl)phthaletel (DEHP), and significant leaching of DEHP can occur.

Drug Administration

IV in a 3- to 24-hour infusion or by an ambulatory infusion pump over 96 hours. Change the ambulatory pump cassette every 24 hours.

To prevent severe hypersensitivity reactions, premedicate

patient with dexamethasone 20 mg PO 12 and 6 hours before paclitaxel; diphenhydramine 50 mg IV 30 to 60 minutes before; and cimetidine 300 mg or ranitidine 50 mg IV 30 to 60 minutes before.

Drug Interaction

◆ Cisplatin and paclitaxel can cause synergistic myelo-suppression and neurotoxicity.
◆ Ketoconazole reduces the effect of paclitaxel.

Side Effects and Toxicities

◆ **Cardiac:** Hypotension, rhythm abnormalities, hypertension, venous thrombosis, ECG abnormalities, complete atrioventricular block
◆ **CNS:** Peripheral neuropathy, syncope, ataxia, arthralgia, myalgia
◆ **Dermatologic:** Injection site reaction, alopecia
◆ **GI:** Nausea and vomiting, diarrhea, mucositis
◆ **Hematologic:** Bone marrow depression, severe neutropenia
◆ **Other:** Hypersensitivity reaction, anaphylaxis, infection

Special Considerations

◆ Contraindicated in patients with previous hypersensitivity, baseline neutropenia of <1500/mm^3, pregnancy, lactation.
◆ Give infusion solution through a 0.22-micron in-line filter using non-PVC tubing.
◆ Severe hypersensitivity reactions require discontinuation of infusion.
◆ Monitor blood counts before, during, and after therapy.
◆ Monitor vital signs before and during infusions.
◆ Perform neurologic examination at baseline and at regular intervals.
◆ Instruct patient on use of contraception.

◆ Pamidronate Disodium

(pam-**ee**'-dro-nayt)   Aredia   Pregnancy Category C

Mechanism of Action

Believed to inhibit bone resorption by blocking the dissolution of calcium phosphate crystals in the bone.

Indications

Osteolytic bone metastases of breast cancer and osteolytic lesions of multiple myeloma; hypercalcemia of malignancy; Paget's disease.

Metabolism/Excretion

Not metabolized; exclusively eliminated by the renal system. Half-life: 16 hours, then 27.3 hours.

Dosage Range

Adult

- ◆ **Osteolytic bone metastasis of breast cancer:** 90 mg as a 2-hour infusion given over 3 to 4 weeks.
- ◆ **Osteolytic bone lesions of multiple myeloma:** 90 mg as a 4-hour infusion on a monthly cycle. Patients with marked Bence-Jones proteinuria and dehydration should be adequately hydrated before the infusion.
- ◆ **Hypercalcemia of malignancy:** For moderate hypercalcemia (corrected serum calcium 12.0 to 13.5 mg/dL), 60 to 90 mg. Give the 60-mg dose as an initial, single-dose infusion over 4 hours; give the 90-mg dose as an initial single-dose infusion over 24 hours. For severe hypercalcemia (corrected serum calcium >13.5 mg/dL), 90 mg given as an initial, single-agent infusion over 24 hours. For hypercalcemic patients who show complete or partial response initially, treatment may be repeated, using the initial dose; 7 days should elapse before retreatment.
- ◆ **Paget's disease:** For patients with moderate to severe conditions, 30 mg/day as a 4-hour infusion given for 3 consecutive days. When clinically indicated, retreatment may be given at the initial dose.

Pediatric

Not labeled for pediatric use.

Drug Preparation/Stability

Reconstitute contents of vial by adding 10 mL sterile water for injection. Preparation is stable for 24 hours at room temperature. The reconstituted solution may be stored under refrigeration at 36° to 46°F for up to 24 hours.

Drug Administration

- ◆ **Osteolytic bone metastasis of breast cancer:** Dilute the recommended dose of 90 mg in 250 mL 0.45% or

0.9% sodium chloride or 5% dextrose injection, and administer as a 2-hour infusion every 3 to 4 weeks.

◆ **Osteolytic bone lesions of multiple myeloma:** Dilute the recommended dose of 90-mg solution in 500 of sterile 0.45% or 0.9% sodium chloride or 5% dextrose injection, and administer as a 4-hour infusion on a monthly cycle.

◆ **Paget's disease:** Dilute the recommended dose of 30 mg in 500 mL sterile 0.45% or 0.9% sodium chloride or 5% dextrose injection, and administer as a 4-hour infusion for 3 consecutive days.

Drug Interaction

Concomitant administration of loop diuretics has had no effect on the calcium-lowering property of pamidronate.

Side Effects and Toxicities

◆ **CNS:** Headache, insomnia
◆ **GI:** Nausea, vomiting, anorexia, constipation, diarrhea
◆ **GU:** Urinary tract infection
◆ **Hematologic:** Anemia, granulocytopenia, thrombocytopenia
◆ **Hypersensitivity:** Allergic reaction characterized by swollen and itchy eyes, runny nose, scratchy throat, and pain at infusion site
◆ **Other:** Fatigue, fever, skeletal pain, transient arthralgias, myalgias

Special Considerations

◆ Monitor serum calcium, electrolytes, phosphate, magnesium, creatinine, and CBC closely.
◆ Monitor patients with pre-existing anemia, leukopenia, or thrombocytopenia closely for the first 2 weeks of treatment.
◆ Do not mix with solutions containing calcium, such as Ringer's solution.
◆ Administer infusion using a dedicated IV line.
◆ Inspect solution for discoloration or particulate manner.

◆ Pegasparagase

(peg-ass-**par**′-a-gase)   Oncaspar   Pregnancy Category C

Mechanism of Action

A derivative of the L-asparaginase enzyme, which destroys

the amino acid asparagine needed for cancer cell proliferation. Inhibits malignant cell production.

Indications

Acute lymphoblastic leukemia in patients hypersensitive to native forms of L-asparaginase.

Metabolism/Excretion

Small amounts are excreted in urine and bile.

Dosage Range

For adults and children with a body surface area of ≥ 0.6 m^2, 2500 IU/m^2 every 14 days. For children with a body surface area of <0.6 m^2, 82.5 IU/kg every 14 days.

Drug Preparation/Stability

Preservative-free 5-mL single-dose vial, 750 IU/mL. Keep vials refrigerated. Discard if left at room temperature for >48 hours or if cloudy, if a precipitate forms, or if frozen. Dilute for IV infusion in 100 mL 5% dextrose or 0.9% sodium chloride injection. IM injection should not exceed 2 mL per dose.

Drug Administration

IV infusion over 1 to 2 hours through a running infusion; IM, rotate administration sites.

Drug Interaction

Nephrotoxic and hepatotoxic drugs increase the risk of nephrotoxicity or hepatotoxicity when concurrently administered with pegasparagase.

Side Effects and Toxicities

- ◆ **Cardiac:** Chest pain, hypotension, hypertension
- ◆ **CNS:** Malaise, confusion, lethargy
- ◆ **GI:** Nausea and vomiting, anorexia, hepatotoxicity
- ◆ **GU:** Tumor lysis syndrome, nephrotoxicity
- ◆ **Hematologic:** Clotting factor depression
- ◆ **Pulmonary:** Respiratory distress
- ◆ **Other:** Pancreatitis, hyperglycemia, fever, hypersensitivity

Special Considerations

- ◆ Contraindicated in patients with history of hemor-

rhagic events with L-asparaginase, previous hypersensitivity, pancreatitis, or history of pancreatitis.
- ◆ Use caution in patients with diabetes.
- ◆ Monitor kidney function, liver function, clotting factors, and serum glucose before and after each dose
- ◆ Can cause contact dermatitis.

◆ Pentostatin

(**pen**′-toe-stah-tin)   Nipent   Pregnancy Category D

Mechanism of Action

An antitumor antibiotic that inhibits the ADA enzyme and causes cell lysis.

Indications

Alpha-interferon–refractory hairy cell leukemia in adults.

Metabolism/Excretion

Metabolized in the liver; excreted in urine.

Dosage Range

- ◆ **Adult:** 4 mg/m^2 IV every other week.
- ◆ **Pediatric:** Safety and effectiveness not established.

Drug Preparation/Stability

10-mg powder for reconstitution for IV administration. Reconstitute with 5 mL sterile water for injection to yield a 2-mg/mL solution. May be further diluted in 25 to 50 mL 5% dextrose or 0.9% sodium chloride injection. Diluted solutions at room temperature must be used within 8 hours.

Drug Administration

IV push or IV piggyback over 20 to 30 minutes.

Drug Interaction

- ◆ Allopurinol used concomitantly may cause skin rashes.
- ◆ Fludarabine used concomitantly may cause fatal pulmonary toxicity.
- ◆ Vidarabine used concomitantly may enhance pentostatin toxicity.

Side Effects and Toxicities

◆ **Dermatologic:** Rash
◆ **GI:** Nausea and vomiting, elevated liver function tests, hepatic disorder
◆ **Hematologic:** Myelosuppression
◆ **GU:** Slight, transient rise in serum creatinine
◆ **Other:** Infection, fever, fatigue

Special Considerations

◆ Contraindicated in patients with previous hypersensitivity, pregnancy, lactation.
◆ Use cautiously with renal failure and myelosuppression.
◆ Avoid administration with fludarabine.
◆ Monitor blood counts and liver and kidney function tests.
◆ Hydrate before pentostatin with 500 to 1000 mL 5% dextrose with 0.9% sodium chloride and after pentostatin with 5% dextrose injection.
◆ Instruct patient on use of contraception.

◆ Pipobroman

(pip-o-**bro**′-man)   Vercyte   Pregnancy Category: Not Available

Mechanism of Action

Unknown; pipobroman is a polyfunctional cytotoxic alkylating agent that is cell cycle–nonspecific.

Indications

Polycythemia vera, chronic granulocytic leukemia.

Metabolism/Excretion

Metabolized in the liver; excreted in urine.

Dosage Range

◆ **Adult:** Initially, 1 mg/kg per day increased to a maximum of 3 mg/kg per day every 30 days; maintenance dose is 0.1 to 0.2 mg/kg per day.
◆ **Pediatric:** Not recommended.

Drug Preparation/Stability
Available in 10- and 25-mg tablets. Store at room temperature.

Drug Administration
PO

Drug Interaction
Information not available.

Side Effects and Toxicities
- ◆ **Dermatologic:** Rash
- ◆ **GI:** Nausea and vomiting, abdominal cramps, diarrhea
- ◆ **GU:** Elevated bilirubin
- ◆ **Hematologic:** Bone marrow suppression
- ◆ **Other:** Secondary malignancy

Special Considerations
Monitor blood counts and serum bilirubin level.

◆ Plicamycin

(plye-kay-**mye'**-sin)   Mithramycin,   Pregnancy Category X
Mithracin

Mechanism of Action
An antitumor antibiotic that binds to DNA and inhibits DNA-directed RNA synthesis. Acts on osteoclasts and blocks the action of parathyroid hormone.

Indications
Testicular carcinoma, hypercalcemia.

Metabolism/Excretion
Metabolized in the liver; excreted in urine.

Dosage Range
Adult
- ◆ **Testicular carcinoma:** 25 to 30 μg/kg per day for 8 to 10 days.
- ◆ **Hypercalcemia:** 25 μg/kg per day for 3 to 4 days.

Pediatric
Safety and effectiveness not established.

Drug Preparation/Stability

Reconstitute 2.5-mg (2,500-μg) vial with 4.9 mL sterile water for injection to prepare a 500-mg/mL solution. Stable for 24 hours at room temperature or 48 hours refrigerated.

Drug Administration

IV infusion in 1 L 5% dextrose injection or 0.9% sodium chloride injection over 4 to 6 hours through a central venous access device.

Drug Interaction

None known

Side Effects and Toxicities

- ◆ **CNS:** Depression, confusion
- ◆ **Dermatologic:** Facial flushing, tissue damage if extravasation occurs.
- ◆ **GI:** Nausea and vomiting, diarrhea, anorexia, stomatitis, hepatotoxicity
- ◆ **Hematologic:** Multiple clotting factor disorders
- ◆ **Other:** Hypophosphatemia, hypokalemia, hypocalcemia, fever

Special Considerations

- ◆ Contraindicated in patients with thrombocytopenia, renal or hepatic dysfunction, coagulation disorders, previous hypersensitivity, electrolyte imbalance, pregnancy, lactation.
- ◆ Monitor blood counts, renal and liver function tests, clotting factors, and electrolytes before, during, and after therapy.
- ◆ Epistaxis may be first indication of bleeding syndrome associated with the onset of a clotting disorder.
- ◆ Educate patient on contraceptive use.

◆ Porfimer Sodium

(**poor**'-fa-mer)   Photofrin   Pregnancy Category C

Mechanism of Action

Acts as a photosensitizer in tissue exposed to light wave lengths >600 nm delivered by a laser to destroy tumor cells.

Indications

Palliation for esophageal cancer refractory to laser therapy.

Metabolism/Excretion

Intracellular metabolism; eliminated at the cellular level.

Dosage Range

♦ **Adult:** 2 mg/kg IV push slowly over 3 to 5 minutes, followed in 40 to 50 hours and 96 to 120 hours with laser therapy.
♦ **Pediatric:** Not used.

Drug Preparation/Stability

75-mg sterile freeze-dried powder vials stored in the dark, refrigerated. Each 75-mg vial is reconstituted with 30 mL 5% dextrose for injection, yielding a concentration of 2.5-mg/mL solution. Reconstituted drug protected from light and stored at room temperature is stable for 24 hours, but use within 4 hours of reconstitution.

Drug Administration

IV push slowly over 3 to 5 minutes.

Drug Interaction

Enhanced photosensitivity with diuretics, sulfonamides, griseofulvin, tetracyclines, phenothiazines.

Side Effects and Toxicities

♦ **Cardiac:** Arrhythmias, hypertension, hypotension, chest pain
♦ **CNS:** Confusion, insomnia
♦ **Dermatologic:** Photosensitivity, severe sunburn
♦ **GI:** Nausea and vomiting, dysphagia, abdominal pain, constipation
♦ **Pulmonary:** Dyspnea, pharyngitis, coughing, fistula, effusion
♦ **Other:** Pain, fever

Special Considerations

♦ Contraindicated in patients with previous hypersensitivity, esophageal fistula, pregnancy, lactation.
♦ Ensure patient has no esophageal fistulas before administration.

◆ Coordinate administration time with laser therapy.
◆ Teach patient to avoid sun exposure and indoor bright light for ≥30 days and to wear protective clothing.
◆ Review medications taken.
◆ Educate patient on use of contraception.
◆ Patient may feel substernal pain from an inflammatory response at the area of treatment; analgesics might be needed.

◆ Procarbazine

(pro-**kar′**-ba-zeen)   Matulane   Pregnancy Category D

Mechanism of Action

Unclear; possible inhibition of DNA, RNA and protein synthesis, and alkylation of DNA. Cell cycle–specific with greatest activity during S phase.

Indications

Hodgkin's disease, brain tumors, multiple myeloma, lymphomas, small cell lung cancer.

Metabolism/Excretion

Metabolized in the liver; excreted in urine.

Dosage Range

◆ **Adult:** Initially, 2 to 4 mg/kg per day PO for 7 days, then 4 to 6 mg/kg per day until maximum response achieved; maintenance, 1 to 2 mg/kg per day.
◆ **Pediatric:** Initially, 50 mg/m^2 per day PO for 7 days, then 100 mg/m^2 per day until maximum response achieved; maintenance, 50 mg/m^2 per day PO. Use in children is not as well established.

Drug Preparation/Stability

50-mg capsule requires no preparation. Stable for 12 years if stored at room temperature in a moisture-free environment. Check expiration date before administration.

Drug Administration

PO

Drug Interaction

◆ CNS depressants concurrently administered with procarbazine may potentiate procarbazine's sedative effects.

◆ Concomitant use of alcohol may cause a disulfiram-like reaction.

◆ Sympathomimetic drugs, tricyclic antidepressants, and foods with tyramine should be avoided because of procarbazine's inhibitory effects on monoamine oxidase.

◆ Concomitant use of digoxin may decrease serum levels and effectiveness of digoxin.

Side Effects and Toxicities

◆ **CNS:** Confusion, lethargy, depression, paresthesias, insomnia, nervousness, ataxia

◆ **Dermatologic:** Alopecia, pruritus, hyperpigmentation

◆ **GI:** Nausea and vomiting, anorexia, diarrhea, constipation, xerostomia, stomatitis

◆ **Hematologic:** Bone marrow depression

◆ **Other:** Fever, pain, diaphoresis

Special Considerations

◆ Monitor blood counts before, during, and after therapy.

◆ Teach patient to avoid the following tyramine-rich foods: wine, cola, cheese, tea, coffee, dark beer, bananas, yogurt.

◆ Instruct patient on use of contraception.

◆ Sargramostim

(sar-**gram'**-oh-stim)   Leukine   Pregnancy Category C

Mechanism of Action

Activates mature granulocytes and macrophages; promotes the proliferation and differentiation of hematopoietic progenitor cells.

Indications

◆ To accelerate neutrophil recovery and reduce the incidence of severe and life-threatening infections after induction chemotherapy in older patients (>55 years) with acute myelogenous leukemia.

◆ Use in mobilization and after transplantation of autologous peripheral blood progenitor cells.

◆ To accelerate myeloid recovery in patients with non-Hodgkin's lymphoma, acute lymphoblastic leukemia, and Hodgkin's disease who are undergoing autologous bone marrow transplantation.

◆ For patients who have undergone allogenic or autologous bone marrow transplantation in whom engraftment is delayed or has failed.

Metabolism/Excretion

Metabolism unknown. Elimination half-life: 12 to 17 minutes, followed by a slower decrease (2 hours) after IV administration. Serum levels peak at 2 hours after SQ injection.

Dosage Range

Adult

◆ **Neutrophil recovery after chemotherapy in acute myelogenous leukemia:** 250 mcg/m^2 per day IV over 4 hours starting roughly on day 11, or 4 days after the completion of induction chemotherapy. Dose can be halved if the neutrophil count exceeds 20,000/mm^3.

◆ **Mobilization and after transplantation of autologous peripheral blood progenitor cells:** 250 mcg/m^2 per day IV over 24 hours or injected daily SQ. Continue until peripheral blood progenitor cell collection is complete. Reduce by half if WBC count is >50,000/mm^3.

◆ **After transplantation of autologous peripheral progenitor cells:** 250 mcg/m^2 per day IV over 24 hours or SQ beginning immediately after infusion of progenitor cells and continuing until neutrophil count is >1500 for 3 consecutive days.

◆ **Myeloid recovery in patients undergoing autologous bone marrow transplantation:** 250 mcg/m^2 per day IV over 2 hours for 21 days starting 2 to 4 hours after the bone marrow infusion and ≥24 hours after the last dose of chemotherapy or radiation therapy. Monitor CBC with differential twice a week during treatment. Withhold or reduce dose by half if neutrophil count exceeds 20,000/mm^3.

◆ **Bone marrow transplantation failure or engraftment delay:** 250 mcg/m^2 per day IV over 2 hours for 14 days. Can repeat dose after 7 days of therapy if engraftment has not occurred. A third cycle of 500 mcg/m^2 per day administered for 14 days may be given after another 7 days of therapy. Withhold or reduce dose by half if neutrophil count exceeds 20,000/mm^3.

Pediatric

Safety and efficacy not established.

Drug Preparation/Stability

Supplied in powder for injection: single-use, preservative-free vial containing 250 or 500 mcg/mL. Reconstitute with 1.0 mL sterile water or bacteriostatic water for injection. Powder diluted with sterile water should be given as soon as possible and within 6 hours after reconstitution. Powder diluted with bacteriostatic water may be stored for up to 20 days at 2° to 8°C (36° to 46°F) before use. Use 0.9% sodium chloride injection to dilute sargramostim for infusion. Discard unused portions. Do not shake or freeze.

Drug Administration

IV administration or SQ injection.

Drug Interaction

Not fully evaluated. Lithium and corticosteroids may potentiate the myeloproliferative effects of sargramostim.

Side Effects and Toxicities

- ◆ **Constitutional:** Fever, malaise, headache, chills, pain, sweats
- ◆ **CNS:** Paresthesia, insomnia, anxiety
- ◆ **GI:** Nausea, diarrhea, vomiting, anorexia, GI disorder, GI hemorrhage, stomatitis, abdominal pain, dyspepsia, constipation
- ◆ **GU:** Urinary tract disorder, kidney function abnormality, hematuria
- ◆ **Hematologic:** Increased glucose, creatinine, BUN, cholesterol, alanine transferase; decreased albumin
- ◆ **Integumentary:** Alopecia, rash, pruritus
- ◆ **Musculoskeletal:** Asthenia, bone pain, arthralgia
- ◆ **Pulmonary and cardiovascular:** Dyspnea, pharyngitis, epistaxis, chest pain, hypertension, tachycardia
- ◆ **Other:** Edema, weight loss, weight gain

Special Considerations

◆ Contraindicated in patients with excessive leukemia myeloid blasts in the bone marrow or peripheral blood; known allergy to sargramostim, yeast-derived products, or any component of the product; concomitant use of chemotherapy and radiation therapy.

◆ Do not use within 24 hours before or after cytotoxic chemotherapy or radiation therapy.

◆ Monitor for respiratory symptoms during or immediately after administration. Rate of infusion may be halved if patient has respiratory symptoms.

◆ Monitor for first-dose reaction characterized by hypotension with flushing and syncope.

◆ Monitor neutrophil and platelet counts twice a week. If neutrophil count exceeds $20,000/mm^3$ or platelet counts exceed $500,000/mm^3$, withhold dose or reduce by half.

◆ Satumomab Pendetide

(sah-**too**′-moe-mab)   OncoScint,   Pregnancy Category C
                          CR/OV

Mechanism of Action

A conjugate from a murine monoclonal antibody that localizes or binds to a tumor-associated antigen (TAG-72).

Indications

To determine the extent and location of extrahepatic malignant disease in patients with known colorectal or ovarian cancer.

Metabolism/Excretion

Elimination pattern with a terminal-phase half-life of 56 ± 14 hours. About 10% of the administered radioisotope dose is excreted in the urine during the 72 hours after IV administration.

Dosage Range

◆ **Adult:** 1 mg radiolabeled with 5 mCi of indium in chloride-111. Each dose is administered IV over 5 minutes. Do not mix with any other medication during administration.

◆ **Pediatric:** Safety and efficacy not established.

Drug Preparation/Stability

Supplied as a kit including one vial containing 1 mg of satumomab pendetide per 2 mL of sodium phosphatase-buffered saline and one 2-mL vial of sodium acetate buffer solution, one sterile 0.22-micron Millex GV filter, prescribing information, and two identification labels. Store upright at 2° to 8°C (36° to 46°F). Do not freeze. Use within 8 hours after radiolabeling.

Drug Administration

IV. Images using a gamma camera should be obtained 48 to 72 hours after injection. Follow-up images can be performed.

Side Effects and Toxicities

Fever

Special Considerations

◆ Contraindicated in patients with known allergy to satumomab pendetide or any other product of murine origins or indium in chloride-111.

◆ Should be given only by physicians or qualified professionals experienced in the safe use and handling of radionuclides.

◆ Although allergic reactions, such as anaphylaxis, have not been observed, medications for the treatment of hypersensitivity reactions should be available during administration.

◆ May result in falsely elevated carcinoembryonic antigen (CEA) and CA-125 tests.

◆ Follow radiation precautions per hospital policy.

◆ Streptozocin

(strep-toe-**zoe**′-sin)   Zanosar   Pregnancy Category C

Mechanism of Action

A nitrosourea alkylating agent that causes cell lysis by impairing DNA synthesis through intrastrand cross-linking of DNA.

Indications

Pancreatic carcinoma, colon carcinoma, carcinoid tumors.

Metabolism/Excretion

Metabolized in the liver; excreted in urine.

Dosage Range

◆ **Adult:** 500 mg/m^2 per day IV for 5 days every 6 weeks or 1 g/m^2 per week IV for 2 weeks; increase next doses if no toxicity or no response; maximum 1.5 g/m^2 per week.
◆ **Pediatric:** Safety and effectiveness not established.

Drug Preparation/Stability

Reconstitute injectable 1-g vial with 9.5 mL 5% dextrose injection or 0.9% sodium chloride injection to yield a solution of 100 mg/mL. Use as soon as possible, but can be kept for up to 12 hours, if refrigerated. Refrigerate 1-g injectable vials and protect from light. Check package label expiration date.

Drug Administration

Slow IV push into a running line of 5% dextrose or 0.9% sodium chloride injection, or IV infusion in up to 500 mL 5% dextrose or 0.9% sodium chloride.

Drug Interaction

Significant hyperglycemic interactions are possible.

Side Effects and Toxicities

◆ **Dermatologic:** Tissue damage secondary to extravasation
◆ **GI:** Nausea and vomiting, diarrhea, elevated liver function tests
◆ **GU:** Nephrotoxicity, renal tubular acidosis
◆ **Hematologic:** Bone marrow depression
◆ **Reproductive:** Infertility likely
◆ **Other:** Insulin-dependent diabetes, hypersensitivity, anaphylaxis, secondary malignancy

Special Considerations

◆ Contraindicated in patients with previous hypersensitivity, bone marrow depression, pregnancy, lactation.
◆ Use with caution in patients with hepatic or renal dysfunction.

◆ Monitor serum glucose before, during, and after therapy because hypoglycemic reactions may occur from the sudden release of insulin.
◆ Monitor liver and renal function tests before, during, and after therapy.
◆ Provide antiemetics as needed.
◆ Discontinue if renal toxicity occurs.

◆ Tamoxifen

(ta-**mox'**-i-fen)　　　Nolvadex　　　Pregnancy Category D

Mechanism of Action

An antiestrogen that competes for estrogen binding sites in breast tissue.

Indications

Axillary node-negative breast cancer in women after total or segmental axillary dissection and breast irradiation; node-positive breast cancer in postmenopausal women after total or segmental mastectomy, breast irradiation, and axillary dissection.

Metabolism/Excretion

Metabolized in the liver; excreted in feces.

Dosage Range

◆ **Adult:** 20 to 40 mg/day PO. Give dosages of >20 mg/day in two divided doses.
◆ **Pediatric:** Safety and effectiveness not established.

Drug Preparation/Stability

Available in 10- and 20-mg tablets stored at room temperature. No preparation required. Check package lot label for expiration date.

Drug Administration

PO

Drug Interaction

◆ Concomitant administration with bromocriptine raises serum levels of tamoxifen.

◆ Increased risk of thromboembolic events when used in combination with antineoplastic cytotoxic agents.

◆ Concomitant use with coumarin-type anticoagulants may increase the anticoagulant effect.

Side Effects and Toxicities

◆ **CNS:** Dizziness, depression, headache, diminished visual acuity, corneal opacity, retinopathy
◆ **Dermatologic:** Skin rash, hot flashes
◆ **GI:** Nausea and vomiting
◆ **GU:** Vaginal bleeding, menstrual irregularities, vaginal discharge
◆ **Hematologic:** Myelosuppression
◆ **Other:** Pain, peripheral edema

Special Considerations

◆ Contraindicated in patients with previous allergy to tamoxifen, pregnancy, lactation.
◆ Monitor blood counts before, during, and after therapy.
◆ Obtain baseline and periodic ophthalmologic examination.
◆ Instruct patient to use a contraceptive.

◆ Temozolomide

(teh-moo-**zoh**′-loh-mide)   Temodar   Pregnancy Category D

Mechanism of Action

Not directly active, but undergoes rapid nonenzymatic conversion to the reactive compound 5-(3-methyltriazen-1-y) imidazole-4-carboxamide (MTIC). The cytotoxic action of MTIC is thought to be due primarily to alkylation of DNA.

Indications

Adult anaplastic astrocytoma that has progressed during or after active treatment with a drug regimen containing a nitrosourea and procarbazine.

Metabolism/Excretion

Spontaneously hydrolyzed at physiologic pH to the active species, MTIC. Rapidly and completely absorbed after oral intake. Mean elimination life: 1.8 hours; eliminated mostly in the urine.

Dosage Range

◆ **Adult:** Initially, 150 mg/m^2 given once a day for 5 days per 28-day cycle. If the absolute neutrophil count at both the nadir and on the day of dosing (day 29 or day 1 of the next cycle) is >1500 and the platelet count exceeds 100,000, the dose may be increased to 200 mg/m^2 for another 5 consecutive days. During treatment, obtain CBC on day 22 or within 48 hours of that day and weekly until the absolute neutrophil count is >1500 and the platelet count exceeds 100,000; do not start the next cycle until these counts are reached. If the absolute neutrophil count falls to ≤1000 and the platelet count is <50,000 during the cycle, decrease the dose by 50 mg/m^2, but not below the lowest recommended dose of 100 mg/m^2.

◆ **Pediatric:** Safety and effectiveness not established.

Drug Preparation/Stability

Store at room temperature.

Drug Administration

PO

Drug Interaction

Administration of valproic acid decreases oral clearance of temozolomide by about 5%. The clinical impact of this reaction is not known.

Side Effects and Toxicities

◆ **GI:** Nausea and vomiting, usually after several cycles of therapy; will resolve within 2 weeks

◆ **Hematologic: Bone marrow suppression, thrombocytopenia and neutropenia are dose-limiting.**

◆ **Other:** Fatigue, headache

Special Considerations

◆ Contraindicated in patients with a history of hypersensitivity to DTIC, because both drugs are metabolized to MTIC.

◆ Obtain initial CBC and on day 22 of the first treatment cycle. Monitor counts weekly until recovery if the absolute neutrophil count falls to <1500 and the platelets are <100,000.

◆ To decrease the risk of nausea, take on an empty stomach, preferably at bedtime.

◆ Premedicate with a 5-HT antagonist to control nausea and vomiting.

◆ Do not open or chew capsules. If capsules are accidentally opened or damaged, avoid inhalation or contact with skin or mucous membranes.

◆ This drug meets the criteria for Medicare's oral anticancer drug benefit, which will minimize coverage issues associated with this drug.

◆ Teniposide

(teh-**nip**'-oh-side)   VM-26, Vumon   Pregnancy Category D

Mechanism of Action

A phase-specific drug that causes DNA strand breakage and the inhibition of type II topoisomerase, which leads to cell death.

Indications

Induction therapy for refractory childhood acute lymphoblastic leukemia.

Metabolism/Excretion

Metabolized in the liver; excreted in urine and bile.

Dosage Range

165 mg/m^2 in combination with cytosine arabinoside 300 mg/m^2 IV two times a week for 8 or 9 doses. Alternatively, 250 mg/m^2 in combination with vincristine 1.5 mg/m^2 IV once a week for 4 to 8 doses and prednisone 40 mg/m^2 PO for 28 days.

Drug Preparation/Stability

50-mg/5-mL injectable ampule. Must be diluted with 5% dextrose injection or 0.9% sodium chloride injection to yield a final concentration of 0.1, 0.2, 0.4, or 1.0 mg/mL. Concentrations of 0.1, 0.2, and 0.4 mg/mL are stable at room temperature for 24 hours after preparation; concentration of 1.0 mg/mL should be given within 4 hours of preparation to prevent precipitation.

Drug Administration

Give using non–DEHP-containing IV administration sets to prevent potential softening and leaking. Administer by slow IV infusion over ≥30 to 60 minutes.

Drug Interaction

Tolbutamide, sodium salicylate, and sulfamethizole displace protein-bound teniposide to plasma proteins, which increase free drug plasma levels, potentiating teniposide toxicity.

Side Effects and Toxicities

- ◆ **Cardiac:** Hypotension with rapid infusion
- ◆ **Dermatologic:** Alopecia, tissue damage secondary to extravasation
- ◆ **GI:** Nausea and vomiting, mucositis, diarrhea, stomatitis, hepatotoxicity
- ◆ **Hematologic:** Bone marrow depression
- ◆ **Other:** Hypersensitivity, anaphylaxis

Special Considerations

- ◆ Contraindicated in patients with previous allergy to teniposide or polyoxyethylated castor oil (Cremophor EL), pregnancy, lactation.
- ◆ Monitor blood counts.
- ◆ Do not give by rapid IV infusion.
- ◆ Monitor vital signs before and during therapy.
- ◆ Check solution before and during administration for precipitation.
- ◆ Instruct patient to use a contraceptive.

◆ Testolactone

(tess-toe-**lak**'-tone)   Teslac   Pregnancy Category X

Mechanism of Action

An androgen estrogen antagonist that impairs tumor growth by suppressing pituitary function.

Indications

Advanced breast carcinoma, refractory anemia.

Metabolism/Excretion

Metabolized in the liver; excreted in urine and feces.

Dosage Range
- ◆ **Adult:** 250 mg four times a day PO.
- ◆ **Pediatric:** Safety and effectiveness not established.

Drug Preparation/Stability
50-mg tablets; no preparation required. Store at room temperature. Check package label for expiration date.

Drug Administration
PO

Drug Interaction
Concomitant use with insulin may alter glucose tolerance.

Side Effects and Toxicities
- ◆ **CNS:** Headache, fatigue, somnolence
- ◆ **Dermatologic:** Skin rashes, alopecia
- ◆ **GI:** Nausea and vomiting
- ◆ **GU:** Fluid retention
- ◆ **Other:** Electrolyte imbalances, mild hirsutism, decreased breast size, edema, clitoral hypertrophy

Special Considerations
- ◆ Use with caution in patients with cardiac or renal dysfunction.
- ◆ Monitor glucose and insulin levels in insulin-dependent diabetics.
- ◆ Obtain baseline serum electrolytes, BUN, creatinine, glucose levels.
- ◆ Monitor vital signs before and during therapy.

◆ Thioguanine

(thye-oh-**gwah**′-neen)   TG,   Pregnancy Category D
6-thioguanine,
Tabloid

Mechanism of Action
An antimetabolite that inhibits purine synthesis by substituting for the nucleotide guanine. S phase–specific.

Indications
Acute lymphocyte leukemia, acute nonlymphocytic leukemia, chronic myelogenous leukemia.

Metabolism/Excretion

Metabolized in the liver; excreted in urine.

Dosage Range

2 mg/kg per day PO, adult and pediatric. If after 4 weeks there is no clinical evidence of improvement, cautiously increase the dosage to 3 mg/kg per day. Total daily dose may be given once daily.

Drug Preparation/Stability

400-mg tablets; no preparation required. Store at room temperature. Check package lot label for expiration date.

Drug Administration

PO

Drug Interaction

Cross-resistant with mercaptopurine.

Side Effects and Toxicities

♦ **GI:** Nausea and vomiting, stomatitis, anorexia
♦ **Hematologic:** Bone marrow depression
♦ **Other:** Hyperuricemia, secondary malignancy

Special Considerations

♦ Contraindicated in patients with previous allergy to thioguanine, pregnancy, lactation, myelosuppression, liver dysfunction.
♦ Best absorbed on an empty stomach.
♦ Administer allopurinol concomitantly to minimize hyperuricemia.
♦ Instruct patient to use a contraceptive.

♦ Thiotepa

| (thy-oh-**tep**′-ah) | Triethylene, Thio-Tepa, TESPA, TSPA | Pregnancy Category D |

Mechanism of Action

An alkylating agent that alters DNA replication, RNA transcription, and nucleic acid formation, resulting in cell death.

Indications

Carcinoma of the bladder, ovaries, and breast; brain tumors; Hodgkin's disease; non-Hodgkin's lymphoma; lymphosarcoma; malignant effusions.

Metabolism/Excretion

Metabolized in the liver; excreted in urine.

Dosage Range

Adult

- ◆ 0.3 to 0.4 mg/kg IV push at 1- to 4-week intervals.
- ◆ **Cytoreduction for brain tumor bone marrow transplant:** 300 mg/m^2 per day for 3 days.
- ◆ **Intracavitary:** 0.6 to 0.8 mg/kg.
- ◆ **Intravesical:** 60 mg once weekly for 4 weeks.

Pediatric

Safety and effectiveness not established.

Drug Preparation/Stability

Add 1.5 mL sterile water to injectable 15-mg vial to yield a concentration of 10 mg/mL. Keep refrigerated and use within 8 hours. Further dilute with 0.9% sodium chloride. To eliminate haze, filter solution through a 0.22-micron filter before administration.

Drug Administration

IV push rapid bolus injection through an infusing IV line; IV infusion in 500 mL 0.9% sodium chloride injection over 3 hours for brain tumor cytoreduction. For intracavitary use, give through an intracavity tube. For intravesical use, dehydrate patient with bladder carcinoma for 8 to 12 hours before administration, then through catheter instill 60 mg in 30 to 60 mL distilled water.

Drug Interaction

Concomitant use with myelosuppressive drugs increases the risk of hematologic toxicity.

Side Effects and Toxicities

- ◆ **CNS:** Dizziness
- ◆ **Dermatologic:** Skin rash, desquamation
- ◆ **GI:** Nausea, vomiting, anorexia, mucositis

◆ **Hematologic:** Bone marrow depression
◆ **Reproductive:** Reduced spermatogenesis, amenorrhea
◆ **Other:** Hypersensitivity reactions, fever

Special Considerations

◆ Contraindicated in patients with previous hypersensitivity to thiotepa, pregnancy, lactation, myelosuppression.
◆ Bone marrow depression may increase with second or third dose.
◆ Monitor blood counts before, during, and after therapy.
◆ Death has occurred from bone marrow depression.
◆ Avoid administration with other myelosuppressive agents.
◆ Instruct patient to use contraception.

◆ Topotecan Hydrochloride

(toe-**poe**'-tee-kan)   Hycamtin   Pregnancy Category D

Mechanism of Action

A semisynthetic derivative of camptothecin, topotecan inhibits the activity of topoisomerase I, an enzyme necessary for DNA replication.

Indications

Metastatic carcinoma of the ovary after failure of initial or subsequent therapy; small cell lung cancer after failure of first-line chemotherapy.

Metabolism/Excretion

Metabolized in the liver. About 30% of the drug is excreted by the kidneys. Renal clearance is an important determinant of topotecan elimination. Half-life: 3 hours.

Dosage Range

◆ **Adult:** 1.5 mg/m² IV for 5 consecutive days every 21 days. At least four courses are recommended, because clinical studies show that the median time for a response is 9 to 12 weeks. In the event of severe neutropenia, reduce the dose by 0.25 mg/m² for the subsequent courses. Alternatively, granulocyte colony-stimulating factor (G-CSF)

may be administered before the subsequent course starting on day 6 (24 hours after the completion of the fifth-
day topotecan dose) before resorting to dose reduction. If
the patient has a creatinine clearance of 20 to 39 mL/min,
reduce the dose to 0.75 mg/mL. No dose requirement is
indicated for patients with hepatic impairment.

◆ **Pediatric:** Safety and efficacy not established.

Drug Preparation/Stability

Available as a 4-mg vial that can be reconstituted with 4 mL
sterile water for injection. Can be further diluted in 0.9%
sodium chloride IV infusion or 5% dextrose IV infusion. Use
reconstituted solution immediately. Protect unopened vials
from light and keep at controlled room temperature (20° to
25°C).

Drug Administration

IV infusion over 30 minutes daily for 5 consecutive days.

Drug Interaction

Concomitant administration of G-CSF can prolong the duration of neutropenia; therefore, G-CSF should be given 24
hours after the fifth dose of topotecan is completed (day 6).
Myelosuppression was more severe if topotecan was given in
combination with cisplatin.

Side Effects and Toxicities

◆ **CNS:** Headache, paresthesia, asthenia
◆ **Cutaneous:** Total alopecia
◆ **GI:** Nausea, vomiting, diarrhea, constipation, abdomi-
nal pain, stomatitis, transient elevation of liver enzymes
◆ **Hematologic: Neutropenia,** leukopenia, thrombo-
cytopenia, anemia

Special Considerations

◆ Monitor bone marrow function before and during
treatment. Give only if patient has adequate bone marrow
reserves, including baseline neutrophil counts of $\geq 1,500$
cells/mm^3 and a platelet count of $\geq 100,000$/mm^3. Do not
give subsequent courses unless neutrophils recover to
>1000 cells/mm^3, platelets recover to 100,000/mm^3, and
hemoglobin levels recover to 9.0 mg/dL (with transfusion
if needed).

◆ Mild erythema and bruising have been reported with extravasation.

◆ Tretinoin

(**tret**'-i-noyn) Retinoic acid, Pregnancy Category D
Vesanoid

Mechanism of Action

Not understood. This natural retinoid may play a role in hematopoiesis and immune function. Inhibits the proliferation of acute promyelocytic leukemia.

Indications

Acute promyelocytic leukemia.

Metabolism/Excretion

Metabolized in the liver; excreted in urine and feces.

Dosage Range

◆ **Adult:** 45 mg/m^2 per day PO in two divided doses. Discontinue 30 days after remission is obtained or after 90 days.
◆ **Pediatric:** Not recommended.

Drug Preparation/Stability

10-mg soft gelatin capsules. Store at room temperature; protect from light. Check package lot label expiration date.

Drug Administration

PO

Drug Interaction

◆ Concomitant use with ketoconazole may increase the risk of tretinoin toxicity.
◆ Concomitant use with vitamin supplements containing vitamin A may increase tretinoin toxicity.

Side Effects and Toxicities

◆ **Cardiac:** Hypotension, congestive heart failure, myocardial infarction
◆ **CNS:** Headache, dizziness, visual changes

◆ **Dermatologic:** Skin erythema, desquamation, cheilitis, photosensitivity
◆ **GI:** Nausea, vomiting, anorexia
◆ **GU:** Renal insufficiency
◆ **Hematologic:** Leukocytosis
◆ **Pulmonary:** Pleural effusion, pulmonary infiltrates
◆ **Other:** Bone and joint pain, elevated triglycerides, elevated liver function tests

Special Considerations

◆ Contraindicated in patients with previous allergy to any retinoid, liver dysfunction, pregnancy, lactation.
◆ Obtain baseline and periodic CBC, liver and renal function tests, and serum triglycerides.
◆ Use contraception during and 2 months after therapy.
◆ Discontinue use if liver function tests are five times greater then the upper-normal range.

◆ Uracil Mustard

(**yoor'**-a-sill)   Pregnancy Category X

Mechanism of Action

An alkylating agent that binds to DNA, inhibits DNA synthesis, and leads to cell death.

Indications

Chronic lymphoblastic leukemia, chronic myelogenous leukemia, non-Hodgkin's lymphoma, mycosis fungoides, polycythemia vera.

Metabolism/Excretion

Metabolized in the liver; excreted in urine.

Dosage Range

Varies based on individual response.
◆ **Adult:** 0.15 mg/kg PO once weekly for 4 weeks.
◆ **Pediatric:** 0.30 mg/kg PO once weekly for 4 weeks.

Drug Preparation/Stability

1-mg capsule. Store at room temperature. Check lot label for expiration date.

Drug Administration

PO

Drug Interaction

Dosage of antigout medications used concomitantly may need to be increased because of elevated serum uric acid levels.

Side Effects and Toxicities

- ◆ **CNS:** Depression, nervousness, irritability
- ◆ **Dermatologic:** Alopecia, dermatitis, pruritus
- ◆ **GI:** Nausea, vomiting, diarrhea, hepatotoxicity
- ◆ **Hematologic:** Myelosuppression, elevated uric acid levels
- ◆ **Reproductive:** Azoospermia, amenorrhea
- ◆ **Other:** Secondary malignancy

Special Considerations

- ◆ Contraindicated in patients with previous reaction to uracil mustard, pregnancy, lactation, leukopenia, thrombocytopenia.
- ◆ Use cautiously with radiation therapy; possible bone marrow depression.
- ◆ Possible use of allopurinol for elevated serum uric acid levels.
- ◆ Obtain baseline and periodic CBC, serum uric acid levels.
- ◆ Encourage PO fluid intake to maintain adequate hydration.
- ◆ Instruct on use of contraception.

◆ Vinblastine

(vin-**blas**'-teen)　　　Velban, VLB　　　Pregnancy Category D

Mechanism of Action

A cell cycle–specific vinca alkaloid that inhibits mitotic spindle formation by binding to tubulin. Most specific for the M phase.

Indications

Hodgkin's lymphoma, lymphoma, testicular carcinoma, Kaposi's sarcoma, mycosis fungoides, breast carcinoma.

Metabolism/Excretion
Metabolized in the liver; excreted in bile.

Dosage Range
◆ Initial therapy: single IV dose once weekly. Guidelines are as follows:

Dose	Adult/Pediatric
1	3.7/2.5 mg/m^2
2	5.5/3.75 mg/m^2
3	7.4/5.0 mg/m^2
4	9.25/6.25 mg/m^2
5	11.1/7.5 mg/m^2

◆ Subsequent doses are increased to a maximum of 18.5 mg/m^2 for adults and 12.5 mg/m^2 for children IV once weekly.
◆ Maintenance therapy: Dosage and duration of therapy are individualized based on response. Maintenance dose is one increment smaller then the dose at which the WBC is reduced to <3000/mm^3. Maintenance dose held until WBC rises to 4000/mm^3.

Drug Preparation/Stability
Dilute injectable 10-mg/mL vial with 0.9% sodium chloride injection preserved with phenol or benzyl alcohol to yield a concentration of 1 mg/mL. Stable for 30 days refrigerated. Protect from light.

Drug Administration
IV push over 1 minute peripherally or through a central access device, or as a dilute IV infusion through a central access device.

Drug Interaction
◆ Phenytoin used in combination with vinblastine and other antineoplastic agents may decrease serum phenytoin levels, predisposing the patient to seizure activity.
◆ Methotrexate used concomitantly with vinblastine may increase methotrexate toxicity.
◆ Mitomycin used concomitantly with vinblastine may cause acute pulmonary reactions.
◆ Incompatible with furosemide and heparin.

Side Effects and Toxicities

◆ **CNS:** Peripheral neuropathy, paresthesias, loss of deep tendon reflexes, jaw pain, autonomic neuropathy manifested by constipation, paralytic ileus, orthostasis, and urinary retention

◆ **Dermatologic:** Alopecia, tissue damage secondary to extravasation

◆ **GI:** Nausea, vomiting, ileus, constipation, stomatitis

◆ **GU:** Polyuria, urinary retention

◆ **Hematologic:** Bone marrow depression

◆ **Pulmonary:** Bronchospasm (acute shortness of breath), more common when given with mitomycin; pulmonary edema

Special Considerations

◆ Contraindicated in patients with pre-existing neurotoxicity, previous sensitivity to vinblastine, pregnancy, lactation, infection.

◆ Obtain baseline and periodic CBC and renal and hepatic function tests.

◆ Obtain baseline neurologic examination.

◆ Administer antiemetics as needed.

◆ Assess for constipation; auscultate for bowel sounds. Suggest prophylactic stool softener.

◆ Patients may report severe pain in the jaw, pharynx, bones, back, or limbs after injection.

◆ Vincristine

(vin-**kris**'-teen)   Oncovin, VCR,   Pregnancy Category D
                    Vincasar

Mechanism of Action

A vinca alkaloid that arrests metaphase by binding microtubule protein to the mitotic spindle. Specific for the S phase.

Indications

Acute lymphocytic leukemia, Wilms tumor, rhabdomyosarcoma, neuroblastoma, Hodgkin's disease, non-Hodgkin's lymphoma.

Metabolism/Excretion

Metabolized in the liver; excreted in urine and feces.

Dosage Range

Adult and pediatric: 1 to 2 mg/m² single IV dose once weekly. Total single dose of 2 mg is seldom exceeded.

Drug Preparation/Stability

Injectable 1 mg/vial = 1 mg/mL; 2 mg/vial = 2 mg/2 mL; 5 mg/vial = 5 mg/5 mL. Stable for 24 hours at room temperature.

Drug Administration

IV push over 1 minute through a peripheral or central line; dilute IV infusion only through a central line.

Drug Interaction

◆ Digoxin used concomitantly with vincristine may decrease serum digoxin levels and the subsequent effects of digoxin.
◆ Mitomycin used concomitantly with vincristine may cause acute pulmonary reactions.

Side Effects and Toxicities

◆ **CNS:** Peripheral neuropathy, paresthesias, numbness, loss of deep tendon reflexes, extraocular muscle paresis
◆ **Dermatologic:** Alopecia, tissue damage secondary to extravasation
◆ **GI:** Nausea, vomiting, anorexia, stomatitis, ileus, constipation, diarrhea
◆ **Other:** Pharyngitis, syndrome of inappropriate antidiuretic hormone (SIADH), hypersensitivity

Special Considerations

◆ Contraindicated in patients with previous sensitivity to vincristine, infection, pregnancy, lactation, neurotoxicity.
◆ Monitor CBC, liver function tests, and serum sodium before and periodically during therapy.
◆ Use prophylactic stool softener regimen.
◆ Instruct patient on use of contraception.

◆ Vindesine

(**vin**'-de-seen)   Eldisine, desacetyl   Pregnancy Category D
vinblastine

Mechanism of Action

A vinca alkaloid that binds to tubulin and alters the microtubular spindle structure, which leads to cell lysis.

Indications

Investigational use for head and neck cancer, esophageal cancer, breast cancer, melanoma, non–small cell lung cancer, lymphoma.

Metabolism/Excretion

Metabolized in the liver; excreted in urine and feces.

Dosage Range

Varies depending on patient and disease.
- ◆ **Adult:** 2.0 to 4.0 mg/m^2 single IV dose once weekly.
- ◆ **Pediatric:** Not recommended.

Drug Preparation/Stability

Reconstitute 10-mg ampule with 10 mL of the provided diluent or 0.9% sodium chloride injection. Reconstituted solution is stable refrigerated for 2 weeks. Unopened ampules are stable refrigerated for 1 year.

Drug Administration

IV push slowly into a peripheral or central line; IV infusion only through a central line.

Drug Interaction

- ◆ Mitomycin concomitantly used with vindesine may cause acute pulmonary reactions.
- ◆ Methotrexate used concomitantly with vindesine may increase methotrexate plasma clearance, reducing the effectiveness of the methotrexate.
- ◆ Concomitant use with other vinca alkaloids is contraindicated because of possible cumulative neurotoxicity.

Side Effects and Toxicities

◆ **CNS:** Paresthesias, muscle weakness, loss of deep tendon reflexes
◆ **Dermatologic:** Tissue damage if extravasated, rash
◆ **GI:** Nausea, vomiting, diarrhea, constipation, ileus
◆ **Hematologic:** Bone marrow suppression

Special Considerations

◆ Contraindicated in patients with previous sensitivity to vindesine, pregnancy, lactation, concomitant use of other vinca alkaloids.
◆ Monitor CBC, liver function tests, and neurologic status before and during therapy.
◆ Suggest prophylactic stool softener.
◆ Instruct patient on use of contraception.

◆ Vinorelbine

(vin-oh-rel-**been**′)   Navelbine   Pregnancy Category D

Mechanism of Action

An antimitotic agent that inhibits microtubule formation by interfering with nucleic acid synthesis.

Indications

Non–small cell lung cancer, breast cancer, ovarian cancer.

Metabolism/Excretion

Metabolized in the liver; excreted in urine and feces.

Dosage Range

◆ **Adult:** 30 mg/m² IV once weekly. Adjust for hematologic toxicity, hepatic dysfunction, or concomitant use with cisplatin for non–small cell lung cancer.
◆ **Pediatric:** Safety and effectiveness not demonstrated.

Drug Preparation/Stability

Dilute 10- and 50-mg vial with 0.9% sodium chloride or 5% dextrose injection to yield a concentration of 1.5 to 3.0 mg/mL. For IV bag dilution, dilute to a concentration of 0.5 to 2.0 mg/mL using a solution of 5% dextrose, 0.9% sodium chloride, 5% dextrose with 0.45% sodium chloride, or lactated Ringer's. Diluted solution is stable for 24 hours. Protect 10- and 50-mg vials from light. Store in refrigerator.

Drug Administration

IV over 6 hours to 10 minutes into a free-flowing IV solution. IV push into a central line. Flush after administration with ≥75 to 125 mL 5% dextrose or 0.9% sodium chloride injection over ≥10 minutes.

Drug Interaction

◆ Mitomycin concomitantly administered with vinorelbine may cause acute pulmonary reactions.
◆ Cisplatin concomitantly used with vinorelbine significantly increases incidence of granulocytopenia.

Side Effects and Toxicities

◆ **Cardiac:** Chest pain, myocardial ischemia
◆ **CNS:** Mild to moderate peripheral neuropathy, loss of deep tendon reflexes
◆ **Dermatologic:** Alopecia, secondary damage if drug extravasates, rash
◆ **GI:** Mild to moderate nausea, constipation, ileus, vomiting, diarrhea, stomatitis, anorexia, transient liver enzyme elevations
◆ **Hematologic:** Bone marrow suppression with severe granulocytopenia
◆ **Pulmonary:** Interstitial pulmonary changes, shortness of breath
◆ **Other:** Fatigue, jaw pain, syndrome of inappropriate diuretic hormone

Special Considerations

◆ Contraindicated in patients with previous sensitivity to vinorelbine, pregnancy, lactation, granulocyte count <1000 cells/mm³.
◆ Follow prophylactic bowel softener regimen.
◆ Obtain baseline and periodic CBC, liver function tests, and serum sodium.
◆ Instruct patient on use of contraception.

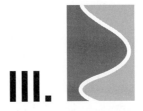

III.

Combination Chemotherapy Regimens

The use of combination chemotherapy is well established. Combining agents have allowed the clinician to achieve maximum cell kill while trying to minimize toxicity to the patient. The drugs that are used exhibit synergy, have different mechanisms of action, and have overlapping toxicities.

Part III is a comprehensive review of combination regimens that are in use today for disease sites as indicated in the tables. It should serve as a general reference or guidelines only, as variations may happen. Dose or cycle modifications of the regimens may happen because of disease progression or toxicity experienced. As ongoing research continues, the clinical utility of the original regimens might be expanded to other cancer sites. For these reasons, the author has decided to alphabetize the regimens instead of the usual classification according to target sites.

ABV

Use:	Kaposi's sarcoma	Cycle: 28 days		
Regimen:	Doxorubicin	40 mg/m^2	IV	Day 1
	Bleomycin	15 units/m^2	IV	Days 1, 15
	Vinblastine	6 mg/m^2	IV	Day 1

ABVD

Use:	Lymphoma (Hodgkin's)			
Regimen:	Doxorubicin	25 mg/m^2	IV	Days 1, 15
	Bleomycin	10 units/m^2	IV	Days 1, 15
	Vinblastine	6 mg/m^2	IV	Days 1, 15
	with			
	Dacarbazine	350–375 mg/m^2	IV	Days 1, 15
	or			
	Dacarbazine	150 mg/m^2	IV	Days 1–5

AC

Use:	Breast cancer	Cycle: 21 days		
Regimen:	Doxorubicin	45–60 mg/m^2	IV	Day 1
	Cyclophosphamide	400–600 mg/m^2	IV	Day 1
Use:	Sarcoma (bony)	Cycle: 28 days		
Regimen:	Doxorubicin	75–90 mg/m^2 total dose CI	CI	Over 96 h
	Cisplatin	95–120 mg/m^2	IV or IA	Day 6

ACE—see CAE

ACE

Use:	Breast cancer	Cycle: 21–28 days		
Regimen:	Cyclophosphamide	200 mg/m^2/day	PO	Days 1–3 or 3–6
	Doxorubicin	40 mg/m^2	IV	Day 1

A-DIC

Use:	Sarcoma (soft tissue)	Cycle: 21 days		
Regimen:	Doxorubicin	45–60 mg/m²	IV	Days 1–5

AP

Use:	Ovarian, endometrial cancer	Cycle: 21 days		
Regimen:	Doxorubicin	50–60 mg/m²	IV	Day 1
	Cisplatin	50–60 mg/m²	IV	Day 1

BCVPP

Use:	Lymphoma (Hodgkin's)	Cycle: 28 days		
Regimen:	Carmustine	100 mg/m²	IV	Day 1
	Cyclophosphamide	600 mg/m²	IV	Day 1
	Vinblastine	5 mg/m²	IV	Day 1
	Procarbazine	50 mg/m²/day	PO	Day 1
	Procarbazine	100 mg/m²/day	PO	Days 2–10
	Prednisone	60 mg/m²/day	PO	Days 1–10

BEP

Use:	Testicular cancer	Cycle: 21 days		
Regimen:	Bleomycin	30 units	IV	Days 2, 9, 16
	Etoposide	100 mg/m²	IV	Days 1–5
	Cisplatin	20 mg/m²	IV	Days 1–5

BIP

Use:	Cervical cancer	Cycle: 21 days		
Regimen:	Bleomycin	30 units	CI	Day 1
	Ifosfamide	5 g/m²	CI	Day 2
	Cisplatin	50 mg/m²	IV	Day 2
	Mesna	8 g/m²	CI over 36 h	Day 2 (with ifosfamide)

BOMP

Use:	Cervical cancer	Cycle: 6 weeks		
Regimen:	Bleomycin	10 units	IM	Weekly
	Vincristine	1 mg/m²	IV	Days 1, 8, 22, 29
	Cisplatin	50 mg/m²	IV	Days 1, 22
	Mitomycin	10 mg/m²	IV	Day 1

CAE (ACE)

Use:	Lung cancer (non–small cell)	Cycle: 21 days		
Regimen:	Cyclophosphamide	1 g/m²	IV	Day 1
	Doxorubicin	45 mg/m²	IV	Day 1
	Etoposide	50 mg/m²	IV	Days 1–5

CAF

Use:	Breast cancer	Cycle: 21 days		
Regimen:	Cyclophosphamide *or*	400–600 mg/m²	IV	Day 1
	Cyclophosphamide *with*	100 mg/m²/day	PO	Days 1–14
	Doxorubicin	40–60 mg/m²	IV	Day 1
	Fluorouracil	400–600 mg/m²	IV	Day 1

CAL–G

Use:	Acute lymphocytic leukemia (ALL)			
Regimen:	Cyclophosphamide	1.2 g	IV	Day 1
	Daunorubicin	45 mg/m²	IV	Days 1–3
	Vincristine	2 mg	IV	Days 1, 8, 15, 22
	Prednisone	60 mg/m²/day	PO	Days 1–21
	with			
	Asparaginase	1000 units/m²	IV	Days 5, 8, 11, 15, 18, 22
	or			
	Pegaspargase	2500 units/m²	IM or IV	Every other week

CAMP

Use:	Lung cancer (non–small cell)	Cycle: 28 days		
Regimen:	Cyclophosphamide	300 mg/m²/day	IV	Days 1, 8
	Doxorubicin	20 mg/m²	IV	Days 1, 8
	Methotrexate	15 mg/m²	IV	Days 1, 8
	Procarbazine	100 mg/m²/day	PO	Days 1–10

CAP

Use:	Lung cancer (non–small cell)	Cycle: 28 days		
Regimen:	Cyclophosphamide	400 mg/m²	IV	Day 1
	Doxorubicin	40 mg/m²	IV	Day 1
	Cisplatin	60 mg/m²	IV	Day 1

CAV (VAC)

Use:	Lung cancer (small cell)	Cycle: 21 days		
Regimen:	Cyclophosphamide	750–1000 mg/m²	IV	Day 1
	Doxorubicin	40–50 mg/m²	IV	Day 1
	Vincristine	1.4 mg/m² (2 mg maximum dose)	IV	Day 1

CAVE

Use:	Lung cancer (small cell)	Cycle: 21–28 days		
Regimen:	Add to CAV:			
	Etoposide	60–100 mg/m²	IV	Days 1–5

CC

Use:	Ovarian cancer	Cycle: 28 days		
Regimen:	Carboplatin	300–500 mg/m²	IV	Day 1
	Cyclophosphamide	600 mg/m²	IV	Day 1

CDDP/VP**

Use:	Brain tumors			
Regimen:	Cisplatin	90 mg/m²	IV	Day 1
	Etoposide	150 mg/m²	IV	Days 2–3

CEV

Use:	Lung cancer (small cell)	Cycle: 21–28 days		
Regimen:	Cyclophosphamide	1 g/m²	IV	Day 1
	Etoposide	50 mg/m²	IV	Day 1
	Etoposide	100 mg/m²	PO	Days 2–5
	Vincristine	1.4 mg/m² (2 mg maximum dose)	IV	Day 1

**Pediatric use

CF

Use:	Adenocarcinoma, head and neck cancer	Cycle: 21–28 days		
Regimen:	Cisplatin	100 mg/m²	IV	Day 1
	Fluorouracil	1 g/m²	CI	Days 1–4 or 5

CF

Use:	Head and neck cancer	Cycle: 21–28 days		
Regimen:	Carboplatin	400 mg/m²	IV	Day 1
	Fluorouracil	1 g/m²	CI	Days 1–4 or 5

CFL

Use:	Head and neck cancer	Cycle: 21–28 days		
Regimen:	Cisplatin	100 mg/m²	IV	Day 1
	Fluorouracil	600–800 mg/m²	CI	Days 1–5
	Calcium leucovorin	200–300 mg/m²	IV	Days 1–5

CFM (CNF/FNC)

Use:	Breast cancer	Cycle: 21 days		
Regimen:	Cyclophosphamide	500 mg/m²	IV	Day 1
	Fluorouracil	500 mg/m²	IV	Day 1
	Mitoxantrone	10 mg/m²	IV	Day 1

CFPT*

Use:	Breast cancer	Cycle: 28 days		
Regimen:	Cyclophosphamide	150 mg/m²	IV	Days 1–5
	Fluorouacil	300 mg/m²	IV	Days 1–5
	Prednisone	10 mg	PO	TID for 1st 7 days of each course
	Tamoxifen	10 mg	PO	BID (continue daily through all courses)

CHAP

Use:	Ovarian cancer	Cycle: 28 days		
Regimen:	Cyclophosphamide *or*	150 mg/m²/day	PO	Days 2–8
	Cyclophosphamide *with*	300–500 mg/m²/day	PO	Day 1
	Altretamine	150 mg/m²/day	PO	Days 2–8
	Doxorubicin	30 mg/m²	IV	Day 1
	Cisplatin	50–60 mg/m²	IV	Day 1

ChLVPP

Use:	Lymphoma (Hodgkin's)	Cycle: 21–28 days		
Regimen:	Chlorambucil	6 mg/m² (10 mg/day maximum dose)	PO	Days 1–14
	Vinblastine	6 mg/m² (10 mg/day maximum dose)	IV	Days 1–8
	Procarbazine	100 mg/m² (150 mg/day max dose)	PO	Days 1–14
	Prednisone	40 mg/m² (25 mg/m²— pediatrics)	PO	Days 1–14

ChlVPP/EVA
Use:	Lymphoma (Hodgkin's)	Cycle: 21–28 days		
Regimen:	See ChlVPP, except chlorambucil, procarbazine, and prednisone days 1–7, vinblastine day 1 only			Days 1–7
	with			
	Etoposide	200 mg/m²	IV	Days 1–3
	Vincristine	2 mg	IV	Day 8
	Doxorubicin	50 mg/m²	IV	Day 8

CHOP
Use:	Lymphoma (non-Hodgkin's)	Cycle: 21 days		
Regimen:	Cyclophosphamide	750 mg/m²	IV	Day 1
	Doxorubicin	50 mg/m²	IV	Day 1
	Vincristine	1.4 mg/m² (2 mg maximum dose)	IV	Day 1
	Prednisone	100 mg/day	PO	Days 1–5

CHOP/BLEO
Use:	Lymphoma (non-Hodgkin's)	Cycle: 14–21 days		
Regimen:	Add to CHOP:			
	Bleomycin	15 units/day	IV	Days 1–5

CISCA
Use:	Bladder cancer	Cycle: 21–28 days		
Regimen:	Cyclophosphamide	650 mg/m²	IV	Day 1
	Doxorubicin	50 mg/m²	IV	Day 1
	Cisplatin	70–100 mg/m²	IV	Day 2

CISCA$_{II}$/VB$_{IV}$
Use:	Germ cell tumors			
Regimen:	Cyclophosphamide	1 g/m²	IV	Days 1–2
	Doxorubicin	80–90 mg/m²	IV	Days 1–2
	Cisplatin	100–120 mg/m²	IV	Day 3
	alternating with			
	Vinblastine	3 mg/m²/day	CI	Days 1–5
	Bleomycin	30 units/day	CI	Days 1–5

CMF
Use:	Breast cancer	Cycle: 21–28 days		
Regimen:	Cyclophosphamide	400–600 mg/m²	IV	Day 1
	or			
	Cyclophosphamide	100 mg/m²	PO	Days 1–14
	with			
	Methotrexate	40–60 mg/m²	IV	Days 1, 8
	Fluorouracil	400–600 mg/m²	IV	Days 1, 8

CMFP
Use:	Breast cancer	Cycle: 28 days		
Regimen:	Cyclophosphamide	100 mg/m²	PO	Days 1–14
	Methotrexate	30–60 mg/m²	IV	Days 1, 8
	Fluorouracil	400–700 mg/m²	IV	Days 1, 8
	Prednisone	40 mg/m²/day	PO	Days 1–14

CMFVP
Use:	Breast cancer	Cycle: 21–28 days		
Regimen:	Add to CMF:			
	Vincristine	1 mg	IV	Days 1–8
	Prednisone	20–40 mg/day	PO	Days 1–7 or 14

CMV

Use:	Bladder cancer	Cycle: 21 days		
Regimen:	Cisplatin	100 mg/m²	IV	Day 2 (at least 12 h after MTX)
	Methotrexate	30 mg/m²	IV	Days 1, 8
	Vinblastine	4 mg/m²	IV	Days 1, 8

COB

Use:	Head and neck cancer	Cycle: 21 days		
Regimen:	Cisplatin	100 mg/m²	IV	Day 1
	Vincristine	1 mg	IV	Days 2, 5
	Bleomycin	30 units/day	CI	Days 2–5

CODE

Use:	Lung cancer (small cell)			
Regimen:	Cisplatin	25 mg/m²	IV	Every week for 9 weeks
	Vincristine	1 mg/m² (2 mg maximum dose)	IV	Weeks 1, 2, 4, 6, 8
	Doxorubicin	25 mg/m²	IV	Weeks 1, 3, 5, 7, 9
	Etoposide	80 mg/m²	IV	Weeks 1, 3, 5, 7, 9

COMLA

Use:	Lymphoma (non-Hodgkin's)	Cycle: 13 weeks		
Regimen:	Cyclophosphamide	1.5 g/m²	IV	Day 1
	Vincristine	1.4 mg/m² (2.5 mg maximum dose)	IV	Days 1, 8, 15
	Methotrexate	120 mg/m²	IV	Days 22, 29, 36, 43, 50, 57, 64, 71
Pediatric regimen:	Leucovorin	25 mg/m²	PO	Every 6 h for 4 doses, 24 h after MTX
	Cytarabine	300 mg/m²	IV	Days 22, 29, 36, 43, 50, 57, 64, 71

COMP**

Use:	Lymphoma (Hodgkin's, pediatric)			
Regimen:	Cyclophosphamide	500 mg/m²	IV	Days 1, 15
	Vincristine	1.4 mg/m² (2 mg maximum dose)	IV	Days 1, 8
	Methotrexate	40 mg/m²	IV	Days 1–2
	Prednisone	40 mg/m²/day	PO	Days 1–15

COP

Use:	Lymphoma (non-Hodgkin's)	Cycle: 21 days		
Regimen:	Cyclophosphamide	400–1000 mg/m²	IV	Day 1
	Vincristine	1.4 mg/m² (2 mg maximum dose)	IV	Day 1
	Prednisone	60 mg/m²	PO	Days 1–5

**Pediatric use

COPE

Use:	Lung cancer (small cell)	Cycle: 21 days		
Regimen:	Cyclophosphamide	750 mg/m²	IV	Day 1
	Vincristine	1.4 mg/m² (2 mg maximum dose)	IV	Day 3
	Cisplatin	20 mg/m²	IV	Days 1–3
	Etoposide	100 mg/m²	IV	Days 1–3

COPP ("C" MOPP)**

Use:	Lymphoma (non-Hodgkin's or Hodgkin's)	Cycle: 28 days		
Regimen:	Cyclophosphamide	500–600 mg/m²	IV	Days 1, 8
	Vincristine	1.4 mg/m² (2 mg maximum dose)	IV	Days 1, 8
	Procarbazine	100 mg/m²	PO	Days 1–14
	Prednisone	40 mg/m²	PO	Days 1–14

CP

Use:	Chronic lymphocytic leukemia (CLL)			
Regimen:	Chlorambucil	0.4 mg/kg/day	PO	Day 1
	Prednisone	100 mg/day	PO	Days 1–7
Use:	Ovarian cancer	Cycle: 21 days		
Regimen:	Cyclophosphamide	600–1000 mg/m²	IV	Day 1
	Cisplatin	50–100 mg/m²	IV	Day 1

CT

Use:	Ovarian cancer	Cycle: 21 days		
Regimen:	Cisplatin	75 mg/m²	IV	Day 1
	Paclitaxel	135 mg/m²	IV	Day 1

CVD

Use:	Malignant melanoma	Cycle: 21 days		
Regimen:	Cisplatin	20 mg/m²	IV	Days 1–5
	Vinblastine	1.6 mg/m²	IV	Days 1–3
	Dacarbazine	800 mg/m²	IV	Day 1

CVI (VIC)

Use:	Lung cancer (non-small cell)	Cycle: 28 days		
Regimen:	Carboplatin	300 mg/m²	IV	Day 1
	Etoposide	60–100 mg/m²	IV	Days 1, 3, 5
	Ifosfamide	1.5 g/m²	IV	Days 1, 3, 5
	Mesna	400 mg	IV bolus	Days 1, 3, 5 (then 1600 mg over 24 h)

CVP

Use:	Lymphoma (non-Hodgkin's), chronic lymphocytic leukemia (CLL)	Cycle: 21 days		
Regimen:	Cyclophosphamide	400 mg/m²	PO	Days 1–5
	Vincristine	1.4 mg/m² (2 mg maximum dose)	IV	Day 1
	Prednisone	100 mg/m²/day	PO	Days 1–5

CVPP

Use:	Lymphoma (Hodgkin's)	Cycle: 28 days		
Regimen:	Lomustine	75 mg/m²/day	PO	Day 1
	Vinblastine	4 mg/m²	IV	Days 1, 8
	Procarbazine	100 mg/m²	PO	Days 1–14
	Prednisone	30 mg/m²	PO	Days 1–14 (cycles 1 and 4 only)

CYVADIC

Use:	Sarcoma (bony or soft tissue)	Cycle: 21 days		
Regimen:	Cyclophosphamide	400–600 mg/m²	IV	Day 1
	Vincristine	1.4 mg/m²	IV	Days 1, 5
	Doxorubicin	40–50 mg/m²	IV	Day 1
	Dacarbazine	200–250 mg/m²	IV	Days 1–5

DA**

Use:	Acute myelocytic leukemia (AML; induction)			
Regimen:	Daunorubicin	45–60 mg/m²/day	CI	Days 1–3
	Cytarabine	100 mg/m²	IV	Every 12 h for 5 to 7 days

DAL

Use:	Acute myelocytic leukemia (AML; induction)			
Regimen:	Cytarabine	3 g/m²	Every 12 h	Days 1–3
	Daunorubicin	45 mg/m²	IV	Days 1, 2
	Asparaginase	6000 units/m²	IV	Day 3 (usually alternated with DAT)

DAT**

Use:	Acute myelocytic leukemia (AML; induction)			
Regimen:	Daunorubicin	45 mg/m²/day	CI	Days 1–3
	Cytarabine	100 mg/m²/day	CI	Days 1–7
	Thioguanine	100 mg/m²/day	PO	Days 1–7

DAV**

Use:	Acute myelocytic leukemia (AML; induction)			
Regimen:	Daunorubicin	30 mg/m²/day	CI	Days 1–3
	Cytarabine	250 mg/m²/day	CI	Days 1–5
	Etoposide	200 mg/m²/day	CI	Days 5–7

**Pediatric use

DCT (DAT, TAD)

Use:	Acute myelocytic leukemia (AML; adult induction)			
Regimen:	Daunorubicin	60 mg/m²	IV	Days 1–3
	Cytarabine	200 mg/m²	IV	Days 1–5
	Thioguanine	100 mg/m²	PO (every 12 h)	Days 1–5

DHAP

Use:	Lymphoma (Hodgkin's)	Cycle: 21–28 days		
Regimen:	Cisplatin	100 mg/m²	CI (over 24 h)	Day 1
	Cytarabine	2 g/m²	IV (every 12 h for 2 doses) (total dose 4 g/m²)	Day 2
	Dexamethasone	40 mg/day	PO or IV	Days 1–4

DI

Use:	Sarcoma (soft tissue)	Cycle: 21 days		
Regimen:	Doxorubicin	50 mg/m²	CI	Day 1
	Ifosfamide	5 g/m²	CI	Day 1
	Mesna	600 mg/m² (IV bolus, then 2.5 g/m²/day)	CI	

DVP

Use:	Acute lymphocytic leukemia (ALL; adult induction)			
Regimen:	Daunorubicin	45 mg/m²	IV	Days 1–3 and 14
	Vincristine	2 mg	IV	Weekly for 4 weeks for
	Prednisone	45 mg/m²/day	PO	28–35 days

DVP**

Use:	Acute lymphocytic leukemia (ALL; pediatric induction)			
Regimen:	Daunorubicin	25 mg/m²	IV	Days 1, 8
	Vincristine	1.5 mg/m² (2 mg maximum dose)	IV	Days 1, 8, 15, 22
	Prednisone	40 mg/m²/day	PO	Days 1–29

EAP

Use:	Gastric, small bowel cancer	Cycle: 21–28 days		
Regimen:	Etoposide	120 mg/m²	IV	Days 4–6
	Doxorubicin	20 mg/m²	IV	Days 1, 7
	Cisplatin	40 mg/m²	IV	Days 2, 8

**Pediatric use

EC

Use:	Lung cancer (small cell)	Cycle: 28 days		
Regimen:	Etoposide *with*	60–100 mg/m²	IV	Days 1–3
	Carboplatin *or*	400 mg/m²	IV	Day 1
	Carboplatin	100–125 mg/m²	IV	Days 1–3

EDAP

Use:	Multiple myeloma			
Regimen:	Etoposide	100–200 mg/m²	CI	Days 1–4
	Dexamethasone	40 mg/m²	IV or PO	Days 1–5
	Cytarabine	1000 mg	IV	Day 5
	Cisplatin	20 mg	CI	Days 1–4

EFP

Use:	Gastric, small bowel cancer	Cycle: 24–28 days		
Regimen:	Etoposide	90 mg/m²	IV	Days 1, 3, 5
	Fluorouracil	900 mg/m²/day	CI	Days 1–5
	Cisplatin	20 mg/m²	IV	Days 1–5

ELF

Use:	Gastric cancer	Cycle: 21 to 28 days		
Regimen:	Etoposide	120 mg/m²	IV	Days 1–3
	Leucovorin	150–300 mg/m²	IV	Days 1–3
	Fluorouracil	500 mg/m²	IV	Days 1–3

EMA 86

Use:	Acute myelocytic leukemia (AML; adult induction)			
Regimen:	Mitoxantrone	12 mg/m²	IV	Days 1–3
	Etoposide	200 mg/m²/day	CI	Days 8–10
	Cytarabine	500 mg/m²/day	CI	Days 1–3 and 8–10

EP

Use:	Adenocarcinoma, small cell lung cancer	Cycle: 21 days		
Regimen:	Etoposide	75–100 mg/m²	IV	Days 1–3
	Cisplatin	75–100 mg/m²	IV	Day 1

ESHAP

Use:	Lymphoma (non-Hodgkin's)	Cycle: 21–28 days		
Regimen:	Methylprednisolone	500 mg/day	IV	Days 1–4
	Etoposide	40–60 mg/m²	IV	Days 1–4
	Cytarabine	2 g/m²	IV	Day 5
	Cisplatin	25 mg/m²/day	CI	Days 1–4

EVA

Use:	Lymphoma (Hodgkin's)	Cycle: 21–28 days		
Regimen:	Etoposide	100 mg/m²	IV	Days 1–3
	Vinblastine	6 mg/m²	IV	Day 1
	Doxorubicin	50 mg/m²	IV	Day 1

FAC

Use:	Breast cancer	Cycle: 21 days		
Regimen:	Fluorouracil	500 mg/m²	IV	Day 1 and bolus on days 4, 5, 8
	Doxorubicin	50 mg/m² (total dose)	Cl	Over 48–96 h starting day 1
	Cyclophosphamide	500 mg/m²	IV	Day 1

FAM

Use:	Adenocarcinoma, gastric cancer	Cycle: 8 weeks		
Regimen:	Fluorouracil	600 mg/m²/day	IV	Days 1, 8, 29, 36
	Doxorubicin	30 mg/m²	IV	Days 1, 29
	Mitomycin	10 mg/m²	IV	Day 1

FAMe

Use:	Gastric cancer	Cycle: 10 weeks		
Regimen:	Fluorouracil	350 mg/m²	IV	Days 1–5 and 36–40
	Doxorubicin	40 mg/m²	IV	Days 1, 36
	Semustine	150 mg/m²	PO	Day 1

FAMTX

Use:	Gastric cancer	Cycle: 28 days		
Regimen:	Fluorouracil	1.5 g/m²	IV	Day 1
	Doxorubicin	30 mg/m²	IV	Day 15
	Methotrexate	1.5 g/m²	IV	Day 1
	Leucovorin	20–25 mg	PO	Every 6 h for 8 doses, 24 h after MTX

FAP

Use:	Gastric	Cycle: 5 weeks		
Regimen:	Fluorouracil	300 mg/²	IV	Days 1–5
	Doxorubicin	40 mg/m²	IV	Day 1
	Cisplatin	60 mg/m²	IV	Day 1

FCE

Use:	Gastric	Cycle: 21 days		
Regimen:	Fluorouracil	900 mg/m²	IV/CI	Days 1–5
	Cisplatin	20 mg/m²	IV	Days 1–5
	Etoposide	90 mg/m²	IV	Days 1, 3, 5

F-CL(FU/LV)

Use:	Colorectal cancer	Cycle: 4–8 weeks		
Regimen:	Fluorouracil	600 mg/m²	IV	Weekly for 6 weeks
	Leucovorin	500 mg/m²	IV	Weekly for 6 weeks
	or			
	Fluorouracil	370–600 mg/m²	IV or Cl	Days 1–5
	Leucovorin	200 mg/m²	IV or Cl	Days 1–5

FEP

Use:	Lung cancer (non–small cell)	Cycle: 21 days		
Regimen:	Fluorouracil	960 mg/m²	Cl	Days 2–4
	Etoposide	80 mg/m²	IV	Days 2–4
	Cisplatin	100 mg/m²	IV	Day 1

FL

Use:	Prostate cancer	Cycle: 28 days		
Regimen:	Flutamide	250 mg	PO	Every 8 h
	with			
	Leuprolide acetate	1 mg	SC	Daily
	or			
	Leuprolide depot	7.5 mg	IM	Every 28 days

FLe

Use:	Colorectal cancer			
Regimen:	Fluorouracil	450 mg/m²	IV	Days 1–5 and day 28 weekly for 48 weeks
	Levamisole	50 mg	PO	Every 8 h days 1–3 every 2 weeks for 1 year

FU/LV—see F-CL

FZ

Use:	Prostate cancer	Cycle: 28 days		
Regimen:	Flutamide	250 mg	PO	Every 8 h
	Goserelin acetate	3.6 mg implant	SC	Every 28 days

HDMTX

Use:	Sarcoma (bony)	Cycle: 2–4 weeks		
Regimen:	Methotrexate	8–12 g/m² (20 g maximum dose)	IV	Day 1
	Leucovorin	15 mg/m²	PO or IV	Every 6 h for 10 doses, 30 h after beginning of 4-h methotrexate infusion

ICE—see MICE

IE

Use:	Sarcoma (soft tissue)	Cycle: 21 days		
Regimen:	Ifosfamide	1.8 g/m²	IV	Days 1–5
	Etoposide	100 mg/m²	IV	Days 1–5
	Mesna	20% of ifosfamide prior to, then 4 and 8 h after ifosfamide		

IfoVP

Use:	Sarcoma (osteo, pediatric)			
Regimen:	Ifosfamide	2 g/m²	IV	Days 1–3
	Etoposide	100 mg/m²	IV	Days 1–3
	Mesna	2 g/m²	IV	Days 1–3

M-2

Use:	Multiple myeloma	Cycle: 5 weeks		
Regimen:	Vincristine	0.03 mg/kg (2 mg maximum dose)	IV	Day 1
	Carmustine	0.5–1 mg/kg	IV	Day 1
	Cyclophosphamide	10 mg/kg	IV	Day 1
	Melphalan	0.25 mg/kg/day	PO	Days 1–4
	Prednisone	1 mg/kg/day	PO	Days 1–7, then tapered over next 14 days

MACOP-B

Use:	Lymphoma (non-Hodgkin's)			
Regimen:	Methotrexate	400 mg/m²	IV	Weeks 2, 6, 10
	Leucovorin	15 mg/m²	PO	Every 6 h for 6 doses, 24 h after MTX
	Doxorubicin	50 mg/m²	IV	Weeks 1, 3, 5, 7, 9, 11
	Cyclophosphamide	350 mg/m²	IV	Weeks 1, 3, 5, 7, 9, 11
	Vincristine	1.4 mg/m²	IV	Weeks 2, 4, 6, 8, 10, 12
	Bleomycin	10 units/m²	IV	Weeks 4, 8, 12
	Prednisone	75 mg/m²	PO for 12 weeks, tapered over last 2 weeks	

MAID

Use:	Sarcoma (soft tissue, bony)	Cycle: 21–28 days		
Regimen:	Mesna	1.5–2.5 g/m²	CI	Days 1–4
	Doxorubicin	15–20 mg/m²	CI	Days 1–3
	Ifosfamide	1.5–2.5 g/m²	CI	Days 1–3
	Dacarbazine	250–300 mg/m²/day	CI	Days 1–3

m-BACOD

Use:	Lymphoma (non-Hodgkin's)	Cycle: 28 days		
Regimen:	Methotrexate	200 mg/²	IV	Days 8, 15 h
	Leucovorin	10 mg/²	PO	Every 6 h for 8 doses, 24 h after MTX
	Bleomycin	4 units/m²	IV	Day 1
	Doxorubicin	45 mg/²	IV	Day 1
	Cyclophosphamide	600 mg/m²	IV	Day 1
	Vincristine	1 mg/m² (2 mg maximum dose)	IV	Day 1
	Dexamethasone	6 mg/m²	PO	Days 1–5

M-BACOD

See m-BACOD, except methotrexate 3 g/m²	IV	Day 14

MBC

Use:	Head and neck cancer	Cycle: 21 days		
Regimen:	Methotrexate	40 mg/m²	IV	Days 1–15
	Bleomycin	10 units/m²	IM	Days 1, 8, 15
	Cisplatin	50 mg/²	IV	Day 4

MC

Use:	Acute myelocytic leukemia (AML; adult induction)	Cycle: 28 days		
Regimen:	Mitoxantrone	12 mg/m²	IV	Days 1–3
	Cytarabine	100–200 mg/m²/day	CI	Days 1–7

MF

Use:	Breast cancer	Cycle: 28 days		
Regimen:	Methotrexate	100 mg/m²	IV	Days 1–8
	Fluorouracil	600 mg/m²	IV	Days 1, 8, given 1 h after MTX
	Leucovorin	10 mg/m²	IV or PO	Every 6 h for 6 doses, 24 h after MTX

MICE (ICE)

Use:	Sarcoma, lung cancer	Cycle: 28 days		
Regimen:	Mesna uroprotection at 20% of ifosfamide doses given by IV immediately before and at 4 and 8 h after ifosfamide infusion			
	Ifosfamide	2 g/m²	IV	Days 1–3
	Carboplatin	300–600 mg/m²	IV	Day 1 or 3
	Etoposide	60–100 mg/m²	IV	Days 1–3

MINE-ESHAP

Use:	Lymphoma (Hodgkin's)	Cycle: 21 days		
Regimen:	Mesna	1.33 g/m²	IV	Days 1–3
	Mesna	500 mg	PO	Four hours after ifosfamide
	Ifosfamide	1.33 g/m²	IV	Day 1–3
	Mitoxantrone	8 mg/m²	IV	Day 1
	Etoposide	65 mg/m²	IV	Days 1–3 Repeat for 6 cycles, then give ESHAP for 3–6 cycles

mini-BEAM

Use:	Lymphoma (Hodgkin's)	Cycle: 4–7 weeks		
Regimen:	Carmustine	60 mg/m²	IV	Day 1
	Etoposide	75 mg/m²	IV	Days 2–5
	Cytarabine	100 mg/m²	IV	Every 12 h, days 2–5
	Melphalan	30 mg/m²	IV	Day 6

MIV

Use:	Lymphoma (non-Hodgkin's)	Cycle: 21 days		
Regimen:	Mitoxantrone	10 mg/m²	IV	Day 1
	Ifosfamide	1.5 g/m²	IV	Days 1–3 with mesna
	Etoposide	150 mg/m²	IV	Days 1–3

MOP

Use:	Brain tumors, pediatrics			
Regimen:	See MOPP without prednisone			

MOPP

Use:	Lymphoma (Hodgkin's)	Cycle: 28 days		
Regimen:	Mechlorethamine	6 mg/m^2	IV	Days 1 and 8
	Vincristine	1.4 mg/m^2 (2 mg maximum dose)	IV	Days 1 and 8
	Procarbazine	100 mg/m^2/day	PO	Days 1–14
	Prednisone	40 mg/m^2/day	PO	Days 1–14

MOPP/ABV

Use:	Lymphoma (Hodgkin's)	Cycle: 28 days		
Regimen:	Mechlorethamine	6 mg/m^2	IV	Day 1
	Vincristine	1.4 mg/m^2 (2 mg maximum dose)	IV	Day 1
	Procarbazine	100 mg/m^2/day	PO	Days 1–7
	Prednisone	40 mg/m^2/day	PO	Days 1–14
	Bleomycin	10 units/m^2	IV	Day 8
	Vinblastine	6 mg/m^2	IV	Day 8
	Doxorubicin	35 mg/m^2	IV	Day 8

MOPP/ABVD

Use:	Lymphoma (Hodgkin's)
Regimen:	Alternate MoP and ABVD regimens every month

MP

Use:	Multiple myeloma	Cycle: 28 days		
Regimen:	Melphalan	8–10 mg/m^2/day	PO	Days 1–4
	Prednisone	40–60 mg/m^2/day	PO	Days 1–7

m-PFL

Use:	Bladder cancer	Cycle: 28 days for 4 cycles		
Regimen:	Methotrexate	60 mg/m^2	IV	Day 1
	Cisplatin	25 mg/m^2	CI	Days 2–6
	Fluorouracil	800 mg/m^2	CI	Days 2–6
	Calcium leucovorin	500 mg/m^2	CI	Days 2–6

MVAC

Use:	Bladder cancer	Cycle: 28 days		
Regimen:	Methotrexate	30 mg/m^2	IV	Days 1, 15, 22
	Doxorubicin	30 mg/m^2	IV	Day 2
	Vinblastine	3 mg/m^2	IV	Days 2, 15, 22
	Cisplatin	70 mg/m^2	IV	Day 2

MVP

Use:	Lung cancer (non–small cell)			
Regimen:	Mitomycin	8 mg/m^2	IV	Days 1, 29, 71
	Vinblastine	4.5 mg/m^2	IV	Days 15, 22, 29, then every 2 weeks
	Cisplatin	120 mg/m^2	IV	Days 1, 29, then every 6 weeks

MVPP

Use:	Hodgkin's disease	Cycle: 4–6 weeks		
Regimen:	Mechlorethamine (nitrogen mustard)	6 mg/m²	IV	Days 1, 8
	Vinblastine	6 mg/m²	IV	Days 1, 8
	Procarbazine	100 mg/m²	PO	Days 1–14
	Prednisone	40 mg/m²	PO	Days 1–14

MTXCP–PDAdr**

Use:	Osteosarcoma			
Regimen:	Methotrexate	12 gm/m²	IV	Weekly for 2–12 weeks
	Calcium leucovorin rescue	15 mg/m²	PO/IV	Every 6 h for 10 doses beginning h 30 after the beginning of the 4-h methotrexate infusion (serum methotrexate levels must be monitored)
	Cisplatin	100 mg/m²	IV	Day 1
	Doxorubicin	37.5 mg/m²	IV	Days 2, 3

MTXCP–PDAdrl**

Use:	Osteosarcoma			
Regimen:	Methotrexate	12 gm/m²	IV	Weekly for 2–12 weeks
	Calcium lecovorin rescue	15 mg/m²	PO/IV	Every 6 h for 10 doses beginning h 30 after the beginning of the 4-h methotrexate infusion (serum methotrexate levels must be monitored)
	Cisplatin	100 mg/m²	IV	Day 1
	Doxorubicin	37.5 mg/m²	IV	Days 2, 3
	Ifosfamide	1.6 mg/m²	IV	Days 1–5

NFL

Use:	Breast cancer	Cycle: 21 days		
Regimen:	Mitoxantrone	12 mg/m²	IV	Day 1
	Calcium leucovorin	300 mg/m²	IV	Days 1–3
	Fluorouracil	350 mg/m²	IV	Days 1–3 given after calcium leucovorin
	or			
	Mitoxantrone	10 mg/m²	IV	Day 1
	Calcium leucovorin	100 mg/m²	IV	Days 1–3
	Fluorouracil	1000 mg/m²	CI	Days 1–3 given after leucovorin

**Pediatric use

NOVP

Use:	Hodgkin's lymphoma	Cycle: 21 days		
Regimen:	Mitoxantrone	10 mg/m²	IV	Day 1
	Vincristine	2 mg/m²	IV	Day 8
	Vinblastine	6 mg/m²	IV	Day 1
	Prednisone	100 mg/m²	PO	Days 1–5

**Pediatric use

NP

Use:	Lung cancer (non–small cell)	Cycle: 6 weeks		
Regimen:	Vinorelbine	30 mg/m²	IV	Every week
	Cisplatin	120 mg/m²	IV	Days 1, 29, then every 6 weeks

OPA**

Use:	Hodgkin's lymphoma			
Regimen:	Vincristine	1.5 mg/m²	IV	Days 1, 8, 15
	Prednisone	60 mg/m²	PO	Days 1–15
	Doxorubicin	40 mg/m²	IV	Days 1, 15

OPPA**

Use:	Hodgkin's lymphoma	Cycle: 28 days		
Regimen:	Vincristine	1.5 mg/m²	IV	Days 1, 8, 15
	Procarbazine	100 mg/m²	PO	Days 1–15
	Prednisone	60 mg/m²	PO	Days 1–15
	Doxorubicin	40 mg/m²	IV	Days 1, 15

PAC

Use:	Ovarian, endometrial cancer	Cycle: 21–28 days		
Regimen:	Cisplatin	50–60 mg/m²	IV	Day 1
	Doxorubicin	45–50 mg/m²	IV	Day 1
	Cyclophosphamide	600 mg/m²	IV	Day 1

PC

Use:	Lung cancer (non–small cell)	Cycle: 21 days		
Regimen:	Paclitaxel	135 mg/m²/day	IV	Day 1
	Carboplatin	dose by Calvert equation to AUC 7.5		Day 1

PCV

Use:	Brain tumor	Cycle: 6–8 weeks		
Regimen:	Lomustine	110 mg/m²/day	PO	Day 1
	Procarbazine	60 mg/m²/day	PO	Days 8–21
	Vincristine	1.4 mg/m² (2 mg maximum dose)	IV	Days 8–29

PFL

Use:	Head and neck, gastric, non–small cell	Cycle: 28 days		
Regimen:	Cisplatin	25 mg/m²/day	CI	Days 1–5
	Fluorouracil	800 mg/m²/day	CI	Days 2–5 or 6
	Leucovorin	500 mg/m²/day	CI	Days 1–5 or 6
	or			
	Cisplatin	100 mg/m²	IV	Day 1
	Fluorouracil	800 mg/m²	CI	Days 1–5
	Calcium leucovorin	100 mg	PO q4h	Days 1–5

**Pediatric use

PFL+IFN

Use:	Head and neck cancer	Cycle: 28 days		
Regimen:	Cisplatin	100 mg/m²	IV	Day 1
	Fluorouracil	640 mg/m²	CI	Days 1–5
	Calcium leucovorin	100 mg	PO (every 4 h)	Days 1–5
	Interferon-alfa-2b	2 × 10⁶ units/m²	SC	Days 1–6

POC**

Use:	Brain tumors	Cycle: 6 weeks		
Regimen:	Prednisone	40 mg/m²	PO	Days 1–14
	Methyl-CCNU	100 mg/m²	PO	Day 2
	Vincristine	1.5 mg/m² (2 mg maximum dose)		Days 1, 8, 15

ProMACE/cytaBOM

Use:	Lymphoma (non-Hodgkin's)	Cycle: 21 days		
Regimen:	Prednisone	60 mg/m²	PO	Days 1–14
	Doxorubicin	25 mg/m²	IV	Day 1
	Cyclophosphamide	650 mg/m²	IV	Day 1
	Etoposide	120 mg/m²	IV	Day 1
	Cytarabine	300 mg/m²	IV	Day 8
	Bleomycin	5 units/m²	IV	Day 8
	Vincristine	1.4 mg/m² (2 mg maximum dose)	IV	Day 8
	Methotrexate	120 mg/m²	IV	Day 8
	Leucovorin	25 mg/m²	PO q6 h for 6 doses, 24 h after MTX	

ProMACE

Use:	Lymphoma (non-Hodgkin's)	Cycle: 28 days		
Regimen:	Prednisone	60 mg/m²	PO	Days 1–14
	Methotrexate	1.5 mg/m²	IV	Day 14
	Leucovorin	50 mg/m²	PO	Every 6 h for 6 doses 24 h after MTX
	Doxorubicin	25 mg/m²	PO	Days 1, 8
	Cyclophosphamide	650 mg/m²	IV	Days 1, 8
	Etoposide	120 mg/m²	IV	Days 1, 8

ProMACE/MOPP

Use:	Lymphoma (Hodgkin's)	Cycle: 28 days
Regimen:	Repeat ProMACE for prescribed cycles, then begin MOPP cycles	

PVB

Use:	Testicular cancer, adenocarcinoma	Cycle: 21–28 days		
Regimen:	Cisplatin	20 mg/m²	IV	Days 1–5
	Vinblastine	0.15–0.4 mg/kg	IV	Day 1 (± day 2)
	Bleomycin	30 units	IV	Day 1 or day 2 weekly

PVDA**

Use:	Acute lymphocytic leukemia (ALL; induction)			
Regimen:	Add to VDA: Prednisone	40 mg/m²/day	PO	Days 1–29

**Pediatric use

PVP-16
Use:	Lung (non–small cell)	Cycle: 21–28 days		
Regimen:	Cisplatin	60–120 mg/m²	IV	Day 1
	Etoposide	50–120 mg/m²	IV	Days 1–3

STANFORD V
Use:	Hodgkin's lymphoma			
Regimen:	Mechlorethamine	6 mg/m²	IV	Weeks 1, 5, 9
	Doxorubicin	25 mg/m²	IV	Weeks 1, 3, 5, 7, 9, 11
	Vinblastine	6 mg/m²	IV	Weeks 2, 4, 6, 8, 10, 12
	Vincristine	1.4 mg/m² (2 mg maximum dose)	IV	Weeks 2, 4, 6, 8, 10, 12
	Bleomycin	5 units/m²	IV	Weeks 2, 4, 6, 8, 10, 12
	Etoposide	60 mg/m²	IV	Days 1–2 on weeks 3, 7, 11
	Prednisone	40 mg/m²	PO	Every other day, tapered over last 15 days

VAC PULSE
Use:	Sarcoma			
Regimen:	Vincristine	2 mg/m² (2 mg maximum)	IV	Weekly for 12 weeks
	Dactinomycin	0.015 mg/kg	IV	Days 1–5, weeks 1, 13
	Cyclophosphamide	10 mg/kg	IV or PO	For 7 days, repeat every 6 weeks

VAC STANDARD
Use:	Sarcoma (soft tissue)			
Regimen:	Vincristine	2 mg/m² (2 mg/week maximum dose)	IV	Weekly for 12 weeks
	Dactinomycin	0.015 mg/kg (0.5 mg/day maximum dose)	IV	Days 1–5, every 3 months
	Cyclophosphamide	2.5 mg/kg/day	PO	Daily for 2 years

VACAdr-IfoVP**
Use:	Sarcoma (bony and soft tissue)			
Regimen:	Vincristine	1.5 mg/m² (2 mg maximum dose)	IV	Days 1, 8, 15
	Dactinomycin	1.5 mg/kg (2 mg maximum dose)	IV	Every other week
	Doxorubicin	60 mg/m²	CI	Day 1
	Cyclophosphamide	1–1.5 g/m²	IV	Day 1
	Ifosfamide	1–6.2 g/m²	IV	Days 1–5
	Etoposide	150 mg/m²	IV	Days 1–5
	(vincristine + dactinomycin alternating with either doxorubicin + cyclophosphamide or ifosfamide + etoposide)			

VAdrC**
Use:	Sarcoma (bony and soft tissue)			
Regimen:	Vincristine	1.5 mg/m² (2 mg maximum dose)	IV	Days 1, 8, 15
	Doxorubicin	35–60 mg/m²	IV	Day 1
	Cyclophosphamide	500–1000 mg/m²	IV	Day 1

**Pediatric use

VAD

Use:	Wilms' tumor (pediatrics)	Cycle: Repeat for a total of 6 months		
Regimen:	Vincristine	1.5 mg/m^2 (2 mg maximum dose)	IV	Weekly for 10 weeks
	with			
	Dactinomycin	0.45 mg/kg		Every 3 weeks
	alternating with			
	Doxorubicin	30 mg/m^2	IV	Every 3 weeks
Use:	Multiple myeloma, leukemia	Cycle: 4–5 weeks		
Regimen:	Vincristine	0.4 mg/m^2/day (2 mg maximum dose)	CI	Days 1–4
	Doxorubicin	9–12 mg/m^2/day	CI	Days 1–4
	Dexamethasone	20 mg/m^2	PO	Days 1–4, 9–12, 17–20

VATH

Use:	Breast cancer	Cycle: 21 days		
Regimen:	Vinblastine	4.5 mg/m^2	IV	Day 1
	Doxorubicin	45 mg/m^2	IV	Day 1
	Thiotepa	12 mg/m^2	IV	Day 1
	Fluoxymestrone	30 mg/day	PO	Daily

VBAP

Use:	Multiple myeloma	Cycle: 21 days		
Regimen:	Vincristine	1 mg/m^2 (2 mg maximum dose)	IV	Day 1
	Carmustine	30 mg/m^2	IV	Day 1
	Doxorubicin	30 mg/m^2	IV	Day 1
	Prednisone	60 mg/m^2/day	PO	Days 1–4

VC

Use:	Lung cancer (non–small cell)	Cycle: 6 weeks		
Regimen:	Vinorelbine	30 mg/m^2	IV	Weekly
	Cisplatin	120 mg/m^2	PO	Days 1, 29

VCAP

Use:	Multiple myeloma	Cycle: 28 days		
Regimen:	Vincristine	1 mg/m^2 (2 mg maximum dose)	IV	Day 1
	Cyclophosphamide	100–125 mg/m^2/day	PO	Days 1–4
	Doxorubicin	25–30 mg/m^2	IV	Day 2
	Prednisone	60 mg/m^2	PO	Days 1–4

VDA[**]

Use:	Acute lymphocytic leukemia (ALL; induction)			
Regimen:	Vincristine	1.5 mg/m^2 (2 mg maximum dose)	IV	Days 1, 8, 15, 22
	Daunorubicin	25 mg/m^2	IV	Days 1, 8
	Asparaginase	10,000 units/m^2	IM	Days 2, 4, 6, 8, 10, 12, 15, 17, 19

VDP

Use:	Malignant melanoma	Cycle: 21–28 days		
Regimen:	Vinblastine	5 mg/m^2	IV	Days 1, 2
	Dacarbazine	150 mg/m^2	IV	Days 1–5
	Cisplatin	75 mg/m^2	IV	Day 5

[**]Pediatric use

VIP

Use:	Testicular cancer	Cycle: 21 days		
Regimen:	Vinblastine *or*	0.11 mg/kg	IV	Days 1–2
	Etoposide *with*	75 mg/m²	IV	Days 1–5
	Ifosfamide	1.2 g/m²	Cl	Days 1–5
	Cisplatin	20 mg/m²	IV	Days 1–5
	Mesna	400 mg/m²	IV	Day 1 (15 min pre-ifosfamide)
	Mesna	1.2 gm/m²	Cl	Days 1–5

VIP-1

Use:	Lung cancer	Cycle: 28 days		
Regimen:	Ifosfamide	1.2 g/m²	IV	Days 1–4 with mesna
	Cisplatin	20 mg/m²	IV	Days 1–4
	Etoposide	37.5 mg/m²	Cl	Days 1–21

VIP-2

Use:	Lung cancer (non–small cell)	Cycle: 28 days		
Regimen:	Ifosfamide	1–1.2 g/m²	IV	Day 1 with mesna
	Cisplatin	100 mg/m²	IV	Days 1, 8
	Etoposide	60–75 mg/m²/day	IV	Days 1–3

VM

Use:	Breast cancer	Cycle: 6–8 weeks		
Regimen:	Mitomycin	10 mg/m²	IV	Days 1, 28 for 2 cycles, then day 1 only
	Vinblastine	5 mg/m²	IV	Days 1, 14, 28, 42 for 2 cycles, then days 1, 21 only

V-TAD

Use:	Acute myelocytic leukemia (AML; induction)			
Regimen:	Etoposide	50 mg/m²	IV	Days 1–3
	Thioguanine	75 mg/m²	PO	Days 1–5 Every 12 h
	Daunorubicin	20 mg/m²	IV	Days 1, 2
	Cytarabine	75 mg/m²/day	Cl	Days 1–5

5 + 2

Use:	Acute myelocytic leukemia (AML; reinduction)			
Regimen:	Cytarabine *with*	100–200 mg/m²/day	Cl	Days 1–5
	Daunorubicin *or*	45 mg/m²	IV	Days 1, 2
	Mitoxantrone	12 mg/m²	IV	Days 1, 2

7 + 3

Use:	AML (induction)			
Regimen:	Cytarabine	100–200 mg/m^2	CI	Days 1–7
	with			
	Daunorubicin	30–45 mg/m^2	IV	Days 1–3
	or			
	Idarubicin	12 mg/m^2	IV	Days 1–3
	or			
	Mitoxantrone	12 mg/m^2	IV	Days 1–3

"8 IN 1"

Use:	Brain tumors			
Regimen:	Methylprednisone	300 mg/m^2	PO	Day 1
	Vincristine	1.5 mg/m^2 (2 mg maximum dose)	IV	Day 1
	Methyl-CCNU	75 mg/m^2	PO	Day 1
	Procarbazine	75 mg/m^2	PO	Day 1
	Hydroxyurea	1.5–3.0 g/m^2	PO	Day 1
	Cisplatin	60–90 mg/m^2	IV	Day 1
	Cytarabine	300 mg/m^2	IV	Day 1
	Cyclophosphamide	300 mg/m^2	IV	Day 1
	or			
	Dacarbazine	150 mg/m^2	IV	Day 1

Adapted with permission from *Facts and Comparisons* (2000), St. Louis, Missouri.

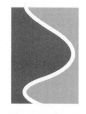

Appendices

Appendices

Appendix A

National Cancer Institute Publications for Cancer Patients and the Public

The National Cancer Institute (NCI) publications are free. There is no handling or shipping charge for orders of twenty or fewer items. These items may consist of twenty copies of one publication or any combination of publications up to a total of twenty items. Orders exceeding twenty publications are considered bulk orders and are charged 10 cents per copy for shipping and handling. The NCI requires that an order of more than twenty items be charged a $5.00 minimum fee. To find out more about the NCI's publication policy, call the Cancer Information Service (CIS) at 1-800-4-CANCER.

▼ English-Language Publications

CANCER PREVENTION

Chew or Snuff is Real Bad for You

Describes the health and social effects of using smokeless tobacco products. Can be used as a poster; it is designed for seventh and eighth graders.

Clearing the Air: A Guide to Quitting Smoking

Designed to help the smoker who wants to quit; offers a variety of approaches to cessation.

5 A DAY Brochures

Easy Entertaining With Fruits and Vegetables

Encourages people to include fruits and vegetables at every course—appetizer, entree, and dessert—when hosting a party.

Eat More Fruits and Vegetables

Provides information about fruits and vegetables that are good sources of vitamins A and C and fiber.

Eat More Salads for Better Health

Gives the fat and calorie content of common salad ingredients. It encourages people to make sure all salad ingredients are healthy choices.

Fast and Easy Fruits and Vegetables for Busy People

Provides suggestions for eating fruits and vegetables daily as part of a busy lifestyle. It offers a guide for microwaving single servings of vegetables.

I Mind Very Much if You Smoke

Explains that secondhand smoke can be a health hazard. It informs the public that secondhand smoke has been classified as a carcinogen by the Environmental Protection Agency.

Smoking Facts and Quitting Tips

Encourages smokers to make changes in everyday behavior that are necessary to quit smoking successfully. It provides practical suggestions to help distract a person from smoking. It encourages smokers who try to quit and fail to try again.

Smoking Facts and Quitting Tips for Black Americans

Discusses the health risks of smoking, who smokes, and why smokers should quit. It also provides quitting tips.

Traditional Foods Can Be Healthy

Encourages Native Americans to reduce dietary fat when preparing traditional foods for their families. It also encourages exercise.

Why Do You Smoke?

Contains a self-test to determine why people smoke and suggests alternatives and substitutes that can help them to stop.

EARLY DETECTION

Cancer Tests You Should Know About: A Guide for People 65 and Over

Describes the cancer tests important for people 65 and older. It informs men and women of the examinations they should be requesting when they see their doctors. It provides a checklist for men and women to record when the cancer tests occur, and it describes the steps to follow should cancer be found.

Chances Are . . . You Need a Mammogram

This a question-and-answer guide for older women on why and how to get regular mammograms and clinical breast examinations.

Get a New Attitude About Cancer: A Guide for Black Americans

Encourages all black adults to get regular checkups from their doctors, to avoid smoking, and to eat less fat and more fruits and vegetables. It informs them of the specific cancers that are the leading causes of cancer death for black men and women.

Questions and Answers About Choosing a Mammography Facility

Lists questions to ask in selecting a quality mammography facility; it also discusses typical costs and coverage. This publication should accompany the brochure, "Are You Age 50 or Over? A Mammogram Could Save Your Life."

Testicular Self-Examination

Contains information about risks and symptoms of testicular cancer and provides instruction on how to perform testicular self-examination.

Understanding Breast Changes: A Health Guide for All Women

Explains how to evaluate breast lumps and other normal breast changes that often occur and are confused with breast cancer. It recommends a regular screening mammography beginning at age 50, a breast exam by a doctor as part of a woman's annual checkup, and monthly breast self-examination for the early detection of breast cancer. This booklet is for all asymptomatic women.

EARLY DETECTION: EASY TO READ

Each brochure has a reading level (RL) rating.

Are You Age 50 or Over? A Mammogram Could Save Your Life (RL-4)

Uses pictures to describe what will happen when a woman goes for a mammogram.

Having a Pelvic Exam and Pap Test (RL-6)

Uses pictures to describe what a woman will experience when getting a Pap test and a pelvic exam.

The Pap Test: It Can Save Your Life!

Explains the importance of getting this test, who should request one, how often it should be done, and where to get the test.

The Pap Test: It Can Save Your Life!

Tells African-Americans the importance of getting a Pap test.

GENERAL CANCER INFORMATION

Bone Marrow Transplantation

Covers current knowledge of bone marrow transplantation as a treatment option for some types of cancer. It explains the different types of transplantation and the complex factors that influence successful treatment.

In Answer to Your Questions About Liver Cancer

Addresses the possible causes of liver cancer and the symptoms, diagnosis, and current treatment options for the disease.

In Answer to Your Questions About Thyroid Cancer

Discusses the types and causes of thyroid cancer, early detection of the disease, and the symptoms, diagnosis, and treatment options.

The Immune System: How It Works

Explains the human immune system for the general public. It describes the sophistication of the body's immune responses, the impact of immune disorders, and the relation of the immune system to cancer therapies, present and future.

What You Need to Know About Cancer

This series of pamphlets discusses symptoms, diagnosis, treatment, emotional issues, and questions to ask the doctor. Includes glossary of terms and other resources.

Bladder	Melanoma
Bone	Moles and dysplastic nevi
Brain	Multiple myeloma
Breast	Non-Hodgkin's lymphoma
Cancer	Oral cancers
Cervix	Ovary
Colon and rectum	Pancreas
Esophagus	Prostate
Hodgkin's disease	Skin
Kidney	Stomach
Larynx	Testes
Lung	Uterus

PATIENT EDUCATION: ADULT

Anticancer Drug Information Sheets

Provide information about side effects of common drugs used to treat cancer, their proper usage, and precautions for patients. The two-sided sheets (English and Spanish) were prepared by the United States Pharmacopeia Convention, Inc., for distribution by the National Cancer Institute.

Advanced Cancer: Living Each Day

Addresses living with a terminal illness, how to cope, and practical considerations for the patient, the family, and friends.

Chemotherapy and You: A Guide to Self-Help During Treatment

In question-and-answer format, addresses problems and concerns of patients receiving chemotherapy. Emphasis is on explanation and self-help.

Eating Hints for Cancer Patients

Includes recipes and suggestions for maintaining optimum nutrition during treatment.

Facing Forward: A Guide for Cancer Survivors

Presents a concise overview of important survivor issues, including ongoing health needs, psychosocial concerns, insurance, and employment. Easy-to-use format includes cancer survivors' experiences, practical tips, record-keeping forms, and resources. It is recommended for cancer survivors, their family, and their friends.

Patient Guide: Managing Cancer Pain

Summarizes information on managing cancer pain; it is published by the Agency for Health Care Policy and Research.

Patient to Patient: Cancer Clinical Trials and You

Provides simple information for patients and families about the clinical trials process. This is a videotape produced in collaboration with the American College of Surgeons Commission on Cancer.

Questions and Answers About Pain Control: A Guide for People with Cancer and Their Families

Discusses pain control using both medical and nonmedical methods. The emphasis is on explanation, self-help, and patient participation.

Radiation Therapy and You: A Guide to Self-Help During Treatment

Addresses concerns of patients receiving forms of radiation therapy. Emphasis is on explanation and self-help.

Taking Time: Support for People with Cancer and the People Who Care About Them

Addresses the feelings and concerns of cancer patients and families. It tells how people with similar concerns have coped.

What Are Clinical Trials About?

Designed for patients who are considering taking part in research for new cancer treatments. It explains clinical trials to patients in easy-to-understand terms and gives them information that will help them decide about participating.

When Cancer Recurs: Meeting the Challenge Again

Details the different types of recurrence, types of treatment, and coping with cancer's return.

PATIENT EDUCATION: EASY TO READ

Get Relief from Cancer (RL-5)

Informs patient that medicine and other treatments almost always can relieve cancer pain. The patient is encouraged to talk to the doctor or nurse as soon as cancer pain begins.

Helping Yourself During Chemotherapy: 4 Steps for Patients

Helps patient understand the importance of telling the doctor about any other medicines the patient is taking, of reporting to the doctor any side effects that occur, and of telling him or her about any emotional problems that arise.

PATIENT EDUCATION: PEDIATRIC

Managing Your Child's Eating Problems During Cancer Treatment

Contains information for parents of children with cancer, about the importance of nutrition, the side effects of cancer and its treatment, ways to encourage your child to eat, and special diets.

Talking with Your Child About Cancer

Addresses the health-related concerns of young people of different ages; it suggests ways to discuss disease-related issues with the child.

When Someone in Your Family Has Cancer

Written for young people whose parent or sibling has cancer, this book includes sections on the disease, its treatment, and emotional concerns.

Young People with Cancer: A Handbook for Parents

Discusses the most common types of childhood cancer, treatment and side effects, and issues that may arise when a child is diagnosed with cancer. Offers medical information and practical tips gathered from parents.

▼ Spanish-Language Publications

CANCER PREVENTION

Datos Consejos Para Dejar de Fumar

Describes the health risks of smoking and tips on how to quit and how to stay quit.

Rompa con el Vicio: Una Guia Para Dejar de Fumar

This is a full-color, self-help smoking cessation booklet prepared specifically for Spanish-speaking Americans.

EARLY DETECTION

Hagase Prueba Pap: Hgalo Hoy . . . Por su Salud y su Familia

Tells women why it is important to get a Pap test. It gives brief, clear information about who needs a Pap test, where to get one, and how often the Pap test should be done.

La Prueba PAP: Un Mtodo Para Diagnosticar el Cancer del Cuello Del Utero

Answers questions about the Pap test, including how often it should be done, the significance of results, and other diagnostic tests and treatments.

Pregunta Para Hacerle su Mdico Sobre el Cancer del Seno

Contains lists of questions that will help a patient ask her doctor about breast cancer. Breast cancer topics covered are early detection, diagnosis, treatment, adjuvant therapy, and reconstruction.

Preguntas Respuestas Sobre de un Centro de Mamografia

Lists questions and answers to ask in selecting a quality mammography facility.

Probablemente . . . Usted Necesita Hacerse un Mamograma

A Spanish question-and-answer guide for older women on the importance of mammography and a clinical breast exam.

¡Tiene 50 Años de Edado o Mas? Un Mamograma Podria Salvarle la Vida

Answers six commonly asked questions about mammography. It encourages all women ages 50 and older to get regular mammograms every 1 to 2 years.

PATIENT EDUCATION

Anticancer Drug Information Sheets

Provides information about side effects of common drugs used to treat cancer, their proper usage, and precautions for patients. The fact sheets were prepared by the United States Pharmacopeia Convention, Inc. for distribution by the National Cancer Institute.

Datos Sobre el Tratamiento de Quimioterapia Contra el Cancer

Provides a brief introduction to cancer chemotherapy.

El Tratamiento de Radioterapia: Guia Para el Paciente Durante el Tratamiento

Addresses the concerns of patients receiving radiation therapy for cancer. Emphasis is on explanation and self-help.

Adapted from *NCI Publications for Cancer Patients and the Public,* National Institutes of Health, National Cancer Institute.

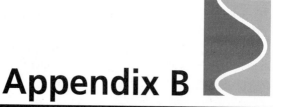

Appendix B

Sample Patient Education Material

▼ Adriamycin® (a-dre-ah-MY-sin)

ALSO KNOWN AS: Doxorubicin, "Adria"

Adriamycin prevents cancer cells from growing by attacking and interfering with DNA, the genetic material in the cell.

HOW IT IS GIVEN:

Intravenously (by vein); the color of the solution is red.

EARLY SIDE EFFECTS:

- Itching, hives, or a red rash can occur at the injection site and along the vein while the drug is being given. This subsides as soon as the injection of the drug is completed.
- Nausea and vomiting can begin one to three hours after the drug is given and last for 24 to 48 hours.
- Urine can be pink or red in color for as long as 48 hours after the treatment.

LATE SIDE EFFECTS:

- A temporary decrease in blood cell counts (white

(continued)

blood cells and platelets) can occur within 10 to 14 days after each treatment.

- Temporary thinning or loss of hair can occur two to four weeks after each treatment.
- Mouth sores can develop within one week after receiving the drug.
- Damage to the heart muscle can occur after a certain dose level is reached. Studies may be done to check heart function.
- Redness of the skin can develop in an area where radiation has previously been given.

CALL YOUR DOCTOR IF YOU:

- have a fever of 100.5°F (38°C) or higher.
- experience pain, redness, swelling, or blistering near the injection site.
- develop mouth sores.
- have black bowel movements, bruising, faint red rash, or any other signs of bleeding.
- have any unexpected, unexplained problems.
- have any questions or concerns.

SPECIAL POINTS:

- Take your antinausea medications as instructed.
- Protect skin from overexposure to the sun. Wear protective clothing and use a sunscreen with an SPF of 15 or greater when in the sun.
- Avoid taking aspirin or products containing aspirin unless prescribed by your doctor.

This information is selective and does not cover all possible side effects; others may occur. Please report any problems to your doctor.

Reprinted with permission from Memorial Sloan-Kettering Cancer Center, New York, NY

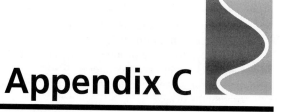

Appendix C

Yellow Pages for Cancer Patients and Caregivers

Agency for Health Care Policy and Research (AHCPR)

AHCPR Publications Clearinghouse
P.O. Box 8547
Silver Spring, MD 20907
800-358-9295
http://www.ahcpr.gov/consumer

This is the only organization in the United States for physicians dedicated to the advancement of hospice or palliative medicine, its practice, research, and education. A compilation of pain management guidelines is available from this agency.

American Association for Cancer Education (AACE)

P.O. Box 601
Smellville, GA 30078-0601
404-329-7612
404-321-4669 (fax)
E-mail: gkrawiec@cancer.org

Provides a forum for health care professionals concerned with the study and improvement of cancer education at the undergraduate, graduate, continuing professional, and para-professional levels.

American Association for Cancer Research (AACR)

Public Ledger Building, Suite 826
150 South Independence Mall West

Philadelphia, PA 19106
215-440-9300
215-440-9313 (fax)
http://www.aacr.org

The association facilitates communication and dissemination of knowledge among scientists and others dedicated to the cancer problem; fosters research in cancer and related biomedical sciences; encourages presentation and discussion of new and important observations in the field; fosters public education, science, education, and training; and advances the understanding of cancer etiology, prevention, diagnosis, and treatment throughout the world.

American Brain Tumor Association (ABTA)

2720 River Road
Suite 146
Des Plaines, IL 60018
847-827-9910 (toll-free)
800-886-2282 (patient line)
847-827-9918 (fax)
http://www.abta.org

Provides written information about brain tumors and their treatments. Services include more than 20 patient education publications, listings of brain tumor support groups, a CONNECTIONS Pen-Pal program, and information about treatment facilities.

American Cancer Society (ACS)

1599 Clifton Road, NE
Atlanta, GA 30329-4251
800-ACS-2345
404-329-7623 (patient services)
512-927-5791 (fax)
(Phone numbers for local units and division are listed in the white pages of the telephone book.)
http://www.cancer.org

Through research, education, and services, ACS not only helps to prevent cancer but also saves lives and diminishes suffering from the disease. Some of the ACS programs and services include the following:

- *Reach to Recovery:* a rehabilitation program for women with breast cancer

- *Ostomy Rehabilitation Program:* a visitation program in which carefully trained volunteers who have successfully adjusted to ostomy surgery visit the newly diagnosed patients
- *International Association of Laryngectomees:* provides information and supportive materials for laryngectomees who wish to offer supportive volunteer services to other people who have undergone a laryngectomy
- *Look Good . . . Feel Better:* a program in which cosmetologists teach cosmetic techniques to patients receiving cancer treatment
- *Lane Adams Award for Nurses and Social Workers:* provides a monetary award for nurses and social workers who demonstrate excellence in caring for people with cancer
- *I Can Cope:* provides information about cancer to patients and families coping with the emotional and physical burdens of the disease
- *Road to Recovery:* provides patients with trained volunteer drivers to transport them to and from treatments

American College of Oncology Administrators (ACDA)

30555 Southfield Road, Suite 150
Southfield, MI 48076
248-540-4310
248-645-0590 (fax)
http://www.pslgroup.com/dg/f7e8e.htm

Promotes the advancement of members' professional standing and personal achievement via continuing education in oncology management, research, strategic planning, and program development.

American College of Radiology (ACR)

1891 Preston White Drive
Reston, VA 22091
Provides a list of accredited mammography programs.

American Foundation for Urologic Disease, Inc.

300 West Pratt Street, Suite 401
Baltimore, MD 21201-2463
410-727-2908
410-528-0050 (fax)
E-mail: admin@afud.org

Dedicated to the prevention and cure of urologic diseases, including prostate and bladder cancer, through the expansion of medical research and the education of the general public and health care professionals.

American Institute for Cancer Research (AICR)

1759 R Street, NW
Washington, DC 20009
202-328-7744 (general information)
800-843-8114 (Nutritional Hotline, publications department)
202-328-7226 (fax)
http://www.aicr.org

Funds research and public education on the prevention and treatment of cancer, focusing particularly on the relationship of diet, nutrition, and cancer.

American Lung Association

1740 Broadway
New York, NY 10019-4374
212-315-8700
http://www.lungusa.org

Provides public education and smoking cessation materials.

American Society for Therapeutic Radiology and Oncology

12500 Fair Lakes Circle, Suite 375
Fairfax, VA 22033-3882
800-962-7886 (toll free)
703-502-7852 (fax)
http://www.astro.org

Extends the benefits of radiation therapy to patients with cancer or other disorders, advances its scientific basis, and provides for the education and professional fellowship of its members.

American Society of Clinical Oncology (ASCO)

225 Reinekers Lane, Suite 650
Alexandria, VA 22314
703-299-0150
703-299-1044 (fax)
http://www.asco.org

Promotes and fosters the exchange of information related to neoplastic diseases for physicians who are academically based or in private practice throughout the United States and other countries.

American Society of Pain Management Nurses (ASPMN)

1550 South Coast Highway, Suite 201
Laguna Beach, CA 92651
714-545-1305
714-545-3643 (fax)
http://www.nursingcenter.com/people/nrgorgs/ASP MN

Dedicated to the constant endeavor of promoting the highest standards of care for patients of all ages experiencing acute, chronic, and malignant pain.

American Society of Plastic and Reconstructive Surgeons

444 East Algonquin Road
Arlington Heights, IL 60055
888-4-PLASTIC
http://www.plasticsurgery.org

Provides written information and a list of certified reconstructive surgeons by geographical area. Caller must provide details on (800) message tape.

Association for Research of Childhood Cancer

P.O. Box 251
Buffalo, NY 14225-0251
716-689-8922

Composed of parents who have lost children to cancer and of people who support cancer research. The association funds the expansion and continuation of research in pediatric cancer centers and provides money for pilot projects in cancer research.

Association for the Care of Children's Health (ACCH)

7910 Woodmont Avenue, Suite 300
Bethesda, MD 20814
301-654-6549

Promotes family-centered care policies and practices that are responsive to the unique development and psychosocial needs of children and youths and their families through international education and advocacy.

Association of Community Cancer Centers (ACCC)

11600 Nebel Street, Suite 201
Rockville, MD 20852
301-984-9496
301-770-1949 (fax)
http://www.accc.cancer.org

Provides a mechanism for the exchange of information among health care professionals who believe that high-quality cancer care should be available in the community.

Association of Nurses in AIDS Care (ANAC)

11250 Roger Bacon Drive, Suite 8
Reston, VA 20190-5202
703-925-0081
703-435-4390 (fax)
http://www.anacnet.org/aids

Founded to foster the professional development of nurses involved in all aspects of HIV care and to promote the health, welfare, and rights of people affected by HIV disease.

Association of Oncology Social Work (AOSW)

1910 East Jefferson Street
Baltimore, MD 21205
410-614-3990
410-614-3991 (fax)
http://www.aosw.org

Composed of professional social workers in oncology. Its functions include advocating sound public and professional programs and policies for patients with cancer.

Association of Pediatric Oncology Nurses (APON)

4700 West Lake Avenue
Glenview, IL 60025-1485
847-375-4727
847-375-4777 (fax)
http://www.apon.org

Dedicated to promoting optimal nursing care for children and adolescents with cancer and their families. Membership in the organization is open to all registered nurses interested in or active in pediatrics or pediatric oncology.

Bone Marrow Transplant Family Support Network

P.O. Box 845
Avon, CT 06001
800-826-9376

Enables families to feel "connected" when coping with the decision to undergo a transplant, with daily routines prior to and following the transplant, and with follow-up care after the transplant.

CancerCare, Inc.

275 Seventh Avenue
New York, NY 10001
800-813-HOPE; 212-302-2400
212-719-0263 (fax)
http://www.cancercareinc.org

Through one-on-one counseling, specialized support groups, educational programs, and telephone contact, CancerCare provides support, guidance, information, and referrals, all free of charge. CancerCare also offers financial assistance for treatment-related costs on a restricted basis.

Cancer Conquerors Foundation

800-238-6479

Committed to teaching patients and families how to cope with cancer.

Cancer Federation, Inc.

711 West Ramsey
P.O. Box 1298
Banning, CA 92220
909-849-HEAL
909-849-0156 (fax)
http://www.cancerfed.com

Supports and funds cancer immunology research programs at hospitals and research centers throughout the United States, offers scholarships to oncology trainees and researchers, and provides referral information to patients with cancer and their families.

Cancer Information Service (CIS)

31 Center Drive MSC2580
Building 31, Room 10A07
Bethesda, MD 20892-2580
800-4-CANCER
800-422-6237
800-332-8615 (TTY)
http://www.cis.nci.gov

Provides accurate, up-to-date information on cancer to patients and their families, health care professionals, and the general public. CIS can provide specific information in English and Spanish about particular types of cancer, information on local trials, and referral to Food and Drug Administration–certified mammography facilities. Each CIS office has access to the NCI treatment database, Physician Data Query (PDQ), which offers callers the most current state-of-the-art treatment and clinical trial information.

CancerFax

National Cancer Institute (NCI) International Cancer Information Center
9030 Old Georgetown Road
Bethesda, MD 20814-1519
301-402-5874 (on fax machine hand set)
800-634-7890 (for technical assistance)

Transmits information on cancer treatment, supportive care, screening and prevention, and selected anticancer drugs, as well as fact sheets for patients and the public and CANCER-LIT Citation and Abstract Digests.

CancerNet™

NCI International Cancer Information Center
9030 Old Georgetown Road
Bethesda, MD 20814-1519
http://cancernet.nic.nih.gov/

Cancer Services on the Internet

Cancer-FAQ, a current list of oncology/cancer services, can be reached on the Internet by pointing to the home page of Medicine Online. The Internet address is:
http://www.meds.com/

Candlelighters Childhood Cancer Foundation

7910 Woodmont Avenue, Suite 460
Bethesda, MD 20814-3015
301-657-8401
800-366-CCCF (800-366-2223)

Provides peer support groups literature, information, help with insurance, employment, and second opinion problems, and referral to local and regional resources.

Centers for Disease Control (CDC) National AIDS Clearinghouse

P.O. Box 6003
Rockville, MD 20849-6003
301-217-0023 (international line)
301-738-6616 (fax)
800-458-5231 (toll-free)
800-243-7012 (TTY/TD/hearing-impaired access)
http://www.cdc.gov/edc.html

Provides primary reference, referral, and publications distribution services for HIV/AIDS information. The clearinghouse acquires, organizes, reviews, updates, and distributes this information.

CHEMOcare

800-55-CHEMO

Educates the public about cancer and its treatment, thereby helping to erase the stigma of the disease. CHEMOcare matches patients with cancer with specially trained volunteers who have successfully gone through their own cancer treatment.

Children's Hospice International

2202 Mt. Vernon Avenue, Suite 3C
Alexandria, VA 22301
1-800-24-CHILD
703-684-0330
703-684-0226 (fax)
http://www.chionline.org

Provides a network of support for children who are dying and their families and serves as a clearinghouse for research programs, support groups, and educational and training programs for the care of children who are terminally ill.

Choice in Dying

1035 30th Street,NW
Washington, DC 20007
202-338-9790 or 800-989-WILL (9455)
202-338-0242 (fax)
http://www.choices.org

Dedicated to fostering communication about complex quality-of-life decisions among individuals, their loved ones, and health care professionals. CID developed the first living will 25 years ago and has distributed approximately 10 million living wills to date. CID is the nation's largest provider of state-specific advance directives.

Combined Health Information Database (CHID)

National Institutes of Health
Box CHID
9000 Rockville Pike
Rockville, MD 20892
301-770-5164 (fax)
http://chid.nih.gov

CHID is a computerized bibliographic database developed and managed by health-related agencies of the U.S. government. It contains references to health information and health education resources, many of which are not referenced in any other computer system or print resource.

The Compassionate Friends

National Office
P.O. Box 3696
Oak Brook, IL 60522-3696
630-990-0010
630-990-0246
http://www.compassionatefriends.org

Supports and aids parents in the positive resolution of grief experienced with the death of a child and fosters the physical and emotional health of bereaved parents and siblings.

Coping

Media America, Inc.
P.O. Box 682268
Franklin, TN 37068-2268
615-790-2400
615-794-0179 (fax)

Nationally distributed consumer magazine for people whose lives have been affected by cancer.

Corporate Angel Network (CAN)

Westchester County Airport
Building 1
White Plains, NY 10604
914-328-1313

Helps patients with cancer bridge the miles between home and needed treatment by providing free plan transportation.

Encore^{plus}

YWCA of the USA Encore^{plus} Program
Office of Women's Health Initiatives
624 9th Street, NW, 3rd Floor
Washington, DC 20001
202-628-3636
202-783-7123 (fax)

Designed to meet the needs of all women and in particular to provide enhanced enabling services to women of color, women of limited income, and older women who do not use appropriate preventive health care services. The comprehensive program model has two basic components: (1) breast and cervical health education and referral to screening and (2) postdiagnosis support that includes a specially designed exercise regimen and peer group support sessions.

Food and Drug Administration

Office of Consumer Affairs, HFE-88
5600 Fishers Lane
Rockville, MD 20857
800-532-4440
http://www.federalregister.com/hpages/fdaz.html

Provides consumers with publications dealing with food-related subjects, cosmetics, general medical information, medical devices, radiologic health, and health fraud.

Gilda Radner Familial Ovarian Cancer Registry

Roswell Park Cancer Institute
Buffalo, NY 14263
1-800-682-7426 (1-800-OVARIAN)
(Monday–Friday, 7 a.m. to 3 p.m.)

**http://www.rpci.med.buffalo.edu/clinic/gynonc/
  grwp.html**

Maintains a registry of families with a history of ovarian and breast cancer. Provides information on advances in screening, treatment, and monitoring for women with a family history of ovarian cancer, including referrals to other support organizations and treatment centers.

Gynecologic Cancer Foundation

401 North Michigan Avenue
Chicago, IL 60611
312-644-6610
312-527-6640 (fax)
http://www.sgo.org/gcf

Administers an aggressive education campaign to disseminate information to the medical community and the public at large about current trends and techniques in gynecologic cancer.

Head and Neck Cancer Information Service

Rush Cancer Institute
Rush-Presbyterian-St. Luke's Medical Center
Suite 863
Chicago, IL 60612
312-563-2322

Staff members of the Head and Neck Cancer Center at Rush-Presbyterian-St. Luke's Medical Center are available to answer questions and review problems pertaining to head and neck cancer.

Hospice Link

Hospice Education Institute
190 Westbrook Road
Essex, CT 06426-1511
800-331-1620; 860-767-1620
860-767-2746 (fax)

Offers information and education about and referrals to hospice and palliative care.

Hospice Nurses Association (HNA)

5512 Northumberland Street
Pittsburgh, PA 15217-1131

412-687-3231
412-687-9095 (fax)

Promotes understanding of the specialty of hospice nursing and the study of hospice nursing research.

International Myeloma Foundation

2120 Stanley Hills Drive
Los Angeles, CA 90046
800-452-CURE
http://www.myeloma.org/imf.html

Promotes education for both physicians and patients regarding myeloma and its treatment and management.

International Society of Nurses in Cancer Care

The Royal College of Nursing
20 Cavendish Square
London WIM OAB
071-495-6119
071-495-6104 (fax)

Advances and disseminates knowledge and understanding of cancer nursing. Membership in the society is open to cancer nursing societies, universities, and institutions involved in cancer care and other entities whose work affects or involves the care of people with cancer.

Intravenous Nurses Society (INS)

Fresh Pond Square, 10 Fawcett Street
Cambridge, MA 02138
617-441-3008

Promotes excellence in intravenous nursing through standards, education, public awareness, and research. INS's ultimate goal is to ensure access to the highest quality, cost-effective care for all individuals requiring intravenous therapies in all practice settings worldwide.
http://www.ins.org

Johanna's On Call to Mend Esteem, Inc.

199 New Scotland Avenue
Albany, NY 12208

Provides preventive, restorative, supportive, and palliative nursing interventions for children, adolescents, and adults with cancer through nursing assessment, image restoration, education, counseling, and referrals to national support organizations.

League of Intravenous Therapy Education (LITE)

P.O. Box 3102
McKeesport, PA 15134-3102
412-678-5025

LITE is the first organization for nurses, pharmacists, and other professionals active in intravenous therapy.

Leukemia Society of America, Inc.

600 Third Avenue
New York, NY 10016
212-573-8484
800-955-4LSA
http://www.leukemia.org

Dedicated to finding the cause of and cure for leukemia and its related disease (lymphoma and multiple myeloma). Services include patient and family support groups, educational materials, and financial assistance for outpatient chemotherapy drugs and therapy, transportation, and transfusions.

Look Good . . . Feel Better (LGFB)

The Cosmetic, Toiletry, and Fragrance Association Foundation
1101 17th Street, NW, Suite 300
Washington, DC 20036
202-331-1770
800-395-LOOK
http://www.lgfb.org

Dedicated to teaching women with cancer (through hands-on experience) beauty techniques that will help to restore their appearance and self-image during chemotherapy and radiation treatment.

LymphEdema Foundation

P.O. Box 834
San Diego, CA 92014-0834
800-LYMPH-DX
800-596-7439

Provides information and resources to people with lymphedema and to health care professionals who treat the condition.

Make-A-Wish Foundation of America

100 West Claredone, Suite 2200
Phoenix, AZ 85013-3518
800-722-WISH
602-279-WISH
602-279-0855 (fax)
http://www.wish.org

The main purpose of this organization is to fulfill the favorite wishes of children with life-threatening or terminal illnesses. The foundation will consider the wish of any child under age 18 and covers all expenses related to granting the wish.

Make Today Count

1235 East Cherokee
Springfield, MO 65804-2263
417-885-2273
800-432-2273

Provides support groups and educational programs as well as brochures and handouts for people with cancer or other life-threatening illness.

The Mary-Helen Mautner Project for Lesbians with Cancer

1707 L Street, NW, Suite 1060
Washington, DC 20036
202-332-5536 (voice/TTY)
202-265-6854 (fax)

Directs services to lesbians with cancer, their partners, and their caregivers. The project provides educational and information to the lesbian community about cancer and educates the health care community about the special concerns of lesbians with cancer and their families. It promotes lesbian health issues on the national and local levels.

National Alliance of Breast Cancer Organizations (NABCO)

9 East 37th Street, 10th Floor
New York, NY 10016
800-719-9154
http://www.nabco.org

Provides assistance and referral to anyone with questions about breast cancer and acts as a voice for the interests and concerns of breast cancer survivors and women at risk.

National Association for Continence (NAFC)

P.O. Box 8310
Spartanburg, SC 29305
864-579-7900
864-579-7902 (fax)
800-BLADDER
http://www.nafc.org

Provides education, advocacy, and support for the public and health professionals about the causes, prevention, diagnosis, treatments, and management alternatives for incontinence.

National Association of Physicians for the Environment (NAPE)

6401 Rockledge Drive, Suite 412
Bethesda, MD 20817
301-571-9791
301-530-8910 (fax)

Works with national medical specialties and subspecialties; with national, state, and local medical societies; and with individual physicians to deal with the impacts of environmental pollutants on the organs, systems, or disease processes best known to them.

National Black Leadership Initiative on Cancer (NBLIC)

6130 Executive Boulevard (EPN 240)
Bethesda, MD 20892
301-496-8589
301-496-8675 (fax)
http://www.uie.edu/UI-Service/programs/UI168.html

Encourages the active participation of community leaders in cancer-related activities and addresses the barriers that limit or prevent access to quality cancer services. Such activities are geared toward accomplishing the overall long-range goal of reducing cancer incidence and mortality rates and increasing survival rates among black Americans.

National Brain Tumor Foundation (NBTF)

785 Market Street, Suite 1600
San Francisco, CA 94103
415-284-0208
800-934-CURE
415-284-0209 (fax)
http://www.braintumor.org/trials.html

Offers information and resources to patients with brain tumors and to their families.

National Breast Cancer Coalition

1707 L Street NW, Suite 1060
Washington, DC 20036
202-296-7477
http://www.natbcc.org

Focuses on action and advocacy to end breast cancer.

National Cancer Institute (NCI) Information Associates Program

9030 Old Georgetown Road
Bethesda, MD 20814-1519
800-NCI-7890 (U.S.)
301-4996-7600 (international)
301-231-6941 (fax)
http://www.nci.nih.gov

Provides easy access to all of NCI's scientific information services for health professionals through one point of contact and for an annual fee.

National Cancer Survivors Day (NCSD) Foundation, Inc.

P.O. Box 682285
Franklin, TN 37068-2285
615-794-3006
615-794-0179 (fax)

NCSD is America's nationwide, annual celebration of life for cancer survivors and their families, friends, and oncology teams. Sunday, June 1, will mark the 10th annual celebration of life. Each celebration is an annual milestone in a survivor's fight against cancer. Ten million cancer survivors live in America.

National Coalition for Cancer Research (NCCR)

Capital Associates, Inc.
426 C Street NE
Washington, DC 20002
202-544-1880
202-543-2565 (fax)

Composed of professional organizations, cancer research centers, and national lay organizations in the United States that are committed to addressing the research and public education efforts necessary to eradicate cancer.

National Coalition for Cancer Survivorship (NCCS)

1010 Wayne Avenue, Suite 505
Silver Spring, MD 20910
301-650-8868
301-565-9670 (fax)

Helps cancer survivors find answers to their questions and attain a better quality of life following diagnosis by linking them to direct service and peer support organizations; addressing financial, professional, legal, and health dilemmas; and participating in and shaping public policy on health care and cancer survivorship research.

National Foundation for Cancer Research (NFCR)

800-321-CURE (free information)

Supports interdisciplinary basic science research in search of a cure for cancer.

National Hispanic Leadership Initiative on Cancer

En Accion Coordinating Center
South Texas Health Research Center
The University of Texas Health Science Center at San Antonio
7703 Floyd Curl Drive
San Antonio, TX 78284-7791
210-614-4496
210-615-0661 (fax)

Empowers Hispanic and Latino populations with the knowledge and the resources they need to prevent and control cancer among their own people through community-based programs.

National Hospice Organization (NHO)

1901 North Moore Street, Suite 901
Arlington, VA 22209
703-243-5900
800-658-8898 (Hospice Hotline)
703-525-5762 (fax)
http://www.nho.org

Advocates for the needs of Americans who are terminally ill. NHO is the only national nonprofit membership organization devoted exclusively to the promotion of hospice care. NHO offers a variety of educational programs, technical assistance, and training curriculums and strives to influence health programs and public policies related to hospice care and the needs of terminally ill people and their families.

National Kidney Cancer Association

708-332-1051
http://www.nkca.org

Provides information to patients and physicians; sponsors and conducts research on kidney cancer; acts as an advocate on behalf of patients with the federal government, insurance companies, and employers; publishes a quarterly newsletter; offers support group meetings in various cities; and holds an annual national convention for patients, families, physicians, and scientists.

National Lymphedema Network (NLN)

2211 Post Street, Suite 404
San Francisco, CA 94115
800-541-3529 (hotline)
415-921-1306 (office)
415-921-2911 (fax)
http://www.wenet.net/-lymhnet/

Disseminates information on the prevention and management of primary and secondary lymphedema to the general public as well as to health care professionals.

National Marrow Donor Program (NMDP)

Coordinating Center
3433 Broadway Street NE, Suite 500
Minneapolis, MN 55413

800-526-7809
800-627-7692 (800-MARROW-2)
612-627-5877
612-627-5899 (fax)
http://www.marrow.org

Focuses on making bone marrow transplants from volunteer unrelated marrow donors available to patients with leukemia and other life-threatening blood diseases.

The National Menopause Foundation, Inc.

222 SW 36th Terrace
Gainesville, FL 32607
800-MENOASK

National Ovarian Cancer Coalition, Inc.

1451 West Cypress Creek Road
Suite 207
Fort Lauderdale, FL 33309
1-888-OVARIAN (toll-free)
954-351-9555
954-351-7655 (fax)
http://www.ovarian.org

Promotes education and awareness throughout the general population and the medical community. NOCC also serves as a resource and referral center for information about ovarian cancer.

National Surgical Adjuvant Breast and Bowel Projects (NSABP)

Operations Center
230 McKee Place, Suite 402
Pittsburgh, PA 15213
412-383-1400
412-383-2221 (fax, administration, and fiscal affairs)
412-383-1388 (fax, medical affairs)

NSABP is a cooperative group that conducts clinical trials in breast and colorectal research.

National Women's Health Network

514 10th Street NW, Suite 400
Washington, DC 20004
202-347-1140

Active in a broad range of women's health issues, including cancer; this health network provides and publishes a newsletter to address these women's issues.

Office of Minority Health Resource Center (OMH-RC)

U.S. Department of Health and Human Services
P.O. Box 37337
Washington, DC 20013-7337

Provides information relating to health resources at the federal, state, and local levels. Target populations are Asians, Pacific Islanders, African-Americans, Hispanics and Latinos, and American Indians and Alaska Natives.

The Oley Foundation

214 Hun Memorial, A23
Albany Medical Center
Albany, NY 12208
518-262-5079
800-776-OLEY
http://www.wizvax.net/oleyfdn

Offers support to consumers of home parenteral or enteral nutrition therapy and their family members. The foundation provides patient and family support group meetings in various locations across the United States and publishes the bimonthly newsletter *Lifeline Letter*.

Oncology Nursing Society (ONS)

501 Holiday Drive
Pittsburgh, PA 15220-2749
412-921-7373
412-921-6565 (fax)
http://www.ons.org

Promotes the highest professional standards of oncology nursing. The society provides support to oncology nurses and encourages study, research, and exchange of information. In addition to guidelines and standards for oncology nursing practice and education, the society publishes a journal, the *Oncology Nursing Forum*, a newsletter, the *ONS News*, which are provided to members and the ONS Online, an Internet-based service for oncology nurses committed to disseminating timely oncology information and continuing education opportunities.

PDQ (Physician Data Query): National Cancer Institute's (NCI) Computerized Data Base for Health Professionals

9030 Old Georgetown Road
Bethesda, MD 20814-1519
800-NCI-7890
301-496-7600 (international)
301-231-6941 (fax)

PDQ is NCI's comprehensive cancer information database that provides access to state-of-the-art cancer treatment information. The database includes summaries of the most common treatment approaches for some 80 types of cancer, ongoing clinical trials that are open to patient entry, and a directory of physicians involved in cancer care and health care organizations that have cancer care programs.

R.A. Bloch Cancer Foundation, Inc.—The Cancer Hotline

4410 Main Street
Kansas City, MO 64111
816-932-8453
816-931-7486 (fax)

Gives people diagnosed with cancer the best possibility of beating the disease as easily as possible through informational resources, peer counseling, medical second opinions, and support groups.

Resource Center for State Cancer Pain Initiatives

3671 Medical Sciences Center
1300 University Avenue
Madison, WI 53706
608-265-4013
608-265-4014 (fax)

Provides information, professional assistance, communications support, referrals, and other services to the growing network of state cancer pain initiatives nationwide.

Ronald McDonald Houses

Ronald McDonald House Charities
One Kroc Drive
Oak Brook, IL 60521
708-575-7070
http://www.rmhomaha.org

Provides places for children and their parents to stay during children's hospital treatment. The houses provide a homelike atmosphere at a reasonable cost and offer the support of other parents and children as well as a management staff.

The Skin Cancer Foundation

245 Fifth Avenue, Suite 2402
New York, NY 10016
212-725-5176
212-725-5751 (fax)
http://www.skincancer.org

Supports skin cancer research and offers patient education materials, including newsletters, books, brochures, pamphlets, posters, slide presentations, and videos.

Society for Biological Therapy (SBT)

P.O. Box 5630
Madison, WI 53705-0630
608-276-6640
http://www.socbiother.com

Committed to investigating, developing, and using biologicals and biological therapy for the treatment of malignant disease.

Society of Gynecological Oncologists

401 North Michigan Avenue
Chicago, IL 60611
312-644-6610
312-527-6640 (fax)
http://www.sgo.org

The society's mission is to improve the care of patients with gynecologic cancer, advance knowledge, and raise standards of practice in gynecologic oncology within the discipline of obstetrics and gynecology, and encourage research in gynecologic oncology.

Society of Surgical Oncology

85 West Algonquin Road #550
Arlington Heights, IL 60005
708-427-1400
http://www.surgonc.org

Ensures the highest quality of comprehensive care for patients with cancer by providing leadership in the broad specialty of surgery.

Susan G. Komen Breast Cancer Foundation

5005 LBJ Freeway, Suite 370
Dallas, TX 75244
214-450-1777
214-450-1710 (fax)
1-800-I'M AWARE
800-462-9273 (national helpline)
http://www.komen.org

Established in 1982, the Komen Foundation is a national volunteer organization working through local chapters and
Race for the Cure events across the country to eradicate
breast cancer as a life-threatening disease by advancing research, education, screening, and treatment.

United Ostomy Association (UOA)

36 Executive Park, Suite 120
Irvine, CA 92714
714-660-8624
800-826-0826
http://www.uoa.org

Provides speakers, literature, and monthly information meetings for people with ostomies. Volunteers, most of whom are
ostomates, will visit patients with ostomies in the hospital or
at home with the consent of the patient's physician.

U.S. Department of Labor Occupational Safety and Health Administration (OSHA)

Directorate of Technical Support
200 Constitution Avenue, NW
Washington, DC 20210
202-219-7047
http://www.osha.org

Involved in the development and enforcement of occupational safety and health standards and strives to ensure safe
and helpful working conditions for every worker in the
United States. The directorate of technical support can provide information regarding work-related hazards and occupational injuries and illnesses.

US TOO International, Inc.

930 North York Road, Suite 50
Hinsdale, IL 60521-2993
800-80-USTOO (800-808-7866)
708-323-1002
708-323-1003 (fax)
http://www.ustoo.org

Provides various types of support for survivors of and patients with prostate cancer. The nonprofit organization offers information and counseling and conducts educational meetings to assist patients in the decision-making process.

We Care Foundation/Camp Dream Street

P.O. Box 3431
Fort Smith, AR 72913
501-441-6292
501-783-6390 (fax)

Provides normal life experiences for children with cancer, their siblings, and their families.

The Wellness Community

2716 Ocean Park Boulevard, Suite 1040
Santa Monica, CA 90405
310-314-2555
http://www.kornet.org/wellness

Has extensive psychosocial support and educational programs to encourage recovery and feeling of wellness.

Women's Cancer Network

2413 West River Road
Grand Island, NY 14072
http://www.wcn.org

Provides support, referral, and resource services to women who have or have had cancer.

Y-ME National Breast Cancer Organization

212 W. Van Buren, Fifth Floor
Chicago, IL 60607-3908
312-986-8338 (office)
800-986-9505 (Hispanic Hotline)
312-986-8228 (24-hour hotline)

800-221-2141 (toll-free hotline, 24 hours)
312-294-8597 (fax)
http://www.y-me.org

Provides information, referral, and emotional support to people concerned about or diagnosed with breast cancer.

Appendix D

National Cancer Institute (NCI) Toxicity Scale

National Cancer Institute Common Toxicity Criteria (CTC)

		Grade			
Toxicity	**0**	**1**	**2**	**3**	**4**
Allergy/Immunology					
Allergic reaction/ hypersensitivity (including drug fever)	None	Transient rash, drug fever <38°C (<100.4°F)	Urticaria, drug fever ≥ 38°C (≥ 100.4°F), and/ or asymptomatic bronchospasm	Symptomatic bronchospasm, requiring parenteral medication(s), with or without urticaria; allergy-related edema/angioedema	Anaphylaxis

Note: Isolated urticaria, in the absence of other manifestations of an allergic or hypersensitivity reaction, is graded in the dermatology/skin category.

| Allergic rhinitis (including sneezing, nasal stuffiness, postnasal drip) | None | Mild, not requiring treatment | Moderate, requiring treatment | — | — |

Continued on next page

National Cancer Institute Common Toxicity Criteria (CTC) *(Continued)*

Toxicity	Grade				
	0	1	2	3	4
Autoimmune reaction	None	Serologic or other evidence of autoimmune reaction but patient is asymptomatic (e.g., vitiligo), all organ function is normal, and no treatment is required	Evidence of autoimmune reaction involving a non-essential organ or function (e.g., hypothyroidism requiring treatment other than immunosuppressive drugs	Reversible autoimmune reaction involving function of a major organ or other toxicity (e.g., transient colitis or anemia), requiring short-term immunosuppressive treament	Autoimmune reaction causing major grade 4 organ dysfunction; progressive and irreversible reaction, long-term administration of high-dose immunosuppressive therapy required

Also consider Hypothyroidism, Colitis, Hemoglobin, Hemolysis

| Serum sickness | None | — | — | Present | — |

Urticaria is graded in the dermatology/skin category if it occurs as an isolated symptom. If it occurs with other manifestations of allergic or hypersensitivity reaction, grade as Allergic reaction/hypersensitivity.

Vasculitis	None	Mild, not requiring treatment	Symptomatic, requiring medication	Requiring steroids	Ischemic changes or requiring amputation
Allergy/Immunology— Other (Specify, _____)	None	Mild	Moderate	Severe	Life-threatening or disabling

Auditory/Hearing

Conductive hearing loss is graded as middle ear/hearing in the Auditory/Hearing category.

Earache is graded in the Pain category.

External auditory canal	Normal	External otitis with erythema or dry desquamation	External otitis with moist desquamation	External otitis with discharge, mastoiditis	Necrosis of the canal, soft tissue, or bone

Note: Changes associated with radiation to external ear (pinnae) are graded under radiation dermatitis in the dermatology/skin category.

Continued on next page

National Cancer Institute Common Toxicity Criteria (CTC) (*Continued*)

Toxicity	Grade				
	0	1	2	3	4
Inner ear/hearing	Normal	Hearing loss on audiometry only	Tinnitus or hearing loss, not requiring hearing aid or treatment	Tinnitus or hearing loss, correctable with hearing aid or treatment	Severe unilateral or bilateral hearing loss (deafness), not correctable
Middle ear/hearing	Normal	Serous otitis without subjective decrease in hearing	Serous otitis or infection requiring medical intervention; subjective decrease in hearing; rupture of tympanic membrane with discharge	Otitis with discharge, mastoiditis, or conductive hearing loss	Necrosis of the canal, soft tissue, or bone
Auditory/Hearing-Other (Specify, _____)	Normal	Mild	Moderate	Severe	Life-threatening or disabling

Blood/Bone Marrow

Bone marrow cellularity	Normal for age	Mildly hypocellular or 25% reduction from normal cellularity for age	Moderately hypocellular or > 25–≤50% reduction from normal cellularity for age or > 2 but < 4 weeks to recovery of normal bone marrow cellularity	Severely hypocellular or > 50–≤ 75% reduction in cellularity for age or 4–6 weeks to recovery of normal bone marrow cellularity	Aplasia or > 6 weeks to to recovery of normal bone marrow cellularity
Normal ranges: children (≤ 18 years)	90% cellularity average			
Younger adults (19–59)	60–70% cellularity average			
Older adults (≥ 60 years)	50% cellularity average			

Note: Grade Bone marrow cellularity only for changes related to treatment not disease.

CD4 count	WNL	< LLN–500/mm^3	200–< 500/mm^3	50–< 200mm^3	< 50mm^3
Haptoglobin	Normal	Decreased	—	Absent	—

Continued on next page

National Cancer Institute Common Toxicity Criteria (CTC) (*Continued*)

Toxicity	0	1	2	3	4
			Grade		
Hemoglobin (Hgb)	WNL	< LLN–10.0 g/dl < LLN–100 g/L < LLN–6.2 mmol/L	8.0–< 10.0 g/dl 80–< 100 g/L 4.9–< 6.2 mmol/L	6.5–< 8.0 g/dl 65–< 80 g/L 4.0–< 4.9 mmol/L	< 6.5 g/dl < 65 g/L < 4.0 mmol/L

Note: The following criteria may be used for leukemia studies or bone marrow infiltrative/myelophthisic process if the protocol so specifies.

Toxicity	0	1	2	3	4
For leukemia studies or bone marrow infiltrative/myelophthisic processes	WNL	10–< 25% decrease from pretreatment	25–< 50% decrease from pretreatment	50–< 75% decrease from pretreatment	≥ 75% decrease from pretreatment
Hemolysis (e.g., immune hemolytic anemia, drug-related hemolysis, other)	None	Only laboratory evidence of hemolysis (e.g., direct antiglobulin test [DAT, Coombs'] schistocytes)	Evidence of red cell destruction and ≥ 2g decrease in hemoglobin, no transfusion	Requiring transfusion and/or medical intervention (e.g., steroids)	Catastrophic consequences of hemolysis (e.g., renal failure, hypotension, bronchospasm, emergency splenectomy)

Also consider Haptoglobin, Hgb.

Leukocytes (total WBC)	WNL	$<$ LLN–3.0 × 10^9/L $<$ LLN–3000/mm^3	≥ 2.0–$<$ 3.0 × 10^9/L ≥ 2000–$<$ 3000/mm^3	≥ 1.0–$<$ 2.0 × 10^9/L ≥ 1000–$<$ 2000/mm^3	$<$ 1.0 × 10^9/L $<$ 1000/mm^3
For BMT studies:	WNL	≥ 2.0–$<$ 3.0 × 10^9/L ≥ 2000–$<$ 3000/mm^3	≥ 1.0–$<$ 2.0 × 10^9/L ≥ 1000–$<$ 2000/mm^3	≥ 0.5–$<$ 1.0 × 10^9/L ≥ 500–$<$ 1000/mm^3	$<$ 0.5 × 10^9/L $<$ 500/mm^3
Note: The following criteria using age, race, and sex normal values may be used for pediatric studies if the protocol so specifies.		≥ 75–$<$ 100% LLN	≥ 50–$<$ 75% LLN	≥ 25–$<$ 50% LLN	$<$ 25% LLN
Lymphopenia	WNL	$<$ LLN–1.0 × 10^9/L $<$ LLN–1000/mm^3	≥ 0.5–$<$ 1.0 × 10^9/L ≥ 500–$<$ 1000/mm^3	$<$ 0.5 × 10^9/L $<$ 500/mm^3	—
Note: The following criteria using age, race, and sex normal values may be used for pediatric studies if the protocol so specifies.		≥ 75–$<$ 100% LLN	≥ 50–$<$ 75% LLN	≥ 25–$<$ 50% LLN	$<$ 25% LLN
Neutrophils/granulocytes (ANC/AGC)	WNL	≥ 1.5–$<$ 2.0 × 10^9/L ≥ 1500–$<$ 2000/mm^3	≥ 1.0–$<$ 1.5 × 10^9/L ≥ 1000–$<$ 1500/mm^3	≥ 0.5–$<$ 1.0 × 10^9/L ≥ 500–$<$ 1000/mm^3	$<$ 0.5 × 10^9/L $<$ 500/mm^3
For BMT:	WNL	≥ 1.0–$<$ 1.5 × 10^9/L ≥ 1000–$<$ 1500/mm^3	≥ 0.5–$<$ 1.0 × 10^9/L ≥ 500–$<$ 1000/mm^3	≥ 0.1–$<$ 0.5 × 10^9/L ≥ 100–$<$ 500/mm^3	$<$ 0.1 × 10^9/L $<$ 100/mm^3
Note: The following criteria may be used for leukemia studies or bone marrow infiltrative/myelophthisic process if the protocol so specifies.					
For leukemia studies or bone marrow infiltrative/myelophthisic process	WNL	10–$<$ 25% decrease from baseline	25–$<$ 50% decrease from baseline	50–$<$ 75% decrease from baseline	≥ 75% decrease from baseline

Continued on next page

National Cancer Institute Common Toxicity Criteria (CTC) (*Continued*)

			Grade		
Toxicity	**0**	**1**	**2**	**3**	**4**
Platelets	WNL	$< \text{LLN}-< 75.0 \times 10^9/\text{L}$ $< \text{LLN}-< 75,000/\text{mm}^3$	$\geq 50.0-< 75.0 \times 10^9/\text{L}$ $\geq 50,000-< 7,500/\text{mm}^3$	$\geq 10.0-< 50.0 \times 10^9/\text{L}$ $\geq 10,000-< 50,000/\text{mm}^3$	$< 10.0 \times 10^9/\text{L}$ $< 10,000/\text{mm}^3$
For BMT:	WNL	$\geq 50.0-< 75.0 \times 10^9/\text{L}$ $\geq 50,000-< 75,000/\text{mm}^3$	$\geq 20.0-< 50.0 \times 10^9/\text{L}$ $\geq 20,000-< 50,000/\text{mm}^3$	$\geq 10.0-< 20.0 \times 10^9/\text{L}$ $\geq 10,000-< 20,000/\text{mm}^3$	$< 10.0 \times 10^9/\text{L}$ $< 10,000/\text{mm}^3$
Note: The following criteria may be used for leukemia studies or bone marrow infiltrative/myelophthisic process if the protocol so specifies.					
For leukemia studies or bone marrow infiltrative/ myelophthisic process	WNL	10–< 25% decrease from baseline	25–< 50% decrease from baseline	50– < 75% decrease from baseline	≥ 75% decrease from baseline
Transfusion: Platelets	None	—	—	Yes	Platelet transfusions and other measures required to improve platelet increment; platelet transfu-

	None	1 platelet transfusion in 24 hours	2 platelet transfusions in 24 hours	≥ 3 platelet transfusions in 24 hours	...sion refractoriness associated with life-threatening bleeding (e.g., HLA or cross-matched platelet transfusions)
For BMT:	None	1 platelet transfusion in 24 hours	2 platelet transfusions in 24 hours	≥ 3 platelet transfusions in 24 hours	Platelet transfusions and other measures required to improve platelet increment; platelet transfusion refractoriness associated with life-threatening bleeding (e.g., HLA or cross-matched platelet transfusions)

Also see Platelets.

Continued on next page

National Cancer Institute Common Toxicity Criteria (CTC) (*Continued*)

Toxicity	Grade				
	0	1	2	3	4
Transfusion: pRBCs	None	—	—	Yes	—
For BMT:	None	≤ 2 u pRBC (≤ *15cc/ kg*) in 24 hours elective or planned	3 u pRBC (*>15 ≤30cc/kg*) in 24 hours elective or planned	≥ 4 u pRBC (*>30cc/ kg*) in 24 hours	Hemorrhage or hemolysis associated with life-threatening anemia: medical intervention required to improve hemoglobin

Also consider Hemoglobin.

Toxicity	0	1	2	3	4
Blood/Bone marrow-Other (Specify, _____)	None	Mild	Moderate	Severe	Life-threatening or disabling
Cardiovascular (Arrhythmia)					
Conduction abnormality/	None	Asymptomatic, not requiring treatment	Symptomatic, but not requiring treatment	Symptomatic and requiring treatment	Life-threatening (e.g., arrhythmia)

atrioventricular heart block	None	(e.g., Mobitz type I second-degree AV block, Wenckebach)		(e.g., Mobitz type II second-degree AV block, third-degree AV block)	associated with CHF, hypotension, syncope, shock
Nodal/junctional arrhythmia/dysrhythmia	None	Asymptomatic, not requiring treatment	Symptomatic, but not requiring treatment	Symptomatic and requiring treatment	Life-threatening (e.g., arrhythmia associated with CHF, hypotension, syncope, shock)
Palpitations	None	Present	—	—	—
Prolonged QTc interval (QTc > 0.48 seconds)	None	Asymptomatic, not requiring treatment	Symptomatic, but not requiring treatment	Symptomatic and requiring treatment	Life-threatening (e.g., arrhythmia associated with CHF, hypotension, syncope, shock)
Sinus bradycardia	None	Asymptomatic, not requiring treatment	Symptomatic, but not requiring treatment	Symptomatic and requiring treatment	Life-threatening (e.g., arrhythmia associated with CHF, hypotension, syncope, shock)

Note: Grade palpitations only in the absence of a documented arrhythmia.

Continued on next page

National Cancer Institute Common Toxicity Criteria (CTC) (*Continued*)

Toxicity	Grade				
	0	1	2	3	4
Sinus tachycardia	None	Asymptomatic, not requiring treatment	Symptomatic, but not requiring treatment	Symptomatic and requiring treatment of underlying cause	associated with CHF, hypotension, syncope, shock)
					—
Supraventricular arrhythmias (SVT/ atrial fibrillation/ flutter)	None	Asymptomatic, not requiring treatment	Symptomatic, but not requiring treatment	Symptomatic and requiring treatment	Life-threatening (e.g., arrhythmia associated with CHF, hypotension, syncope, shock)

Syncope (fainting) is graded in the Neurology category.

Toxicity	0	1	2	3	4
Vasovagal episode	None	—	Present without loss of consciousness	Present with loss of consciousness	—

Ventricular arrhythmia (PVCs/bigeminy/trigeminy/ventricular tachycardia)	None	Asymptomatic, not requiring treatment	Symptomatic, but not requiring treatment	Symptomatic and requiring treatment	Life-threatening (e.g., arrhythmia associated with CHF, hypotension, syncope, shock)
Cardiovascular/Arrhythmia-Other (Specify, _____)	None	Asymptomatic, not requiring treatment	Symptomatic, but not requiring treatment	Symptomatic, and requiring treatment of underlying cause	Life-threatening (e.g., arrhythmia associated with CHF, hypotension, syncope, shock)
Cardiovascular (General)					
Acute vascular leak syndrome	Absent	—	Symptomatic, but not requiring fluid support	Respiratory compromise or requiring fluids	Life-threatening requiring pressor support and/or ventilatory support
Cardiac—ischemia/infarction	None	Nonspecific T-wave flattening or changes	Asymptomatic, ST- and T-wave changes suggesting ischemia	Angina without evidence of infarction	Acute myocardial infarction

Continued on next page

National Cancer Institute Common Toxicity Criteria (CTC) (*Continued*)

Toxicity	Grade				
	0	1	2	3	4
Cardiac left ventricular funtion	Normal	Asymptomatic decline of resting ejection fraction of ≥ 10% but < 20% of baseline value; shortening fraction ≥ 24% but < 30%	Asymptomatic but resting ejection fraction below LLN for laboratory or decline of resting ejection fraction ≥ 20% of baseline value; < 24% shortening fraction	CHF responsive to treatment	Severe or refractory CHF or requiring intubation

CNS cerebrovascular ischemia is graded in the neurology category.

| Cardiac troponin I (cTnI) | Normal | — | — | Levels consistent with unstable angina as defined by the manufacturer | Levels consistent with myocardial infarction as defined by the manufacturer |
| Cardiac troponin T (cTnT) | Normal | ≥ 0.03–< 0.05 ng/mL | ≥ 0.05–< 0.1 ng/mL | ≥ 0.1–< 0.2 ng/mL | ≥ 0.2 ng/mL |

Edema	None	Asymptomatic, not requiring therapy	Symptomatic, requiring therapy	Symptomatic edema limiting function and unresponsive to therapy or requiring drug discontinuation	Anasarca (severe generalized edema)
Hypertension	None	Asymptomatic, transient increase by > 20 mmHg (diastolic) or to > 150/100* if previously WNL; not requiring treatment	Recurrent or persistent or symptomatic increase by > 20 mm Hg (diastolic) or to > 150/100* if previously WNL; not requiring treatment	Requiring therapy or more intensive therapy than previously	Hypertensive crisis

*Note: For pediatric patients, use age- and sex-appropriate normal values > 95th percentile ULN.

Hypotension	None	Changes, but not requiring therapy (including transient orthostatic hypotension)	Requiring brief fluid replacement or other therapy but not hospitalization; no physiologic consequences	Requiring therapy and sustained medical attention, but resolves without persisting physiologic consequences	Shock (associated with acidemia and impairing vital organ function due to tissue hypoperfusion)

Also consider Syncope (fainting).

Angina or MI is graded as Cardiac-ischemia/infarction in the cardiovascular (general) category.

For pediatric patients, systolic BP 65 mm Hg or less in infants up to 1 year old and 70 mm Hg or less in children older than 1 year of age, use two successive or three measurements in 24 hours.

Continued on next page

National Cancer Institute Common Toxicity Criteria (CTC) (*Continued*)

Toxicity	Grade				
	0	1	2	3	4
Myocarditis	None	—	—	CHF responsive to treatment	Severe or refractory CHF
Operative injury of vein/artery	None	Primary suture repair for injury, but not requiring transfusion	Primary suture repair for injury, requiring transfusion	Vascular occlusion requiring surgery or bypass for injury	Myocardial infarction; resection of organ (e.g., bowel, limb)
Pericardial effusion/pericarditis	None	Asymptomatic effusion, not requiring treatment	Pericarditis (rub, ECG changes, and/or chest pain)	Physiologic consequences resulting from symptoms	Tamponade (drainage or pericardial window required)
Peripheral arterial ischemia	None	—	Brief episode of ischemia managed non-surgically and without permanent deficit	Requiring surgical intervention	Life-threatening or with permanent functional deficit (e.g., amputation)

Adverse Event	None	Mild	Moderate	Severe	Life-threatening
Phlebitis (superficial)	None	—		Present	—

Injection site reaction is graded in the dermatology/skin category.

Thrombosis/embolism is graded in the cardiovascular (general) category.

Syncope (fainting) is graded in the neurology category.

Adverse Event	None	Mild	Moderate	Severe	Life-threatening
Thrombosis/embolism	None	—	Deep vein thrombosis, not requiring anticoagulant therapy	Deep vein thrombosis, requiring anticoagulant therapy	Embolic event, including pulmonary embolism

Vein/artery operative injury is graded as Operative injury of vein/artery in the cardiovascular (general) category.

Adverse Event	None	Mild	Moderate	Severe	Life-threatening
Visceral arterial ischemia (nonmyocardial)	None	—	Brief episode of ischemia managed nonsurgically and without permanent deficit	Requiring surgical intervention	Life-threatening or with permanent functional deficit (e.g., resection of ileum)
Cardiovascular/General—Other (Specify, _____)	None	Mild	Moderate	Severe	Life-threatening or disabling

Continued on next page

National Cancer Institute Common Toxicity Criteria (CTC) (*Continued*)

Toxicity	Grade				
	0	1	2	3	4
Coagulation					
Note: See the hemorrhage category for grading the severity of bleeding events.					
DIC (disseminated intravascular coagulation)	Absent	—	—	Laboratory findings present with no bleeding	Laboratory findings and bleeding
Also grade Platelets.					
Note: Must have increased fibrin split products or D-dimer in order to grade as DIC.					
Fibrinogen	WNL	$\geq 0.75 - < 1.0 \times$ LLN	$\geq 0.5 - < 0.75 \times$ LLN	$\geq 0.25 - < 0.5 \times$ LLN	$< 0.25 \times$ LLN
Note: The following criteria may be used for leukemia studies or bone marrow infiltrative/myelophthisic process if the protocol so specifies.					
For leukemia studies	WNL	$< 20\%$ decrease from pretreatment value or LLN	$\geq 20 - < 40\%$ decrease from pretreatment value or LLN	$\geq 40 - < 70\%$ decrease from pretreatment value or LLN	< 50 mg%
Partial thromboplastin time (PTT)	WNL	$> $ ULN $- \leq 1.5 \times$ ULN	$> 1.5 \leq 2 \times$ ULN	$> 2 \times$ ULN	—

Phlebitis is graded in the cardiovascular (general) category.

	WNL	> ULN–≤ 1.5 × ULN	> 1.5–≤ 2 × ULN	> 2 × ULN	—
Prothrombin time (PT)	WNL	> ULN–≤ 1.5 × ULN	> 1.5–≤ 2 × ULN	> 2 × ULN	—

Thrombosis/embolism is graded in the cardiovascular (general) category.

Thrombotic microangiopathy (e.g., thrombotic thrombocytopenic purpura/TTP or hemolytic uremic syndrome/HUS)	Absent	Evidence of RBC destruction (schistocytosis) without clinical consequences	—	Laboratory findings present without clinical consequences	Laboratory findings and clinical consequences (e.g., CNS hemorrhage/bleeding or thrombosis/embolism or renal failure) requiring therapeutic intervention
For BMT:	—	—	Evidence of RBC destruction with elevated creatinine (≤ 3 × ULN)	Evidence of RBC destruction with creatinine (> 3 × ULN) not requiring dialysis	Evidence of RBC destruction with renal failure requiring dialysis and/or encephalopathy

Continued on next page

433

National Cancer Institute Common Toxicity Criteria (CTC) (*Continued*)

			Grade		
Toxicity	**0**	**1**	**2**	**3**	**4**
Also consider Hemoglobin (Hgb), Platelets, Creatinine. *Note: Must have microangiopathic changes on blood smear (e.g., schistocytes, helmet cells, red cell fragments).*					
Coagulation—Other (Specify, _____)	None	Mild	Moderate	Severe	Life-threatening or disabling
Constitutional Symptoms					
Fatigue (lethargy, malaise, asthenia)	None	Increased fatigue over baseline, but not altering normal activities	Moderate (e.g., decrease in performance status by 1 ECOG level *or* 20% Karnofsky or *Lansky*) *or* causing difficulty performing some activities	Severe (e.g., decrease in performance status by ≥ 2 ECOG levels *or* 40% Karnofsky or *Lansky*) *or* loss of ability to perform some activities	Bedridden or disabling

Fever (in the absence of neutropenia, where neutropenia is defined as AGC $< 1.0 \times 10^9$/L)	None	38.0–39.0°C (100.4–102.2°F)	39.1–40.0°C (102.3–104.0°F)	> 40.0°C (> 104.0°F) for < 24hrs	> 40.0°C (> 104.0°F) for > 24hrs

Also consider Allergic reaction/hypersensitivity.
Note: The temperature measurements listed above are oral or tympanic.

Hot flashes/flushes are graded in the endocrine category.

Rigors, chills	None	Mild, requiring symptomatic treatment (e.g., blanket) or non-narcotic medication	Severe and/or prolonged, requiring narcotic medication	Not responsive to narcotic medication	—
Sweating (diaphoresis)	None	Mild and occasional	Frequent or drenching	—	—
Weight gain	< 5%	5–< 10%	10–< 20%	≥ 20%	—

Also consider Ascites, Edema, Pleural effusion.

Continued on next page

National Cancer Institute Common Toxicity Criteria (CTC) (*Continued*)

Toxicity	Grade				
	0	1	2	3	4
Weight gain—veno-occlusive disease (VOD)					≥ 10% or fluid retention resulting in pulmonary failure
Note: The following criteria are to be used ONLY for weight gain associated with VOD.	< 2%	≥ 2–< 5%	≥ 5–< 10%	≥ 10% or as ascites	
Weight loss Also consider Vomiting, Dehydration, Diarrhea.	< 5%	5–< 10%	10–< 20%	≥ 20%	
Constitutional Symptoms-Other (Specify, _____)	None	Mild	Moderate	Severe	Life-threatening or disabling
Dermatology/Skin					
Alopecia	Normal	Mild hair loss	Pronounced hair loss	—	—

Bruising (in absence of grade 3 or 4 thrombocytopenia)	None	Localized or in dependent area	Generalized	—	—

Note: Bruising resulting from grade 3 or 4 thrombocytopenia is graded as Petechiae/purpura and Hemorrhage/bleeding with grade 3 or 4 thrombocytopenia in the Hemorrhage category, not in the Dermatology/Skin category.

Dermatitis, focal (associated with high-dose chemotherapy and bone marrow transplant)	None	Faint erythema or dry desquamation	Moderate to brisk erythema or a patchy moist desquamation, mostly confined to skin folds and creases; moderate edema	Confluent moist desquamation, ≥ 1.5 cm diameter, not confined to skin folds; pitting edema	Skin necrosis or ulceration of full thickness dermis; may include spontaneous bleeding not induced by minor trauma or abrasion
Dry skin	Normal	Controlled with emollients	Not controlled with emollients	—	—
Erythema multiforme (e.g., Stevens-	Absent	—	Scattered, but not generalized eruption	Severe or requiring IV fluids (e.g., general-	Life-threatening (e.g., exfoliative

Continued on next page

National Cancer Institute Common Toxicity Criteria (CTC) (*Continued*)

Toxicity	0	1	2	3	4
				Grade	
Johnson syndrome, toxic epidermal necrolysis)				ized rash or painful stomatitis)	or ulcerating dermatitis or requiring enteral or parenteral nutritional support)
Flushing	Absent	Present	—	—	—
Hand-foot skin reaction	None	Skin changes or dermatitis without pain (e.g., erythema, peeling)	Skin changes with pain, not interfering with function	Skin changes with pain, interfering with function	—
Injection site reaction	None	Pain or itching or erythema	Pain or swelling, with inflammation or phlebitis	Ulceration or necrosis that is severe or prolonged, or requiring surgery	—
Nail changes	Normal	Discoloration or ridging (koilonychia) or pitting	Partial or complete loss of nail(s) or pain in nailbeds	—	—

438

Petechiae is graded in the Hemorrhage category.

	None	Painless erythema	Painful erythema	Erythema with desquamation	
Photosensitivity	None				—
Pigmentation changes (e.g., vitiligo)	None	Localized pigmentation changes	Generalized pigmentation changes	—	—
Pruritus	None	Mild or localized, relieved spontaneously or by local measures	Intense or widespread, relieved spontaneously or by systemic measures	Intense or widespread and poorly controlled despite treatment	—

Purpura is graded in the Hemorrhage category.

	None	Painless erythema	Painful erythema	Erythema with desquamation	
Radiation dermatitis	None	Faint erythema or dry desquamation	Moderate to brisk erythema or a patchy moist desquamation mostly confined to skin folds and creases; moderate edema	Confluent moist desquamation, ≥ 1.5 cm diameter, not confined to skin folds; pitting edema	Skin necrosis or ulceration of full thickness dermis; may include bleeding not induced by minor trauma or abrasion

Note: Pain associated with radiation dermatitis is graded separately in the Pain category as Pain due to radiation.

Continued on next page

439

National Cancer Institute Common Toxicity Criteria (CTC) (*Continued*)

Toxicity	0	1	2	3	4
			Grade		
Radiation recall reaction (reaction following chemotherapy in the absence of additional radiation therapy that occurs in a previous radiation port)	None	Faint erythema or dry desquamation	Moderate to brisk erythema or a patchy moist desquamation, mostly confined to skin folds and creases; moderate edema	Confluent moist desquamation, ≥ 1.5 cm diameter, not confined to skin folds; pitting edema	Skin necrosis or ulceration of full thickness dermis; may include bleeding not induced by minor trauma or abrasion
Rash/desquamation	None	Macular or papular eruption or erythema without associated symptoms	Macular or papular eruption or erythema with pruritus or other associated symptoms covering < 50% of body surface or localized desquamation or other lesions covering < 50% of body surface area	Symptomatic generalized erythroderma or macular, papular, or vesicular eruption or desquamation covering ≥ 50% of body surface area	Generalized exfoliative dermatitis or ulcerative dermatitis

	None				Surface area generalized exfoliative dermatitis or ulcerative dermatitis or bullous formation
For BMT:	None	Macular or papular eruption or erythema covering < 25% of body surface area without associated symptoms	Macular or papular eruption or erythema with pruritus or other associated symptoms covering ≥ 25–< 50% of body surface or localized desquamation or other lesions covering ≥ 25–< 50% of body surface area	Symptomatic generalized erythroderma or symptomatic macular, papular, or vesicular eruption, with bullous formation, or desquamation covering ≥ 50% of body	Surface area generalized exfoliative dermatitis or ulcerative dermatitis or bullous formation

Also consider Allergic reaction/hypersensitivity.
Erythema multiforme (Stevens-Johnson syndrome) is graded separately as Erythema multiforme.

Urticaria (hives, welts, wheals)	None	Requiring no medication	Requiring PO or topical treatment or IV medication or steroids for < 24 hours	Requiring IV medication or steroids for ≥ 24 hours	—
Wound—infectious	None	Cellulitis	Superficial infection	Infection requiring IV antibiotics	Necrotizing fasciitis
Wound—noninfectious	None	Incisional separation	Incisional hernia	Fascial disruption without evisceration	Fascial disruption with evisceration

Continued on next page

National Cancer Institute Common Toxicity Criteria (CTC) (*Continued*)

			Grade		
Toxicity	0	1	2	3	4
Dermatology/Skin-Other (Specify, ____)	None	Mild	Moderate	Severe	Life-threatening or disabling
Endocrine					
Cushingoid appearance (e.g., moon face with or without buffalo hump, centripetal obesity, cutaneous striae) Also consider Hyperglycemia, Hypokalemia.	Absent	—	Present	—	—
Feminization of male	Absent	—	—	Present	—
Gynecomastia	None	Mild	Pronounced or painful	Pronounced or painful and requiring surgery	—

	None	Mild or no more than 1 per day	Moderate and greater than 1 per day		
Hot flashes/flushes	None	Mild or no more than 1 per day	Moderate and greater than 1 per day	—	—
Hypothyroidism	Absent	Asymptomatic, TSH elevated, no therapy given	Symptomatic or thyroid replacement treatment given	Patient hospitalized for manifestations of hypothyroidism	Myxedema coma
Masculinization of female	Absent	—	—	Present	—
SIADH (syndrome of inappropriate anti-diuretic hormone)	Absent	—	—	Present	—
Endocrine-Other (Specify, _____)	None	Mild	Moderate	Severe	Life-threatening or disabling

Amylase is graded in the Metabolic/Laboratory category.

Gastrointestinal

	None	Loss of appetite	Oral intake significantly decreased	Requiring IV fluids	Requiring feeding tube or parenteral nutrition
Anorexia	None	Loss of appetite	Oral intake significantly decreased	Requiring IV fluids	Requiring feeding tube or parenteral nutrition

Continued on next page

443

National Cancer Institute Common Toxicity Criteria (CTC) (*Continued*)

Toxicity	Grade				
	0	1	2	3	4
Ascites (non-malignant)	None	Asymptomatic	Symptomatic, requiring diuretics	Symptomatic, requiring therapeutic paracentesis	Life-threatening physiologic consequences
Colitis	None	—	Abdominal pain with mucus and/or blood in stool	Abdominal pain, fever, change in bowel habits with ileus or peritoneal signs, and radiographic or biopsy documentation	Perforatin or requiring surgery or toxic mega-colon

Also consider Hemorrhage/bleeding with grade 3 or 4 thrombocytopenia, Hemorrhage/bleeding without grade 3 or 4 thrombocytopenia, Melena/GI bleeding/hematochezia, Rectal bleeding/hematochezia, Hypotension.

Toxicity	Grade				
	0	1	2	3	4
Constipation	None	Requiring stool softener or dietary modification	Requiring laxatives	Obstipation requiring manual evacuation or enema	Obstruction or toxic megacolon
Dehydration	None	Dry mucous membranes and/or diminished skin turgor	Requiring IV fluid replacement (brief)	Requiring IV fluid replacement (sustained)	Physiologic consequences requiring intensive care, hemodynamic collapse

Also consider Hypotension, Diarrhea, Vomiting, Stomatitis/pharyngitis (oral/pharyngeal mucositis).

Diarrhea patients without colostomy:	None	Increase of < 4 stools/day over pretreatment	Increase of 4–6 stools/day, or nocturnal stools	Increase of ≥ 7 stools/day or incontinence; or need for parenteral support for dehydration	Physiologic consequences requiring intensive care; or hemodynamic collapse
Patients with colostomy:	None	Mild increase in loose, watery colostomy output compared with pretreatment	Moderate increase in loose, watery colostomy output compared with pretreatment, but not interfering with normal activity	Severe increase in loose, watery colostomy output compared with pretreatment, interfering with normal activity	Physiologic consequences, requiring intensive care; or hemodynamic collapse
For BMT	None	> 500–≤ 1000mL of diarrhea/day	> 1000–≤ 1500mL of diarrhea/day	> 1500mL of diarrhea/day	Severe abdominal pain with or without ileus
For Pediatric BMT:		*> 5–≤ 10 ml/kg of diarrhea/day*	*> 10–≤ 15 ml/kg of diarrhea/day*	*> 15 ml/kg of diarrhea/day*	—

Also consider Hemorrhage/bleeding with grade 3 or 4 thrombocytopenia, Hemorrhage/bleeding without grade 3 of 4 thrombocytopenia, Pain, Dehydration, Hypotension.

Continued on next page

National Cancer Institute Common Toxicity Criteria (CTC) (*Continued*)

Toxicity	0	1	2	3	4
			Grade		
Duodenal ulcer (requires radiographic or endoscopic documentation)	None	—	Requiring medical management or non-surgical treatment	Uncontrolled by outpatient medical management; requiring hospitalization	Perforation or bleeding, requiring emergency surgery
Dyspepsia/heartburn	None	Mild	Moderate	Severe	—
Dysphagia, esophagitis, odynophagia (painful swallowing)	None	Mild dysphagia, but can eat regular diet	Dysphagia, requiring predominantly pureed, soft, or liquid diet	Dysphagia, requiring IV hydration	Complete obstruction (cannot swallow saliva) requiring enteral or parenteral nutritional support, or perforation

Note: If toxicity is radiation-related, grade under either Dysphagia—esophageal related to radiation or Dysphagia—pharyngeal related to radiation.

Adverse Event				
Dysphagia—*esophageal* related to radiation	None	Mild dysphagia, but can eat regular diet	Dysphagia, requiring predominantly liquid, pureed, or soft diet	Dysphagia requiring feeding tube, IV hydration, or hyper-alimentation	Complete obstruction (cannot swallow saliva); ulceration with bleeding not induced by minor trauma or abrasion or perforation

Also consider Pain due to radiation, Mucositis due to radiation.

Note: Fistula is graded separately as Fistula—esophageal.

Adverse Event				
Dysphagia—*pharyngeal* related to radiation	None	Mild dysphagia, but can eat regular diet	Dysphagia, requiring predominantly pureed, soft, or liquid diet	Dysphagia, requiring feeding tube, IV hydration, or hyper-alimentation	Complete obstruction (cannot swallow saliva); ulceration with bleeding not induced by minor trauma or abrasion or perforation

Also consider Pain due to radiation, Mucositis due to radiation.

Note: Fistula is graded separately as Fistula—pharyngeal.

Continued on next page

National Cancer Institute Common Toxicity Criteria (CTC) (*Continued*)

Toxicity	Grade				
	0	1	2	3	4
Fistula—esophageal	None	—	—	Present	Requiring surgery
Fistula—intestinal	None	—	—	Present	Requiring surgery
Fistula—pharyngeal	None	—	—	Present	Requiring surgery
Fistula—rectal/anal	None	—	—	Present	Requiring surgery
Flatulence	None	Mild	Moderate		
Gastric ulcer (requires radiographic or endoscopic documentation)	None		Requiring medical management or nonsurgical treatment	Bleeding without perforation, uncontrolled by outpatient medical management, requiring hospitalization or surgery	Peforation or bleeding, requiring emergency surgery

Also consider Hemorrhage/bleeding with grade 3 or 4 thrombocytopenia, Hemorrhage/bleeding without grade 3 or 4 thrombocytopenia.

Gastritis	None	—	Requiring medical management or non-surgical treatment	Uncontrolled by out-patient medical management, requiring hospitaliza-tion or surgery	Life-threatening bleeding, requiring emer-gency surgery

Also consider Hemorrhage/bleeding with grade 3 or 4 thrombocytopenia, Hemorrhage/bleeding without grade 3 or 4 thrombocytopenia.

Hematemesis is graded in the Hemorrhage category.

Hematochezia is graded in the Hemorrhage category as Rectal bleeding/hematochezia.

Ileus (or neuro-constipation)	None	—	Intermittent, not requiring intervention	Requiring nonsurgical intervention	Requiring surgery
Mouth dryness	Normal	Mild	Moderate	—	—

Mucositis

Note: Mucositis not due to radiation is graded in the Gastrointestinal category for specific sites: Colitis, Esophagitis, Gastritis, Stomatitis/pharyngitis (oral/pharyngeal mucositis), and Typhlitis; or the Renal/Genitourinary category for Vaginitis.

Radiation-related mucositis is graded as Mucositis due to radiation.

Continued on next page

National Cancer Institute Common Toxicity Criteria (CTC) (*Continued*)

Toxicity	Grade				
	0	1	2	3	4
Mucositis due to radiation	None	Erythema of the mucosa	Patchy pseudomembranous reaction (patches generally ≦ 1.5 cm in diameter and noncontiguous)	Confluent pseudomembranous reaction (contiguous patches generally > 1.5 cm in diameter)	Necrosis or deep ulceration; may include bleeding not induced by minor trauma or abrasion

Also consider Pain due to radiation.

Note: Grade radiation mucositis of the larynx here.

Dysphagia related to radiation is also graded as *either* Dysphagia—esophageal related to radiation *or* Dysphagia—pharyngeal related to radiation, depending on the site of treatment.

Toxicity	Grade				
Nausea	None	Able to eat	Oral intake significantly decreased	No significant intake, requiring IV fluids	—

Toxicity	Grade				
Pancreatitis	None	—	—	Abdominal pain with pancreatic enzyme elevation	Complicated by shock (acute circulatory failure)

Also consider Hypotension.

Note: Asymptomatic amylase and Amylase are graded in the Metabolic/Laboratory category.

Pharyngitis is graded in the Gastrointestinal category as Stomatitis/pharyngitis (oral/pharyngeal mucositis).

Proctitis	None	Increased stool frequency, occasional blood-streaked stools, or rectal discomfort (including hemorrhoids), not requiring medication	Increased stool frequency, bleeding, mucus discharge, or rectal discomfort requiring medication, anal fissure	Increased stool frequency/diarrhea, requiring parenteral support; rectal bleeding, requiring transfusion; or persistent mucus discharge, necessitating pads	Perforation, bleeding or necrosis or other life-threatening complication requiring surgical intervention (e.g., colostomy)

Also consider Hemorrhage/bleeding with grade 3 or 4 thrombocytopenia, Hemorrhage/bleeding without grade 3 or 4 thrombocytopenia. and Pain due to radiation.

Note: Fistula is graded separately as Fistula—rectal/anal.

Proctitis occurring more than 90 days after the start of radiation therapy is graded in the RTOG/EORTC Late Radiation Morbidity Scoring Scheme.

Salivary gland changes	None	Slightly thickened saliva/may have slightly altered taste (e.g., metallic); additional fluids may be required	Thick, ropy, sticky saliva; markedly altered taste; alteration in diet required	—	Acute salivary gland necrosis
Sense of smell	Normal	Slightly altered	Markedly altered	—	—

Continued on next page

National Cancer Institute Common Toxicity Criteria (CTC) (*Continued*)

Toxicity	Grade				
	0	1	2	3	4
Stomatitis/pharyngitis (oral/pharyngeal mucositis)	None	Painless ulcers, erythema, or mild soreness in the absence of lesions	Painful erythema, edema, or ulcers but can eat or swallow	Painful erythema, edema, or ulcers requiring IV hydration	Severe ulceration or requires parenteral or enteral nutritional support or prophylactic intubation
For BMT:	None	Painless ulcers, erythema, or mild soreness in the absence of lesions	Painful erythema, edema, or ulcers but can swallow	Painful erythema edema, or ulcers preventing swallowing or requiring hydration or parenteral (or enteral) nutritional support	Severe ulceration requiring prophylactic intubation or resulting in documented aspiration pneumonia

Note: Radiation-related mucositis is graded as Mucositis due to radiation.

Taste disturbance (dysgeusia)	Normal	Slightly altered	Markedly altered	—	—
Typhlitis (inflammation of the cecum)	None	—	—	Abdominal pain, diarrhea, fever, or radiographic documentation	Perforation, bleeding or necrosis or other life-threatening complication requiring surgical intervention (e.g., colostomy)

Also consider Hemorrhage/bleeding with grade 3 or 4 thrombocytopenia, Hemorrhage/bleeding without grade 3 or 4 thrombocytopenia, Hypotension, Febrile/neutropenia.

Vomiting	None	1 episode in 24 hours over pretreatment	2–5 episodes in 24 hours over pretreatment	≥ 6 episodes in 24 hours over pretreatment; or need for IV fluids	Requiring parenteral nutrition; or physiologic consequences requiring intensive care; hemodynamic collapse

Also consider Dehydration.

Continued on next page

National Cancer Institute Common Toxicity Criteria (CTC) (Continued)

Toxicity	Grade			
	0	1	2	3	4
Weight gain is graded in the Constitutional Symptoms category.				
Weight loss is graded in the Constitutional Symptoms category.				
Gastrointestinal—Other (Specify, _____)	None	Mild	Moderate	Severe	Life-threatening or disabling

Hemorrhage

Note: Transfusion in this section refers to pRBC infusion.

For *any* bleeding with grade 3 or 4 platelets (< 50,000), *always* grade Hemorrhage/bleeding with grade 3 or 4 thrombocytopenia. Also consider platelets, transfusion-pRBC, and transfusion-platelets in addition to the grade that incorporates the site or type of bleeding.

If the site or type of hemorrhage/bleeding is listed, also use the grading that incorporates the site of bleeding: CNS hemorrhage/bleeding, Hematuria, Hematemesis, Hemoptysis, Hemorrhage/bleeding with surgery, Melena/lower GI bleeding, Petechiae/purpura (Hemorrhage/bleeding into skin), Rectal bleeding/hematochezia, Vaginal bleeding.

If the platelet count is ≥ 50,000 and the site or type of bleeding is listed, grade the specific site. If the site or type is *not* listed and the platelet count is ≥ 50,000, grade Hemorrhage/bleeding without grade 3 or 4 thrombocytopenia and specify the site or type in the Other category.

Hemorrhage/bleeding with grade 3 or 4 thrombocytopenia	None	Mild without transfusion	—	Requiring transfusion	Catastrophic bleeding requiring major nonelective intervention

Also consider Platelets, Hemoglobin, Transfusion-platelet, Transfusion-pRBCs.

Note: This toxicity must be graded for any bleeding with grade 3 or 4 thrombocytopenia. Also grade the site or type of hemorrhage/bleeding. If the site is not listed, grade as Other in the Hemorrhage category.

Hemorrhage/bleeding without grade 3 or 4 thrombocytopenia	None	Mild without transfusion	—	Requiring transfusion	Catastrophic bleeding requiring major nonelective intervention

Also consider Platelets, Hemoglobin, Transfusion-platelet, Transfusion-pRBCs.

Note: Bleeding in the absence of grade 3 or 4 thrombocytopenia is graded here only if the specific site or type of bleeding is not listed elsewhere in the Hemorrhage category. Also grade as Other in the Hemorrhage category.

CNS hemorrhage/bleeding	None	—	—	Bleeding noted on CT or other scan with no clinical consequences	Hemorrhagic stroke or hemorrhagic vascular event (CVA) with neurologic signs and symptoms

Continued on next page

National Cancer Institute Common Toxicity Criteria (CTC) (*Continued*)

Toxicity	Grade				
	0	1	2	3	4
Epistaxis	None	Mild without transfusion	—	Requiring transfusion	Catastrophic bleeding, requiring major nonelective intervention
Hematemesis	None	Mild without transfusion	—	Requiring transfusion	Catastrophic bleeding, requiring major nonelective intervention
Hematuria (in the absence of vaginal bleeding)	None	Microscopic only	Intermittent gross bleeding, no clots	Persistent gross bleeding or clots; may require catheterization or instrumentation, or transfusion	Open surgery or necrosis or deep bladder ulceration
Hemoptysis	None	Mild without transfusion	—	Requiring transfusion	Catastrophic bleeding,

					requiring major nonelective intervention
Hemorrhage/ bleeding associated with surgery	None	Mild without transfusion	—	Requiring transfusion	Catastrophic bleeding, requiring major nonelective intervention

Note: Expected blood loss at the time of surgery is not graded as a toxicity.

Melena/GI bleeding	None	Mild without transfusion	—	Requiring transfusion	Catastrophic bleeding, requiring major nonelective intervention
Petechiae/purpura (hemorrhage/ bleeding into skin or mucosa)	None	Rare petechiae of skin	Petechiae or purpura in dependent areas of skin	Generalized petechiae or purpura of skin or petechiae of any mucosal site	—
Rectal bleeding/ hematochezia	None	Mild without transfusion or medication	Persistent, requiring medication (e.g., steriod suppositories)	Requiring transfusion	Catastrophic bleeding, requiring major

Continued on next page

National Cancer Institute Common Toxicity Criteria (CTC) (*Continued*)

Toxicity	Grade				
	0	1	2	3	4
			and/or break from radiation treatment		nonelective intervention
Vaginal bleeding	None	Spotting, requiring < 2 pads per day	Requiring ≥ 2 pads per day, but not requiring transfusion	Requiring transfusion	Catastrophic bleeding, requiring major nonelective intervention
Hemorrhage-Other (Specify site, _____)	None	Mild without transfusion	—	Requiring transfusion	Catastrophic bleeding, requiring major nonelective intervention
Hepatic					
Alkaline phosphatase	WNL	> ULN–2.5 × ULN	> 2.5–5.0 × ULN	> 5.0–20.0 × ULN	> 20.0 × ULN

Bilirubin	WNL	> ULN–1.5 × ULN	> 1.5–3.0 × ULN	> 3.0–10.0 × ULN	> 10.0 × ULN

Bilirubin—graft-versus-host disease (GVHD)

Note: The following criteria are used only for bilirubin associated with graft-versus-host disease.

	Normal	≥ 2–< 3 mg/100 mL	≥ 3–< 6 mg/100 mL	≥ 6–< 15 mg/100 mL	≥ 15 mg/100 mL
GGT (g-Glutamyl transpeptidase)	WNL	> ULN–2.5 × ULN	> 2.5–5.0 × ULN	> 5.0–20.0 × ULN	> 20.0 × ULN
Hepatic enlargement	Absent	—	—	Present	—

Note: Grade Hepatic enlargement only for changes related to VOD or other treatment-related toxicity.

Hypoalbuminemia	WNL	< LLN–3 d/dL	≥ 2–< 3 g/dL	< 2 g/dL	—
Liver dysfunction/ failure (clinical)	Normal	—	—	Asterixis	Encephalopathy or coma

Note: Documented viral hepatitis is graded in the Infection category.

Portal vein flow	Normal	—	Decreased portal vein flow	Reversal/retrograde portal vein flow	—
SGOT (AST) (serum glutatmic oxaloacetic transaminase)	WNL	> ULN–2.5 × ULN	> 2.5–5.0 × ULN	> 5.0–20.0 × ULN	> 20.0 × ULN

Continued on next page

National Cancer Institute Common Toxicity Criteria (CTC) (*Continued*)

Toxicity	Grade				
	0	1	2	3	4
SGPT (ALT) (serum glutamic pyruvic transaminase)	WNL	> ULN–2.5 × ULN	> 2.5–5.0 × ULN	> 5.0–20.0 × ULN	> 20.0 × ULN
Hepatic—Other (Specify, _____)	None	Mild	Moderate	Severe	Life-threatening or disabling
Infection/Febrile Neutropenia					
Catheter-related infection	None	Mild, no active treatment	Moderate, localized infection, requiring local or oral treatment	Severe, systemic infection, requiring IV antibiotic or antifungal treatment or hospitalization	Life-threatening sepsis (e.g., septic shock)

Febrile neutropenia (fever of unknown origin without clinically or microbiologically documented infection) (ANC < 1.0 × 10⁹/L, fever ≥ 38.5°C)	None	—	Life-threatening sepsis (e.g., (septic shock)

Note: Hypothermia instead of fever may be associated with neutropenia and is graded here.

Infection (documented clinically or microbiologically) with grade 3 or 4 neutropenia (ANC < 10.0 × 10⁹/L)	None	—	Life-threatening sepsis (e.g., septic shock)

Note: Hypothermia instead of fever may be associated with neutropenia and is graded here. In the absence of documented infection with grade 3 or 4 neutropenia, grade as Febrile neutropenia.

Infection with unknown ANC	None	—	Life-threatening sepsis (e.g., septic shock)

Note: This toxicity criterion is used in the rare case when ANC in unknown.

Continued on next page

461

National Cancer Institute Common Toxicity Criteria (CTC) (*Continued*)

Toxicity	0	1	2	3	4
			Grade		
Infection without neutropenia	None	Mild, no active treatment	Moderate, localized infection, requiring local or oral treatment	Severe, systemic infection, requiring IV antibiotic or antifungal treatment, or hospitalization	Life-threatening sepsis (e.g., septic shock)
Infection/Febrile Neutropenia-Other (Specify, ____)	None	Mild	Moderate	Severe	Life-threatening or disabling
Wound-infectious is graded in the Dermatology/Skin category.					
Lymphatics	Normal	Mild lymphedema	Moderate lymphedema requiring compression; lymphocyst	Severe lymphedema limiting function; lymphocyst requiring surgery	Severe lymphedema limiting function with ulceration
Lymphatics-Other (Specify, ____)	None	Mild	Moderate	Severe	Life-threatening or disabling

		Metabolic/Laboratory		
Acidosis (metabolic or respiratory)	Normal	pH < normal, but ≥ 7.3	—	pH < 7.3	pH < 7.3 with life-threatening physiologic consequences
Alkosis (metabolic or respiratory)	Normal	pH > normal, but ≤ 7.5	—	pH > 7.5	pH > 7.5 with life-threatening physiologic consequences
Amylase	WNL	> ULN–1.5 × ULN	> 1.5–2.0 × ULN	> 2.0–5.0 × ULN	> 5.0 × ULN
Bicarbonate	WNL	< LLN–16 mEq/dL	11–15 mEq/dL	8–10 mEq/dL	< 8 mEq/dL
CPK (creatine phosphokinase)	WNL	> ULN–2.5 × ULN	> 2.5–5 × ULN	> 5–10 × ULN	> 10 × ULN
Hypercalcemia	WNL	> ULN–11.5 mg/dL > ULN–2.9 mmol/L	> 11.5–12.5 mg/dL > 2.9–3.1 mmol/L	> 12.5–13.5 mg/dL > 3.1–3.4 mmol/L	> 13.5 mg/dL > 3.4 mmol/L
Hypercholesterolemia	WNL	> ULN–300 mg/dL > ULN–7.75 mmol/L	> 300–400 mg/dL > 7.75–10.34 mmol/L	> 400–500 mg/dL > 10.34–12.92 mmol/L	> 500 mg/dL > 12.92 mmol/L

Continued on next page

463

National Cancer Institute Common Toxicity Criteria (CTC) *(Continued)*

Toxicity	Grade				
	0	1	2	3	4
Hyperglycemia	WNL	> ULN–160 mg/dL > ULN–8.9 mmol/L	> 160–250 mg/dL > 8.9–13.9 mmol/L	> 250–500 mg/dL > 13.9–27.8 mmol/L	> 500 mg/dL > 27.8 mmol/L or ketoacidosis
Hyperkalemia	WNL	> ULN–5.5 mmol/L	> 5.5–6.0 mmol/L	> 6.0–7.0 mmol/L	> 7.0 mmol/L
Hypermagnesemia	WNL	> ULN–3.0 mg/dL > ULN–1.23 mmol/L	—	> 3.0–8.0 mg/dL > 1.23–3.30 mmol/L	> 8.0 mg/dL > 3.30 mmol/L
Hypernatremia	WNL	> ULN–150 mmol/L	> 150–155 mmol/L	> 155–160 mmol/L	> 160 mmol/L
Hypertriglyceridemia	WNL	> ULN–2.5 × ULN	> 2.5–5.0 × ULN	> 5.0–10 × ULN	> 10 × ULN
Hyperuricemia	WNL	> ULN–≤ 10 mg/dL ≤ 0.59 mmol/L without physiologic consequences	—	> ULN–≤ 10 mg/dL ≤ 0.59 mmol/L with physiologic consequences	> 10 mg/dL > 0.59 mmol/L

Also consider Tumor lysis syndrome, Renal failure, Creatinine, Potassium.

| Hypercalcemia | WNL | < LLN–8.0 mg/dL
< LLN–2.0 mmol/L | 7.0–< 8.0 mg/dL
1.75–< 2.0 mmol/L | 6.0–< 7.0 mg/dL
15.–< 1.75 mmol/L | < 6.0 mg/dL
< 1.5 mmol/L |

Hypoglycemia	WNL	< LLN–55 mg/dL < LLN–3.0 mmol/L	40–< 55 mg/dL 2.2–< 3.0 mmol/L	30–< 40 mg/dL 1.7–< 2.2 mmol/L	< 3.0 mg/dL 1.7 mg/dL
Hypokalemia	WNL	< LLN–3.0 mmol/L	—	2.5–< 3.0 mmol/L	< 2.5 mmol/L
Hypomagnesemia	WNL	< LNN–1.2 mg/dL < LLN–0.5 mmol/L	0.9–< 1.2 mg/dL 0.4–< 0.5 mmol/L	0.7–< 0.9 mg/dL 0.3–< 0.4 mmol/L	< 0.7 mg/dL < 0.3 mmol/L
Hyponatremia	WNL	< LLN–130 mmol/L	—	120–< 130 mmol/L	< 120 mmol/L
Hypophosphatemia	WNL	< LNN–2.5 mg/dL < LLN–0.8 mmol/L	≥ 2.0–< 2.5 mg/dL ≥ 0.6–< 0.8 mmol/L	≥ 1.0–< 2.0 mg/dL ≥ 0.3–< 0.6 mmol/L	< 1.0 mg/dL < 0.3 mmol/L
Hypothyroidism is graded in the Endocrine category.					
Lipase	WNL	> ULN–1.5 × ULN	> 1.5–2.0 × ULN	> 2.0–5.0 × ULN	> 5.0 × ULN
Metabolic/Laboratory-Other (Specify,____)	None	Mild	Moderate	Severe	Life-threatening or disabling
Musculoskeletal					
Arthralgia is graded in the Pain category.					
Arthritis	None	Mild pain with inflammation,	Moderate pain with inflammation,	Severe pain with inflammation,	Disabling

Continued on next page

National Cancer Institute Common Toxicity Criteria (CTC) (*Continued*)

Toxicity	0	Grade			
		1	2	3	4
		erythema or joint swelling but not interfering with function	erythema or joint swelling interfering with function, but not interfering with activities of daily living	erythema or joint swelling and interfering with activities of daily living	
Muscle weakness (not due to neuropathy)	Normal	Asymptomatic with weakness on physical exam	Symptomatic and interfering with function, but not intering with activities of daily living	Symptomatic and interfering with activities of daily living	Bedridden or disabling

Myalgia is graded in the Pain category.

| Myositis (inmflammation/damage of muscle | None | Mild pain, not interfering with function | Pain interfering with function, but not interfering with activities of daily living | Pain interfering with function and interfering with activities of daily living | Bedridden or disabling |

Also condier CPK.

Note: Myositis implies muscle damage (i.e., elevated CPK).

Osteonecrosis (avascular necrosis)	None	Asymptomatic and detected by imaging only	Symptomatic and interfering with function but not interfering with activities of daily living	Symptomatic and interfering with activities of daily living	Symptomatic; or disabling
Musculoskeletal-Other (Specify, _____)	None	Mild	Moderate	Severe	Life-threatening or disabling

Neurology

Aphasia, receptive and/or expressive, is graded under Speech impairment in the Neurology category.

Arachnoiditis/ meningismus/ radiculitis	Absent	Mild pain not interfering with function	Moderate pain interfering with function but not interfering with activities of daily living	Severe pain interfering with activities of daily living	Unable to function or perform activities of daily living; bedridden; paraplegia

Also consider Headache, Vomiting, Fever.

Ataxia (incoordination)	Normal	Asymptomatic but abnormal on physical exam, and not interfering with function	Mild symptoms interfering with funtion but not interfering with activities of daily living	Moderate symptoms interfering with activities of daily living	Bedridden or disabling

Continued on next page

National Cancer Institute Common Toxicity Criteria (CTC) (*Continued*)

			Grade		
Toxicity	**0**	**1**	**2**	**3**	**4**
CNS cerebrovascular ischemia	None	—	—	Transient ischemic event or attack (TIA)	Permanent event (e.g., cerebral vascular accident)
CNS hemorrhage/bleeding is graded in the Hemorrhage category.					
Cognitive disturbance/learning problems	None	Cognitive disability; not interfering with work/school performance; preservation of intelligence	Cognitive disability; interfering with work/school performance; decline of 1 SD (Standard Deviation) or loss of developmental milestones	Cognitive disability; resulting in significant impairment of work/school performance; cognitive decline > 2 SD	Inability to work/frank mental retardation
Confusion	Normal	Confusion or disorientation of attention deficit of brief duration; resolves spontaneously with no sequelae	Confusion or disorientation or attention deficit interfering with function, but not interfering with activities of daily living	Confusion or delirium interfering with activities of daily living	Harmful to others or self; requiring hospitalization

Cranial neuropathy is graded in the Neurology category as Neuropathy-cranial.

	Normal	—	Present	Toxic psychosis
Delusions	Normal	—	Present	Toxic psychosis
Depressed level of consciousness	Normal	Somnolence or sedation not interfering with function	Somnolence or sedation interfering with function, but not interfering with activities of daily living	Obtundation or stupor; difficult to arouse; interfering with activities of daily living	Coma

Syncope (fainting) is graded in the Neurology category.

	None	Not interfering with function	Interfering with function, but not interfering with activities of daily living	Interfering with activities of daily living	Bedridden or disabling
Dizziness/ light-headedness	None	Not interfering with function	Interfering with function, but not interfering with activities of daily living	Interfering with activities of daily living	Bedridden or disabling

Dysphasia, receptive and/or expressive, is graded under Speech impairment in the Neurology category.

	None	Mild involuntary movements not interfering with function	Moderate involuntary movements interfering with function, but not interfering with activities of daily living	Severe involuntary movements or torticollis interfering with activities of daily living	Bedridden or disabling
Extrapyramidal/ involuntary movement/ restlessness	None	Mild involuntary movements not interfering with function	Moderate involuntary movements interfering with function, but not interfering with activities of daily living	Severe involuntary movements or torticollis interfering with activities of daily living	Bedridden or disabling
Hallucinations	Normal	—	Present	Toxic psychosis

Continued on next page

National Cancer Institute Common Toxicity Criteria (CTC) (*Continued*)

| | Grade | | | | |
Toxicity	0	1	2	3	4
Headache is graded in the Pain category.					
Insomnia	Normal	Occasional difficulty sleeping not interfering with function	Difficulty sleeping interfering with function, but not interfering with activities of daily living	Frequent difficulty sleeping, interfering with activities of daily living	

Note: This toxicity is graded when insomnia is related to treatment. If pain or other symptoms interfere with sleep, do NOT grade as insomnia.

| Irritability (children < 3 years of age) | Normal | Mild; easily consolable | Moderate; requiring increased attention | Severe; inconsolable | — |
| Leukoencephalopathy-associated radiological findings | None | Mild increase in SAS (subarachnoid space) and/or mild ventriculomegaly; and/or small (+/− multiple) focal T2 hyperintensities involving periventricular white matter or < 1/3 of | Moderate increase in SAS; and/or moderate ventriculomegaly; and/or focal T2 hyperintensities extending into centrum ovale; or involving 1/3 to 2/3 of susceptible areas of cerebrum | Severe increase in SAS; severe ventriculomegaly; near total white matter T2 hyperintensities or diffuse low attenuation (CT); focal white matter necrosis (cystic) | Severe increase in SAS; severe ventriculomegaly; diffuse low attenuation with calcificatin (CT); diffuse white matter necrosis (MRI) |

susceptible areas of cerebrum

Memory loss	Normal	Memory loss not interfering with function	Memory loss interfering with function but not interfering with activities of daily living	Memory loss interfering with activities of daily living	Amnesia
Mood alteration—anxiety/agitation	Normal	Mild mood alteration not interfering with function	Moderate mood alteration interfering with function, but not interfering with activities of daily living	Severe mood alteration interfering with activities of daily living	Suicidal ideation or danger to self
Mood alteration—depression	Normal	Mild mood alteration not interfering with function	Moderate mood alteration interfering with function, but not interfering with activities of daily living	Severe mood alteration interfering with activities of daily living	Suicidal ideation or danger to self
Mood alteration—euphoria	Normal	Mild mood alteration not interfering with function	Moderate mood alteration interfering with function, but not interfering with activities of daily living	Severe mood alteration interfering with activities of daily living	Danger to self

Continued on next page

National Cancer Institute Common Toxicity Criteria (CTC) (*Continued*)

| | Grade | | | | |
Toxicity	0	1	2	3	4
Neuropathic pain is graded in the Pain category.					
Neuopathy—cranial	Absent	—	Present, interfering with activities of daily living	Present, interfering with activities of daily living	Life-threatening, disabling
Neuropathy—motor	Normal	Subjective weakness but no objective findings	Mild objective weakness interfering with function, but not interfering with activities of daily living	Objective weakness interfering with activities of daily living	Paralysis
Neuropathy—sensory	Normal	Loss of deep tendon reflexes or paresthesia (including tingling), but not interfering with function	Objective sensory loss or paresthesia (including tingling), interfering with function, but not interfering with activities of daily living	Sensory loss paresthesia interfering with activities of daily, living permanent sensory	Loss that interferes with function
Nystagmus	Absent	Present	—	—	—

Also consider Vision—double vision.

Personality/behavioral	Normal	Change, but not disruptive to patient or family	Disruptive to patient or family	Disruptive to patient and family; requiring mental health intervention	Harmful to others or self; requiring hospitalization
Pyramidal tract dysfunction (e.g., tone, hyperreflexia, positive Babinski, fine motor coordination)	Normal	Asymptomatic with abnormality on physical examination	Symptomatic or interfering with function, but not interfering with activities of daily living	Interfering with activities of daily living	Bedridden or disabling; paralysis
Seizure(s)	None	—	Seizure(s) self-limited and consciousness is preserved	Seizure(s) in which consciousness is altered	Seizures of any type that are prolonged, repetitive, or difficult to control (e.g., status epilepticus, intractable epilepsy)
Speech impairment (e.g., dysphasia or aphasia)	Normal	—	Awareness of receptive or expressive dysphasia, not impairing ability to communicate	Receptive or expressive dysphasia, impairing ability to communicate	Inability to communicate

Continued on next page

473

National Cancer Institute Common Toxicity Criteria (CTC) (*Continued*)

Toxicity	0	1	2	3	4
			Grade		
Syncope (fainting)	Absent			Present	—
Also consider Cardiovascular (Arrhythmia), Vasovagal episode, CNS cerebrovascular ischemia.					
Tremor	None	Mild and brief or intermittent but not interfering with function	Moderate tremor interfering with function but not interfering with activities of daily living	Severe tremor interfering with activities of daily living	—
Vertigo	None	Not interfering with function	Interfering with function but not interfering with activities of daily living	Interfering with activities of daily living	Bedridden or disabling
Neurology-Other (Specify, _____)	None	Mild	Moderate	Severe	Life-threatening or disabling
Ocular/Visual					
Cataract	None	Asymptomatic	Symptomatic, partial visual loss	Symptomatic, visual loss requiring	—

				treatment or interfering with function	
Conjunctivitis	None	Abnormal ophthalmologic changes, but asymptomatic or symptomatic without visual impairment (i.e., pain and irritation)	Symptomatic and interfering with function, but not interfering with activities of daily living	Symptomatic and interfering with activities of daily living	—
Dry eye	None	Mild, not requiring treatment	Moderate or requiring artificial tears	—	—
Glaucoma	None	Increase in intraocular pressure but no visual loss	Increase in intraocular pressure with retinal changes	Visual impairment	Unilateral or bilateral loss of vision (blindness)
Keratitis (corneal inflammation/corneal ulceration)	None	Abnormal ophthalmologic changes but asymptomatic or symptomatic without visual impairment (i.e., pain and irritation)	Symptomatic and interfering with function, but not interfering with activities of daily living	Symptomatic and interfering with activities of daily living	Unilateral or bilateral loss of vision (blindness)

Continued on next page

National Cancer Institute Common Toxicity Criteria (CTC) (*Continued*)

Toxicity	Grade				
	0	1	2	3	4
Tearing (watery eyes)	None	Mild, not interfering with function	Moderate; interfering with function but not interfering with activities of daily living	Interfering with activities of daily living	—
Vision—blurred vision	None	—	Symptomatic and interfering with function, but not interfering with activities of daily living	Symptomatic and interfering with activities of daily living	—
Vision—double vision (diplopia)	Normal	—	Symptomatic and interfering with function, but not interfering with activities of daily living	Symptomatic and interfering with activities of daily living	—
Vision—flashing lights/floaters	Normal	Mild, not interfering with function	Symptomatic and interfering with function, but not interfering with activities of daily living	Symptomatic and interfering with activities of daily living	—

Vision—night blindness (nyctalopia)	Normal	Abnormal electro-retinography but asymptomatic	Symptomatic and interfering with function, but not interfering with activities of daily living	Symptomatic and interfering with activities of daily living	—
Vision—photophobia	Normal	—	Symptomatic and interfering with function, but not interfering with activities of daily living	Symptomatic and interfering with activities of daily living	—
Ocular/Visual-Other (Specify, _____)	Normal	Mild	Moderate	Severe	Unilateral or bilateral loss of vision (blindness)

Pain

Abdominal pain or cramping	None	Mild pain not interfering with function	Moderate pain; pain or analgesics interfering with function, but not interfering with activities of daily living	Severe pain; pain or analgesics severely interfering with activities of daily living	Disabling

Continued on next page

National Cancer Institute Common Toxicity Criteria (CTC) (*Continued*)

			Grade		
Toxicity	0	1	2	3	4
Arthralgia (joint pain)	None	Mild pain not interfering with function	Moderate pain; pain or analgesics interfering with function, but not interfering with activities of daily living	Severe pain; pain or analgesics severely interfering with activities of daily living	Disabling
Arthritis (joint pain with clinical signs of inflammation) is graded in the Musculoskeletal category.					
Bone pain	None	Mild pain not interfering with function	Moderate pain; pain or analgesics interfering with function, but not interfering with activities of daily living	Severe pain; pain or analgesics severely interfering with activities of daily living	Disabling
Chest pain (noncardiac and nonpleuritic)	None	Mild pain not interfering with function	Moderate pain; pain or analgesics interfering with function, but not interfering with activities of daily living	Severe pain; pain or analgesics severely interfering with activities of daily living	Disabling

	None	Mild	Moderate	Severe	Disabling
Dysmenorrhea	None	Mild pain not interfering with function	Moderate pain; pain or analgesics interfering with function, but not interfering with activities of daily living	Severe pain; pain or analgesics severely interfering with activities of daily living	Disabling
Dyspareunia	None	Mild pain not interfering with function	Moderate pain interfering with sexual activity	Severe pain preventing sexual activity	—

Dysuria is graded in the Renal/Genitourinary category.

	None	Mild	Moderate	Severe	Disabling
Earache (otalgia)	None	Mild pain not interfering with function	Moderate pain; pain or analgesics interfering with function, but not interfering with activities of daily living	Severe pain; pain or analgesics severely interfering with activities of daily living	Disabling
Headache	None	Mild pain not interfering with function	Moderate pain; pain or analgesics interfering with function, but not interfering with activities of daily living	Severe pain; pain or analgesics severely interfering with activities of daily living	Disabling

Continued on next page

479

National Cancer Institute Common Toxicity Criteria (CTC) *(Continued)*

			Grade		
Toxicity	0	1	2	3	4
Hepatic pain	None	Mild pain not interfering with function	Moderate pain; pain or analgesics interfering with function, but not interfering with activities of daily living	Severe pain; pain or analgesics severely interfering with activities of daily living	Disabling
Myalgia (muscle pain)	None	Mild pain not interfering with function	Moderate pain; pain or analgesics interfering with function, but not interfering with activities of daily living	Severe pain; pain or analgesics severely interfering with activities of daily living	Disabling
Neuropathic pain (e.g., jaw pain, neurologic pain, phantom limb pain, post infectious neuralgia, or painful neuropathies)	None	Mild pain not interfering with function	Moderate pain; pain or analgesics interfering with function, but not interfering with activities of daily living	Severe pain; pain or analgesics severely interfering with activities of daily living	Disabling

Pain due to radiation	None	Mild pain not interfering with function	Moderate pain; pain or analgesics interfering with function, but not interfering with activities of daily living	Severe pain; pain or analgesics severely interfering with activities of daily living	Disabling
Pelvic pain	None	Mild pain not interfering with function	Moderate pain; pain or analgesics interfering with function, but not interfering with activities of daily living	Severe pain; pain or analgesics severely interfering with activities of daily living	Disabling
Pleuritic pain	None	Mild pain not interfering with function	Moderate pain; pain or analgesics interfering with function, but not interfering with activities of daily living	Severe pain; pain or analgesics severely interfering with activities of daily living	Disabling
Rectal or perirectal pain (proctalgia)	None	Mild pain not interfering with function	Moderate pain; pain or analgesics interfering with function, but not interfering with activities of daily living	Severe pain; pain or analgesics severely interfering with activities of daily living	Disabling

Continued on next page

481

National Cancer Institute Common Toxicity Criteria (CTC) (*Continued*)

Toxicity	0	1	2	3	4
			Grade		
Tumor pain (onset or exacerbation of tumor pain due to treatment)	None	Mild pain not interfering with function	Moderate pain; pain or analgesics interfering with function, but not interfering with activities of daily living	Severe pain; pain or analgesics severely interfering with activities of daily living	Disabling
Tumor flare is graded in the Syndrome category.					
Pain-Other (Specify, _____)	None	Mild	Moderate	Severe	Disabling
			Pulmonary		
Adult Respiratory Distress Syndrome (ARDS)	Absent	—	—	—	Present
Apnea	None	—	—	Present	Requiring intubation

Carbon monoxide diffusion capacity (DL_{co})	$\geq 90\%$ of pre-treatment or normal value	$\geq 75-< 90\%$ of pretreament or normal value	$\geq 50-< 75\%$ of pretreatment or normal value	$\geq 25-< 50\%$ of pretreatment or normal value	$< 25\%$ of pre-treatment or normal value
Cough	Absent	Mild, relieved by nonprescription medication	Requiring narcotic antitussive	Severe cough or coughing spasms, poorly controlled or unresponsive to treatment	—
Dypsnea (shortness of breath)	Normal	—	Dyspnea on exertion	Dyspnea at normal level of activity	Dyspnea at rest or requiring ventilator support
Forced Expiratory Volume (FEV_1)	$\geq 90\%$ of pre-treatment or normal value	$\geq 75-< 90\%$ of pretreatment or normal value	$\geq 50-< 75\%$ of pretreatment or normal value	$\geq 25-< 50\%$ of pretreatment or normal value	$< 25\%$ of pre-treatment or normal value
Hiccoughs (hiccups, singultus)	None	Mild, not requiring treatment	Moderate, requiring treatment	Severe, prolonged, and refractory to treatment	—

Continued on next page

National Cancer Institute Common Toxicity Criteria (CTC) (*Continued*)

Toxicity	0	1	2	3	4
			Grade		
Hypoxia	Normal	—	Decreased O_2 saturation with exercise	Decreased O_2 saturation at rest, requiring supplemental oxygen	Decreased O_2 saturation, requiring pressure support (CPAP) or assisted ventilation
Pleural effusion (nonmalignant)	None	Asymptomatic and not requiring treatment	Symptomatic, requiring diuretics	Symptomatic, requiring O_2 or therapeutic thoracentesis	Life-threatening (e.g., requiring intubation)
Pneumonitis/ pulmonary infiltrates	None	Radiographic changes but asymptomatic or symptoms not requiring steroids	Radiographic changes and requiring steroids or diuretics	Radiographic changes and requiring oxygen	Radiographic changes and requiring assisted ventilation

Pleuritic pain is graded in the Pain category.

	None	No intervention required	Chest tube required	Sclerosis or surgery required	Life-threatening
Pneumothorax	None	No intervention required	Chest tube required	Sclerosis or surgery required	Life-threatening

Pulmonary embolism is graded as Thrombosis/embolism in the Cardiovascular (General) category.

	None	Radiographic changes, but asymptomatic or symptoms not requiring steroids	Requiring steroids or diuretics	Requiring oxygen	Requiring assisted ventilation
Pulmonary fibrosis	None	Radiographic changes, but asymptomatic or symptoms not requiring steroids	Requiring steroids or diuretics	Requiring oxygen	Requiring assisted ventilation

Radiation-related pulmonary fibrosis is graded in the RTOG/EORTC Late Radiation Morbidity Scoring Scheme—Lung.

	Normal	Mild or intermittent hoarseness	Persistent hoarseness, but able to vocalize; may have mild to moderate edema	Whispered speech, not able to vocalize, may have marked edema	Marked dyspnea/stridor requiring tracheostomy or intubation
Voice changes/ stridor/larynx (e.g., hoarseness, loss of voice, laryngitis)	Normal	Mild or intermittent hoarseness	Persistent hoarseness, but able to vocalize; may have mild to moderate edema	Whispered speech, not able to vocalize, may have marked edema	Marked dyspnea/stridor requiring tracheostomy or intubation

Cough from radiation is graded as cough in the Pulmonary category.

Radiation-related hemoptysis from larynx/pharynx is graded as Grade 4 Mucositis due to radiation in the Gastrointestinal category.

Radiation-related hemoptysis from the thoracic cavity is graded at Grade 4 Hemoptysis in the Hemorrhage category.

	None	Mild	Moderate	Severe	Life-threatening or disabling
Pulmonary-Other (Specify, _____)	None	Mild	Moderate	Severe	Life-threatening or disabling

Continued on next page

National Cancer Institute Common Toxicity Criteria (CTC) *(Continued)*

Toxicity	0	1	2	3	4
			Renal/Genitourinary		
Bladder spasms	Absent	Mild symptoms, not requiring intervention	Symptoms requiring antispasmodic	Severe symptoms requiring narcotic	—
Creatinine	WNL	> ULN–1.5 × ULN	> 1.5–3.0 × ULN	> 3.0–6.0 × ULN	> 6.0 × ULN
Note: Adjust to age-appropriate levels for pediatric patients.					
Dysuria (painful urination)	None	Mild symptoms requiring no intervention	Symptoms relieved with therapy	Symptoms not relieved despite therapy	—
Fistula or GU fistula (e.g., vaginal, vesicovaginal)	None	—	—	Requiring intervention	Requiring surgery
Hemoglobinuria	—	Present	—	—	—
Hematuria (in the absence of vaginal bleeding) is graded in the Hemorrhage category.					

Grade

Incontinence	None	With coughing, sneezing, etc.	Spontaneous, some control	No control (in the absence of fistula)	—
Operative injury to bladder and/or ureter	None	—	Injury of bladder with primary repair	Sepsis, fistula, or obstruction requiring secondary surgery; loss of one kidney; injury requiring anastomosis or reimplantation	Septic obstruction of both kidneys or vesicovaginal fistula requiring diversion
Proteinuria	Normal or < 0.15 g/24 hours	1+ or 0.15–1.0g/24 hours	2+ to 3+ or 1.0–3.5 g/24 hours	4+ or > 3.5 g/24 hours	Nephrotic syndrome

Note: If there is an inconsistency between absolute value and uristix reading, use the absolute value for grading.

Renal failure	None	—	—	Requiring dialysis, but reversible	Requiring dialysis and irreversible
Ureteral obstruction	None	Unilateral, not requiring surgery	—	Bilateral, not requiring surgery	Stent, nephrostomy tube, or surgery

Continued on next page

National Cancer Institute Common Toxicity Criteria (CTC) (*Continued*)

Toxicity	Grade				
	0	1	2	3	4
Urinary electrolyte wasting (e.g., Fanconi's syndrome, renal tubular acidosis)	None	Asymptomatic, not requiring treatment	Mild, reversible, and manageable with oral replacement	Reversible but requiring IV replacement	Irreversible, requiring continued replacement

Also consider Acidosis, Bicarbonate, Hypocalcemia, Hypophosphatemia.

Toxicity	Grade				
	0	1	2	3	4
Urinary frequency/urgency	Normal	Increase in frequency or nocturia up to 2 × normal	Increase > 2 × normal but < hourly	Hourly or more with urgency, or requiring catheter	—
Urinary retention	Normal	Hesitancy or dribbling, but no significant residual urine; retention occurring during the immediate postoperative period	Hesitancy requiring medication or occasional in/out catheterization (< 4 × per week), or operative bladder atony requiring indwelling catheter beyond immediate postoperative period but for < 6 weeks	Requiring frequent in/out catheterization (≥ 4 × per week) or urological intervention (e.g., TURP, suprapubic tube, urethrotomy)	Bladder rupture

Urine color change (not related to other dietary or physiologic cause e.g., bilirubin, concentrated urine, hematuria)	Normal	Asymptomatic, change in urine color	—	—	—

Vaginal bleeding is graded in the Hemorrhage category.

Vaginitis (not due to infection)	None	Mild, not requiring treatment	Moderate, relieved with treatment	Severe, not relieved with treatment, or ulceration not requiring surgery	Ulceration requiring surgery
Renal/Genitourinary-Other (Specify, ___)	None	Mild	Moderate	Severe	Life-threatening or disabling

Secondary Malignancy

Secondary Malignancy-Other (Specify type, ___) excludes metastatic tumors	None	—	—	Present	—

Continued on next page

National Cancer Institute Common Toxicity Criteria (CTC) (*Continued*)

Toxicity	0	1	2	3	4
			Grade		
			Sexual/Reproductive Function		
Dyspareunia is graded in the Pain category.					
Dysmenorrhea is graded in the Pain category.					
Erectile impotence	Normal	Mild (erections impaired but satisfactory)	Moderate (erections impaired, unsatisfactory for intercourse)	No erections	—
Female sterility	Normal	—	Sterile	—	—
Feminization of male is graded in the Endocrine category.					
Irregular menses (change from baseline)	Normal	Occasionally irregular or lengthened interval, but continuing menstrual cycles	Very irregular, but continuing menstrual cycles	Persistent amenorrhea	—

Libido	Normal	Decrease in interest	Severe loss of interest	—	—
Male infertility	—	—	Oligospermia (low sperm count)	Azoospermia (no sperm)	—
Masculinization of female is graded in the Endocrine category.					
Vaginal dryness	Normal	Mild	Requiring treatment and/or interfering with sexual function, dyspareunia	—	—
Sexual/Reproductive Function–Other (Specify, _____)	None	Mild	Moderate	Severe	Disabling

Syndromes (not included in previous categories)

Acute vascular leak syndrome is graded in the Cardiovascular (General) category.

ARDS (Adult Respiratory Distress Syndrome) is graded in the Pulmonary category.

Autoimmune reactions are graded in the Allergy/Immunology category.

Continued on next page

491

National Cancer Institute Common Toxicity Criteria (CTC) (*Continued*)

			Grade		
Toxicity	0	1	2	3	4

DIC (disseminated intravascular coagulation) is graded in the Coagulation category.

Fanconi's syndrome is graded as Urinary electrolyte wasting in the Renal/Genitourinary category.

Renal tubular acidosis is graded as Urinary electrolyte wasting in the Renal/Genitourinary category.

Stevens-Johnson syndrome (erythema multiforme) is graded in the Dermatology/Skin category.

SIADH (syndrome of inappropriate antidiuretic hormone) is graded in the Endocrine category.

Thrombotic microangiopathy (e.g., thrombotic thrombocytopenic purpura/TTP or hemolytic uremic syndrome/HUS) is graded in the Coagulation category.

Tumor flare	None	Mild pain not interfering with function	Moderate pain; pain or analgesics interfering with function, but not interfering with activities of daily living	Severe pain; pain or analgesics interfering with function and interfering with activities of daily living	Disabling

Also consider Hypercalcemia.

Note: Tumor flare is characterized by a constellation of symptoms and signs in direct relation to initiation of therapy (e.g., antiestrogens/androgens or additional hormones). The symptoms/signs include tumor pain, inflammation of visible tumor, hypercalcemia, diffuse bone pain, and other electrolyte disturbances.

	None	Mild	Moderate	Severe	Life-threatening or disabling
Tumor lysis syndrome	Absent	—	—	Present	—

Also consider Hyperkalemia, Creatinine.

Urinary electrolyte wasting (e.g., Fanconi's syndrome, renal tubular acidosis) is graded under the Renal/Genitourinary category.

	None	Mild	Moderate	Severe	Life-threatening or disabling
Syndromes-Other (Specify, _____)	None	Mild	Moderate	Severe	Life-threatening or disabling

Note: From National Cancer Institute Common Toxicity Criteria, Version 2.0 [Online], revised March 23, 1998. Available: http://ctep.info.nih.gov/CTC3/ctc.htm (1999, January 20).

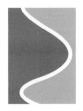

INDEX

Page numbers followed by the letter *f* indicate figures; page numbers followed by *t* indicate tabular material

Food and Drug Administration (FDA), 43, 44
Forced Expiratory Volume (FEV$_1$), 483*t*
Free radicals, 146
FRY scale, 165
5-FU. *See* 5-Fluorouracil
FUDR (Floxuridine), 258–260

Gap phases, 4–5, 5*f*
Gastric cancer, 361, 362, 363, 369
Gastric ulcers, 448*t*
Gastritis, 449*t*
Gastrointestinal toxicity
    anorexia, 107–108, 449*t*
    of biologic response modifiers, 37*t*–38*t*
    constipation, 111–112, 450*t*
    criteria for, 443*t*–454*t*
    diarrhea, 112–113, 451*t*
    emetogenic potential of agents, 103*t*–106*t*
    GI bleeding, 457*t*
    management and patient education, 101, 102*t*, 105–107, 106*t*
    mucositis, 108–109, 110*t*, 111, 450*t*
    nausea and vomiting, 98–101, 99*t*
G-CSF. *See* Granulocyte colony-stimulating factor
Gemcitabine (Gemzar), 104*t*, 265–267
Gene therapy, 33
Genitourinary system toxicity. *See* Renal toxicity
Geriatric patients, 168
Germ cell tumors, 357
GGT (g-Glutamyl transpeptidase), 459*t*
Glaucoma, 475*t*
Glucocorticoids, 11
Glucose levels, 464*t*
GM-CSF. *See* Granulocyte macrophage colony-stimulating factor
GM-CSF/IL-3 fusion protein (PIXY 321), 28
Goal setting, 169
Gonadal dysfunction, 137
Gonadotropin inhibitors, 11
Goserelin acetate (Zoladex), 267–270, 364
Granisetron (Kytril), 102*t*
Granulocyte colony-stimulating factor (G-CSF), 28–29
    clinical applications, 17*t*–18*t*
    indications/administration/side effects of, 256–258
Granulocyte macrophage colony-stimulating factor (GM-CSF), 28, 29
    clinical applications, 18*t*
    indications/administration/side effects, 326–329
Granulocytes, 114*t*, 119, 421*t*
Granulocytopenia, 118
Growth fraction, 8, 11–12
Gynecomastia, 442*t*

Hair follicles, 93
Hair loss. *See* Alopecia
Hallucinations, 469*t*
Hand-foot syndrome, 94–95, 438*t*
Haptoglobin, 419*t*
Headaches, 479*t*

Head and neck cancer, 356, 358, 365, 369, 370
Hearing toxicity criteria, 417*t*–418*t*
Heartburn, 446*t*
Hematemesis, 456*t*
Hematochezia, 457*t*
Hematocrit (Hct), 114*t*
Hematologic malignancies, 108
Hematologic toxicity
    anemia, 118–119
    of biologic response modifiers, 38*t*
    myelosuppression, 113–115, 116*t*–117*t*, 118
    neutropenia, 119–121
    thrombocytopenia, 121–122
Hematopoiesis, 26, 27*f*, 28, 113, 115*f*
Hematopoietic growth factors
    action of, 26, 27*f*, 28, 113
    applications of, 18*t*, 23*t*–24*t*
    cellular sources, 23*t*–24*t*
    erythropoietin, 29–30
    granulocyte colony-stimulating factor, 28–29
    granulocyte macrophage colony-stimulating factor, 29
Hematuria, 456*t*
Hemoglobin (Hgb), 114*t*, 420*t*
Hemoglobinuria, 486*t*
Hemolysis, 420*t*
Hemoptysis, 456*t*
Hemorrhage, toxicity criteria, 454*t*–458*t*
Hepatic enlargement, 459*t*
Hepatic pain, 480*t*
Hepatic pumps, 60–61, 61*f*
Hepatocellular dysfunction, 122
Hepatotoxicity, 122–123
    agents causing, 122*t*
    of biologic response modifiers, 39*t*
    criteria for, 458*t*–460*t*
Herceptin (Trastuzumab), 18*t*, 19
Hexalen. *See* Altretamine
Hexamethylmelamine. *See* Altretamine
Hiccoughs (hiccups), 483*t*
Hives, 441*t*
Home care, 171–174
Homeostasis, 4
Hormone antagonists, 11
Hormones, 11
Hospital administrators, 53
Hot flashes/flushes, 443*t*
Hyaluronidase (Wydase), 150*t*, 157
Hybridoma technology, 13, 14*f*
Hycamtin (Topotecan hydrochloride), 104*t*, 340–342
Hydrea. *See* Hydroxyurea
Hydroxyurea (Hydrea)
    acral erythema, 94
    classification of, 11
    in combination regimens, 374
    cutaneous toxicity of, 91*t*
    emetic risk of, 105*t*
    indications/administration/side effects, 270–272
    myelosuppressive effect of, 117*t*
Hypercalcemia, 463*t*, 464*t*
Hypercholesterolemia, 463*t*
Hyperkalemia, 464*t*